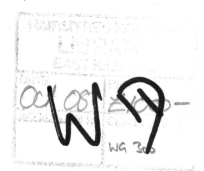

Rebuilding the Infarcted Heart

Rebuilding the Infarcted Heart

Edited by

Kai C Wollert MD
Division of Molecular and Translational Cardiology
Department of Cardiovascular Medicine
Hannover University Medical School
Hannover, Germany

Loren J Field PhD
Herman B Wells Center for Pediatric Research
Division of Pediatric Cardiology and
the Krannert Institute of Cardiology
Indiana University School of Medicine
Indianapolis, IN, USA

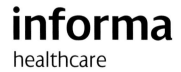

informa
healthcare

First published in the United Kingdom in 2007 by Informa Healthcare, Telephone House, 69-77 Paul Street, London EC2A 4LQ. Informa Healthcare is a trading division of Informa UK Ltd. Registered Office: 37/41 Mortimer Street, London W1T 3JH. Registered in England and Wales number 1072954.

Tel: +44 (0)20 7017 5000
Fax: +44 (0)20 7017 6699
Email: info.medicine@tandf.co.uk
Website: www.informahealthcare.com

A CIP record for this book is available from the British Library.

Library of Congress Cataloging-in-Publication Data

Data available on application

ISBN-10: 0 415 41942 7
ISBN-13: 978 0 415 41942 6

Distributed in North and South America by
Taylor & Francis
6000 Broken Sound Parkway, NW, (Suite 300)
Boca Raton, FL 33487, USA
Within Continental USA
Tel: 1 (800) 272 7737; Fax: 1 (800) 374 3401
Outside Continental USA
Tel: (561) 994 0555; Fax: (561) 361 6018
Email: orders@crcpress.com

Distributed in the rest of the world by
Thomson Publishing Services
Cheriton House
North Way
Andover, Hampshire SP10 5BE, UK
Tel: +44 (0)1264 332424
Email: tps.tandfsalesorder@thomson.com

Composition by C&M Digitals (P) Ltd, Chennai, India
Printed and bound in India by Replika Press Pvt Ltd

Contents

List of Contributors

Philip Barnett PhD
Heart Failure Research Center
Academic Medical Center
University of Amsterdam
Amsterdam
The Netherlands

Sophie Bekkers MD
Department of Cardiology
Heart Lung Centre
University Medical Center Utrecht
Utrecht
The Netherlands

Nirat Beohar MD
Division of Cardiology
Feinberg School of Medicine
Northwestern University
Chicago, IL
USA

Peter R Brink PhD
Department of Physiology and Biophysics
Stony Brook State University
Stony Brook, NY
USA

Ira S Cohen MD PhD
Department of Physiology and Biophysics
Stony Brook State University
Stony Brook, NY
USA

Wangde Dai MD
Heart Institute, Good Samaritan Hospital
Keck School of Medicine
University of Southern California
Los Angeles, CA
USA

Pieter A Doevendans MD
Department of Cardiology
Heart Lung Centre
University Medical Center Utrecht
Utrecht
The Netherlands

Sergey V Doronin PhD
Department of Physiology and Biophysics
Stony Brook State University
Stony Brook, NY
USA

Loren J Field PhD
Herman B Wells Center for Pediatric Research
Division of Pediatric Cardiology and the
Krannert Institute of Cardiology
Indiana University School of Medicine
Indianapolis, IN
USA

Glen R Gaudette PhD
Department of Biomedical Engineering
Worcester Polytechnic Institute
Worcester, MA
USA

Lior Gepstein MD PhD
Bruce Rappaport Faculty of Medicine
Technion-Israel Institute of Technology
Haifa
Israel

Marie-José Goumans MD
Department of Cardiology
Heart Lung Centre
University Medical Center Utrecht
Utrecht
The Netherlands

Preface

The infarcted heart heals by scar formation, and large myocardial infarctions typically result in heart failure. Although cardiomyocyte cell cycle activity is present at the border zone of an infarct, and adult stem cells with the capacity to transform into various cardiac cell types and to secrete cardioprotective cytokines have been identified, the endogenous repair mechanisms in the adult heart are not sufficient to reverse the damage after large myocardial infarctions. These observations, however, suggest that it may be feasible to develop interventions aimed at enhancing these processes, and, in effect, to rebuild the infarcted heart. While aspects of this concept are currently being tested in pre-clinical studies as well as in clinical trials, much remains to be learned about the biological basis of cardiac repair and regeneration.

This book brings together a panel of renowned experts to share their experiences and ideas on this rapidly evolving field in Cardiovascular Medicine. We would like to take the opportunity to thank all of the authors for their valuable input into this project. We hope that readers from both basic science and clinical science backgrounds will find the book useful. We anticipate that ongoing research into the basic foundations of stem cell biology and cell cycle control, and the possible clinical applications of cell therapy, may lead to new treatments for congestive heart failure patients.

Kai C Wollert and Loren J Field
Hannover and Indianapolis

chapter 1

Origins of Cardiac Differentiation and Morphogenesis

Philip Barnett, Antoon FM Moorman, and Maurice JB van den Hoff

Introduction

Owing to the negligible ability of the adult heart to replace damaged myocardium, an intense search has been initiated to find progenitor cells that can be used as a replacement therapy. Despite large research projects and huge investments, controversy remains as to the interpretation and efficiency of regeneration or transplantation strategies within the damaged heart. What is, however, clear is that the regenerative capacity of the "normal" adult human myocardium is insufficient to maintain cardiac function upon loss of cardiomyocytes. Moreover, irrespective of the source of cells introduced into the damaged heart, cardiomyocyte differentiation is in no way sufficient to replace dysfunctional myocardium. Trials carried out so far have often noted a certain level of physiological improvement, though the exact nature and reason for this has not yet been identified. From an optimistic point of view, it is defendable to conclude that replacement therapy is a viable approach to cure the diseased heart. One means of advancing these replacement therapies to a point where it should be plausible to efficiently replenish the diseased heart with functional viable cardiomyocytes is by advancing our current knowledge on the cellular and signaling pathways involved in cardiogenesis. Although developmental biologists have identified many individual components of this intricate process, our understanding of the integration of the various components is limited. In this chapter we will discuss the formation of the developing heart,

with respect to the different cell types that contribute to the heart and the main signaling pathways involved in cardiogenesis (Figure 1.1).

First Wave of Myocardium Formation

Within the third week of human development the process of gastrulation is initiated, a process during which mesodermal cells are formed and make their first contributions to the heart. The earliest signals that recruit mesodermal cells into the cardiac lineage are, therefore, likely to be preceded by signals regulating gastrulation and the formation of mesoderm. Developmental studies have shown that an instructive/inductive signal from the hypoblast is required for the specification of cardiac progenitors.[1–3] This notion was substantiated by the finding that a specific human embryonic stem cell line, which in contrast to many others does not spontaneously differentiate into beating heart muscle cells, could give rise to such cells when cocultured with a visceral endoderm-like cell line.[4] Although these and other studies have not yet identified the paracrine factor or factors providing the endoderm-derived signal, activins,[5,6] bone morphogenetic proteins (BMPs),[6–8] fibroblast growth factors (FGFs),[8,9] and Wnt[10–12] have been suggested as likely candidates. Neither FGFs nor BMPs have been shown to be able to substitute for the visceral endoderm-like cell line in inducing spontaneously contracting cardiomyocytes,[4] whereas FGFs and/or BMPs were found to

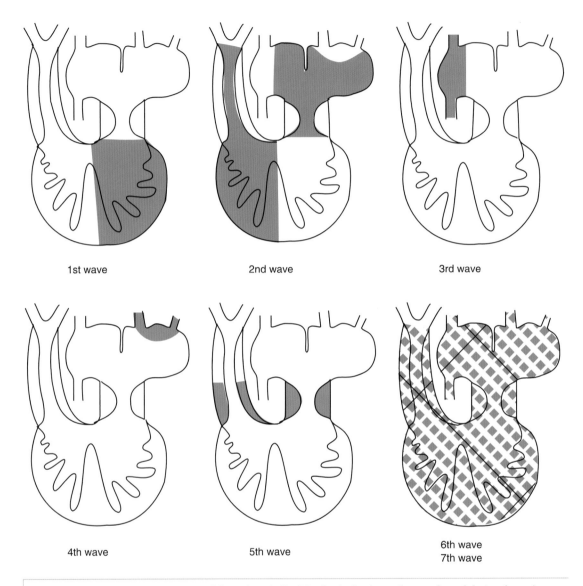

1st wave   2nd wave   3rd wave

4th wave   5th wave   6th wave
7th wave

Figure 1.1   *Schematic representation of the regions (red) of the developing heart that are formed during the various waves of myocardium formation.*

stimulate cardiomyogenesis in other stem cell studies.[13–16] Although induction of heart muscle cell formation in embryonic stem cells results in spontaneously contracting cardiomyocytes, a more detailed analysis of the electrophysiological properties of these cells revealed that they retain an early primary heart tube phenotype.[17] This feature then limits their applicability for transplanta-tion or regeneration, as a ventricular-like pheno-type would obviously be much more desirable. It should also be appreciated: (1) that visceral endo-derm does not contribute to the embryo proper, which might underlie the fact that in the adult heart, cardiogenesis of transplanted cells is not induced; (2) that, concomitant with the forma-tion of mesoderm, the definitive endoderm is also formed; (3) that pure cell populations cannot be isolated from early developing embryos to test the hypothesis in vitro; and (4) that functional disruption of these genes in mice was found to be non-informative regarding heart development, as test mice either die during gastrulation prior to the induction of cardiomyogenesis or are viable due to some form of functional redundancy.

Newly formed mesodermal cells find themselves in a Wnt-expression domain, preventing them from initiating the cardiac gene expression program. These cells are often referred to a non-precardiac mesoderm. With the anterolateral migration of the mesodermal cell, Wnt signaling is neutralized by Dickkopf family members and/or crescent.[10,11] Although these cells, referred to as precardiac mesoderm, have not yet truly initiated the cardiac gene program as such, stimulation with BMPs and/or FGFs induces the expression of one of the earliest cardiac marker genes *Nkx2–5*. In the normal developing embryo the cardiac gene program is initiated when the mesodermal cells arrive anterolaterally at the periphery of the embryo, forming the so-called bilateral heart-forming regions, classic heart field, or primary heart field. As development proceeds the mesoderm separates into a parietal and a splanchnic layer due to the formation of the intraembryonic coelomic cavity. The precardiac mesodermal cells segregate with the visceral layer.[18] In vivo and in vitro experiments suggest that BMPs and FGFs are crucial in the onset, restriction, and maintenance of the cardiac gene program in the heart-forming regions.[8,10,11,19–21] In the visceral layer a subset of the precardiac mesodermal cells dislodge from their epithelial context and form mesenchymal cells in between the precardiac mesoderm and the endoderm. From these cells, the endocardial inner lining of myocardium will be formed.[22] The factors inducing the formation of endocardium are unknown, as yet.

With subsequent development the embryo starts to fold, bringing the heart-forming regions together along the ventral midline, where they cranially fuse and start to form a linear heart tube. The linear heart tube proceeds to bend rightwards,[23] and at the outer curvature of this loop the primitive embryonic ventricle starts to form. Ventricular development becomes evident when trabeculations start to form at embryonic day (ED) 8 of mouse development and Hamilton and Hamburger (HH) stage 12 of chicken development (for review see reference 24). The inducer of ventricular chamber-formation myocardium is not yet known. However, based on knockout mice, myocardially expressed BMP10,[25] endocardially expressed angiopoietin 1,[26] or endocardially expressed Tie2 receptor[27] are all potential candidates. Interestingly, if serum response factor (SRF) is deleted specifically from the cardiomyocytes,[28] or if the Tbx TBX2 is ectopically overexpressed throughout the forming primary heart tube,[29] ventricular formation is not observed.

Second Wave of Myocardium Formation

The primary heart field gives rise to the initial heart tube, in which at the outer curvatures the working myocardium of the future left systemic ventricle and of the atria differentiate. This early embryonic heart is very reminiscent of the tubular heart found in lower vertebrates, such as the fish. The fish heart is composed of a single ventricle and atrium separated by a valved atrioventricular canal. Blood enters the heart via the sinus venosus and exits via an unseptated outflow tract to enter the ventral aorta. A single systemic blood circuit then suffices for blood supply and oxygenation before returning to the heart. It is further interesting to note at this point that the heart of amphibians such as the frog possesses septated atria, which both drain into a single or univentricle. In line with this, the molecular marker Hand1, which is largely restricted to the left systemic ventricle in mice,[30,31] displays uniform expression throughout the univentricle in *Xenopus*.[32] Moreover, a marker for the right ventricle in mice, Hand2, is not expressed during *Xenopus* cardiac development.[33,34] For higher vertebrates with separated pulmonary and systemic circuits, the primary heart tube must derive a second ventricle and divide its outflow tract to supply both these systems. From an evolutionary point, study of both the lower and the higher vertebrate cardiopulmonary systems continues to provide key discoveries in the cardiophysiology of all vertebrates.

So, if the primary heart field provides the foundations for the systemic half of the heart, how is the pulmonary half of the heart formed? Already in the 1970s, before the real evolvement of molecular biological techniques, it was hypothesized that a population of cells existed, distinct from those involved in the makeup of the primary heart tube, but making a contribution to heart development at a later secondary stage. Electron microscopy studies by Viragh and Challice[35] revealed a population of splanchnic epithelial cells contributing to the heart at both its venous and its arterial pole. Initial lineage tracing studies by de la Cruz et al using labeling techniques showed that the initial heart tube elongates by recruitment of cells to both its poles.[36] More recent studies using chicken embryos demonstrated that indeed the outflow tract is derived from cells located at the cranial side of the heart.[37,38] Though both studies showed a cranially located cardiac progenitor pool, the location of the cells and the extent of contributions differ. One of several mouse lines, in which the *lacZ* transgene under control of the myosin light chain promoter was randomly integrated,[39] showed staining in the right ventricle, outflow tract, and an adjacent cell population extending into the dorsal pericardial wall and the mesodermal core of the pharyngeal arches. Further analysis of this transgene revealed that integration of this *lacZ* transgene cassette had occurred in a region of the genome involved in the specification of this late cardiac contribution. Sequence analysis revealed that the cassette had integrated approximately 114 kb upstream of the gene encoding FGF10. Contribution of this cell population to the heart at a later stage could be assumed from the fact that these cells in the anterior heart field were β-galactosidase positive and expressed *lacZ* and *Fgf10* mRNA, whereas they were only β-galactosidase positive within the outflow tract. This field of cells has received the name anterior heart field, and now constitutes a part of the secondary heart field. Interestingly, mice homozygous null for *Fgf10* possess no direct heart phenotype, dying immediately after birth due to pulmonary insufficiency.[40]

The same group that defined the anterior heart field has since been able to observe and note apparent differential growth phases of cells contributing to the heart tube.[41] This approach, named a retrospective clonal analysis, makes use of a rare reverse mutational event occurring in the *lacZ* gene. A mutated form of *nlacZ*, known as *nlaacZ*, encodes a non-functional β-galactosidase protein. A very rare, but spontaneously occurring mitotic recombination event of the *nlaacZ* integrated transgene gives rise to a functional *lacZ* gene.[42] For this purpose the *nlaacZ* gene was targeted to the α-cardiac actin locus which is expressed throughout the myocardium of the heart. At ED 8.5 in the mouse, clonally related β-galactosidase positive cells could be identified on basis of their regionalization within the heart tube. From these patterns a clear distinction could be made between cells arising from an initial dispersive proliferative growth during early heart development and cells contributing to differing extents to both ventricles, atria, and atrioventricular canal. Further, cells of the primary heart field, basically considered the first lineage, contribute to the venous pole and the primitive left ventricle. In contrast, those of the anterior heart field, part of the secondary heart field, contribute to the outflow tract and right ventricle but not the primitive left ventricle. Cells from a second growth phase which follow a more oriented coherent cell growth with low intermingling also contribute to most compartments. However, it was subsequently demonstrated that this secondary heart field as a whole actually contributed much more widely to the heart, even reaching as far as the atria, than was originally thought.[43] These findings indicate that the second wave of myocardium formation is not limited to the cranial side of the heart but also contributes myocardium to the caudal side, sometimes referred to as the posterior heart field. Collectively, the cells that contribute to the primary heart tube belong to the first lineage, and cells that are subsequently added to both poles of the heart belong to the second lineage, i.e. both the anterior/secondary heart field and the posterior heart field. The fact that most compartments of the heart receive contributions from both the first and the second lineages indicates two keys facts in heart development: first, that both the first and second lineages are derived from a common precursor, and second, that true clonal identity of heart components is achieved much later than was originally believed. The idea that cellular specification for compartmentalization is strictly assigned in a segmental fashion along the forming primary heart tube now starts to fall short in the light of these new lineage tracing studies. One can now start to envision the first and second lineages simply as a definition of two groups of cells from a single progenitor pool separated only by the timing of segregation from the common progenitor pool, the distinction of which lies only in the method and/or marker chosen to identify it at a given moment. Underscoring this concept is the fact that, to date, no proteins or mRNAs have been identified whose expression specifically recognizes either field, and it is unknown whether cells are developmentally restricted within each field. Thus, rather than indicating a distinct molecular identity, the concept of the anterior, secondary, or posterior heart field is currently a teleologic one. Perhaps it would be simpler in terms of definition to consider the heart arising from a single progenitor lineage which can be subdivided into sublineages.

Definition of the boundaries of the second lineage came from the examination of mice null for a LIM-homeodomain transcription factor Islet 1 (*Isl1*) which revealed a severely abnormal heart phenotype. Originally studied for its role in neurogenesis, it was shown that the *Isl1* knockout mice were observed to die around ED 10.5, displaying little advance in development beyond ED 9.5. A disruption of the dorsal aorta and embryonic vasculature was the suggested cause of this arrested development and embryonic death.[44] Reexamination of these mutant embryos by Cai et al in 2003[45] revealed the true extent of malformation. Hearts were noted as displaying severe right ventricular and outflow tract underdevelopment, as well as ventricular and atrial defects. The use of

Isl1–Cre labeling techniques demonstrated the extent of the "second lineage", as approximately 97% of cells in the outflow tract, 92% in the right ventricle, fewer than 20% in the left ventricle, and 70% in the right atrium stained blue for β-galactosidase activity. Like cells from the first lineage, second lineage cells must also differentiate into endocardial and myocardial cells; this subdivision has, as yet, not been evaluated. Further, *Isl1*–/–cells could be shown to have lost the ability to migrate to the heart. In regions of *Isl1* expression, *Isl1*–/– mice also displayed loss of certain growth factors including BMP4, BMP7, and the anterior heart field marker FGF10.

Though the potential use of *Isl1* as a marker for undifferentiated cardiac progenitors cells of at least a large subset of the second lineage cannot be doubted, the contribution of *Isl1* expressing ancestors to the left ventricle does, however, seem to present somewhat of an anomaly compared to the previously described work using retrospective clonal analysis, which suggested that there was no contribution of the second lineage to the primitive left ventricle. This idea is supported by the discovery of an *Mef2c* enhancer element which was able to drive *Mef2c* expression in, and only in, cells of the anterior heart field, whereas during normal development *Mef2c* is expressed in the whole embryonic heart. Examination of the sequence of this enhancer element, which when fused to *lacZ* showed β-galactosidase enzyme activity only in the right ventricle and outflow tract, revealed the presence of GATA and *Isl1* binding sites. Expression from this enhancer promoter construct becomes less as the embryo ages.[46] On the basis of these studies, a clearer spatiotemporal study of *Isl1* may be required before it can be truly labeled as a marker of cells of the second lineage.

It has been reported[47] that a very small proportion of *Isl1* expressing cells remain in the myocardium and could represent a source of cardiac progenitor cells derived or left over from the second lineage. When isolated from postnatal rat hearts, a fraction of these cells displayed the ability to further differentiate into working cardiomyocytes displaying active intracellular Ca^{2+} transients. These experiments made use of mice possessing a tamoxifen inducible Cre system knocked in to the *Isl1* locus and then crossed with R26R *lacZ* mice. Injection of tamoxifen at ED 17 and isolation of postnatal hearts revealed the expression of a small number of cells in the outflow tract and right atrium. Further, the in vitro induction of postnatally derived hearts with tamoxifen also led to the induction of β-galactosidase in a fraction of the isolated cells. More recently, Moretti et al[48] have been able to demonstrate that *Isl1* expressing cells can be isolated from embryos, cultured, and then further selected on the basis of *Is1l*, *Nkx2-5*, and *flk1* expression to derive a potential cardiac progenitor cell capable of differentiating into both the heart muscle and endocardial lineages. However, it still remains to be shown that cells with these properties can actually be isolated from adult hearts, which could represent a source of cardiac progenitor cells for stem cell therapy applications.

Third Wave of Myocardium Formation

As discussed above, the second wave of myocardium formation contributes in part to atrial development. However, the addition of myocardium to the venous pole of the heart is far more extensive, and at the caudal site of the heart a third wave of myocardium, possessing a unique molecular signature, provides the myocardium formed along the cardinal veins at the caudal border of the heart.

In chickens, *Tbx18* positive mesodermal cells adjacent to the caudal border of the heart were found to contribute to the myocardium and the developing proepicardium. In the formed myocardium, the expression of *Tbx18* ceases and the proepicardial *Tbx18* expression is sustained.[49] Analogous with the first wave of myocardium formation, a cooperative interaction between BMP and FGF signaling seems to underlie these lineage decisions.[50,51] The proepicardium gives rise to the epicardium, the subepicardial mesenchyme, the coronaries, and the cardiac (adventitial, interstitial, and subendocardial)

fibroblasts, but does not derive cardiomyocytes.[52-55] In vitro analysis showed that, upon attachment of the proepicardial cells to the myocardium, the proepicardial cells lose the capacity to differentiate into heart muscle cells.[50] In a recent study in which adult human epicardial cells were transduced in culture with myocardin, these cells were found to be able to differentiate into smooth muscle cell,[56] and transduction of neonatal cardiac fibroblasts with MyoD induced differentiation of the skeletal myocyte lineage.[57,58] If the proper factors could be identified it might be possible to reprogram cardiac fibroblasts into heart muscle cells. Interestingly, in zebrafish, in which the ventricle can regenerate upon resection of the apex, the formation of coronary vessels was found to be essential for proper regeneration.[59]

Mice deficient for *Tbx18* fail to correctly form the sinus horns and caval myocardium, but atrial and pulmonary development appears normal.[60] As in chickens, the *Tbx18* expressing population of cells is located at the caudal side of the heart tube and is associated spatially with precursor cells of the septum transversum and of the proepicardium. This population of cells is *Isl1* negative, and the formed myocardium was found to be *Nkx2-5* negative, underscoring our suggestion of a third wave of myocardium formation. Furthermore, the association of this cardiac progenitor pool with the septum transversum progenitors positions them lateral and cranial to the cardiac crescent of the germinal disc before embryonic folding, which is in contrast to the medial location of the progenitors of the second wave of myocardium formation.

Fourth Wave of Myocardium Formation

The origin and formation of the pulmonary vein is a contentious topic. The current view is that the pulmonary vein is formed by vasculogenesis in the mesenchyme surrounding the lung buds[61] during early development, and enters via the dorsal mesocardium into the future left atrium.[62,63] From Camegie stage (CS) 13 onward in the human,[64] ED 14 in the mouse,[65] and HH stage 25 in the chicken,[66] a myocardial sleeve develops around the vein. The sleeve extends from the left atrium onto the adventitial surface of the pulmonary vein.[67,68] These cells have been shown to express similar myocardial markers to those of the flanking atria, which has led to the hypothesis that myocardialization of the pulmonary vein has its origins in atrial myocardium.[68] Alternatively, mesodermal cells surrounding the pulmonary veins may differentiate into myocardium. This is based on the observation that pulmonary myocardium can be observed as far as the fifth bifurcation in some animals, and that a pattern of smooth muscle expression precedes myosin heavy chain expression during development.[65,69,70]

In contrast to mice, which possess a single pulmonary atrial return vein, humans[71] possess four veins that drain into the left atrium. The myocardial sleeves surrounding these veins reach at most up to their entry into the lungs. Although this does seem to suggest that pulmonary myocardium is less extensive in humans, it should be appreciated that, within the confines of the entering pulmonary veins, smooth-walled myocardium is present. The pulmonary vein appears to be taken up into the atrium during envelopment by heart muscle cells. Concomitant with absorption of the pulmonary vein, the pulmonary myocardium contributes to the smooth-walled myocardium of the left atrium and multiple entry sites of the pulmonary vein into the left atrium are created.

To date, the only transgenic strain in which the pulmonary vein is not formed is the FGF10 knockout mouse.[40,72] In these mice, lung buds fail to develop. Because the lung veins are formed by vasculogenesis of mesoderm cells in the lung buds, the absence of lung veins is probably a secondary effect. In several mouse strains, anomalous pulmonary venous return has been reported.[73,74] This phenotype, however, is related to the entry side of the pulmonary vein into the heart and, therefore, to left–right positional information rather than to the formation of the pulmonary myocardium per se.

Fifth Wave of Myocardium Formation

The heart is septated into a right pulmonary and a left systemic half by the formation of a muscular atrial septum and a muscular ventricular septum, and what remains is septated by the endocardial cushions. These cushions are formed in the remnants of the primary heart tube, or in other words in the regions that flank the forming ventricles and atria. The cushions not only divide the atrioventricular canal and the outflow tract (OFT) into two halves and connect to the atrial and ventricular septum, but also contribute to the mitral, tricuspid, and semilunar valves. The cushions are initially acellular but become mesenchymal with subsequent development. This mesenchyme is mainly derived from the endocardial layer, and in a small part from epicardium in the atrioventricular canal. In the OFT the cushions are predominantly populated by mesenchyme of the cardiac neural crest, and to a lesser extent from the endocardium. Upon fusion of the cushions the atrioventricular septum and the outflow septum are derived. In the adult heart, however, most of the septa are myocardial, indicating that the initial mesenchymal septa have to be converted into myocardial structures. In vitro and in vivo experiments suggest that muscularization of the mesenchymal septa is achieved by both myocardialization and differentiation of cushion mesenchyme into heart muscle cells. Myocardialization refers to migration of existing flanking heart muscle into the cushion mesenchyme.[75-77] The relative contribution of both processes is not known, and might differ between locations in the heart and between species.

Immunohistochemical analysis of the muscularizing outlet septum showed that smooth muscle markers precede the expression of myocardial markers,[65] and calponin H1 specifically stains the cells at the interface between mesenchyme and myocardium.[78] In vitro experiments using OFT explants derived from chicken or mouse embryos showed that BMPs and/or FGFs are necessary but not sufficient to induce myocardialization in vitro.[76,77,79,80] Experiments using the two-component Cre–*loxP* system to identify the cell type that differentiates into cardiomyocytes

addition, PGCs express *Stella*, a gene that is detected exclusively in lineage-restricted germ cells.[11,12] The *Stella* positive nascent germ cells exhibit repression of *Hox* genes. In addition, *Stella* is also expressed in undifferentiated ESCs, suggesting that *Stella* may be crucial for the retention of pluripotency.[11,12] Transcriptional repression of *Hox* genes and chromatin modifications block mouse PGCs from following somatic differentiation programs, and may be key to initiating a lasting transcriptional profile compatible with totipotency (see reference 28 for an excellent review of the preservation of the totipotency in germ cells).

In 1992, two laboratories reported that when PGCs are cultured with a mixture of membrane associated and soluble stem cell factor (SCF), LIF, and basic fibroblast growth factor (bFGF), PGCs continue to divide in culture and give rise to lines of undifferentiated cells. These cells have been termed embryonic germ cells (EGCs) to distinguish them from ESCs (Figure 2.3).[29,30] Human PGCs exposed to the same growth factors also form EGCs that are pluripotent.[31]

Each of the growth factors required for EGCs activates unique signal transduction pathways, but there is also considerable overlap in the downstream effectors that are activated. The c-Kit receptor, a tyrosine kinase receptor for SCF, is expressed by PGCs, promoting cell proliferation and survival signals in response to SCF during fetal PGC migration.[32] Some studies have suggested that membrane-bound SCF may mediate PGC adhesion to somatic cells and provide cues to guide their migration, and soluble SCF may act as a survival factor or a mitogen for PGCs.

Activation of the signaling component of the LIF receptor, gp130, is required for PGC survival in vivo and in vitro. Binding of ligand to the LIF receptor complex causes gp130 to associate with the Janus kinases (Jaks), which in turn transduce intracellular signals via the signal transducers and activation of transcriptions (Stats). PGCs are severely depleted in gp130 knockout mice, and treatment of cultured PGCs with a blocking gp130 antibody causes apoptosis. Therefore, gp130-mediated signaling is required for PGC survival, and together with c-Kit signaling promotes PGC proliferation.[33] It is not clear how bFGF affects PGC growth. However, once EGCs are established, they no longer require bFGF and SCF for their growth, but they still require feeder cells and LIF.

Like ESCs, EGCs are able to self-renew in vitro for a long time. They express *Oct4*, *Nanog*, and *Sox2*, and are positive for alkaline phosphatase (ALP) and stage-specific antigen 1 (SSEA1). Using the hanging drop method, EGCs can form embryoid bodies in vitro and differentiate into all derivates of the three embryonic germ layers, including functional cardiomyocytes. After injection into early blastocysts, they are able to contribute to chimeras and populate the germline. They can also give rise to teratomas when transferred to appropriate ectopic sites. This suggests that EGCs are very similar in their properties to the ESCs. The major difference is that the epigenetic state of imprinted genes in PGCs from which EGCs are derived is different from those in the ICM from which ESCs are derived. Pluripotent mouse EGCs can be derived from day 8.5 germ cells of both sexes, but from day 12.5 male cells only. EGCs are derived from PGCs isolated throughout the period during which imprint erasure is believed to take place: before migration (day 8.0–8.5), during migration (day 9.5–10.5), or after entering the genital ridge (day 11.5–12.5). Labosky and colleagues found differences in methylation of region 2 of the imprint gene *Igf2r* between ESCs and EGCs.[34] They also found some degree of imprint erasure in EGCs derived from day 8.5 PGCs, and more in EGCs derived from day 11.5 PGCs.[30] However, it is known that the methylation status of EGCs does not necessarily represent that of the germ cells from which they are derived. It has been suggested that the methylation differences between different EGC lines may not pre-exist before the lines are established, but instead are the result of a difference in their response to in vitro culture. It is also known that in vitro culture of ESCs and EGCs generally induces genetic and epigenetic changes including aberrant genomic imprinting, which can lead to morphological or functional abnormalities in the embryo or offspring.[35,36] The instability of these embryonic germline cells probably reflects their embryonic origin, which is susceptible to subtle changes in the maternal environment. Human EGCs are derived from the gonadal ridge and adjacent mesentery of 5–11-week embryos, at a time and location that mouse studies would predict complete erasure of imprints. Surprisingly, the epigenetic mark and preferential expression of imprinting genes are not erased in differentiated cells derived from human EGCs. In addition, human EGC-derived cells show the absence of epigenetic instability or epigenetic heterogeneity in comparison to the mouse.[37] This information is critical for their possible safe clinical use in the future. Interestingly, Onyango and his colleagues also found that mouse EGCs acquire preferential allele expression after in vitro differentiation.[37]

As mentioned above, spermatogonial stem cells (SSCs, the germline stem cells in the male) are developed from gonocytes after birth during early neonatal development. In the testis, only SSCs, not other germ cells, can self-renew. Therefore, they are responsible for maintaining spermatogenesis throughout life in the male. Since female germ cells are believed to be not capable of self-renewal after birth, SSCs are the only stem cells in the adult that continue to proliferate and are capable of transmitting genetic information to the next generation under normal circumstances. The SSCs are a subset of single cells (A_{single} or A_s), which are located along the basement membrane of seminiferous tubules in the mouse testis.[18] Although they are present in low numbers in the testis (0.02–0.03% of the total testicular cell population), these cells divide continuously and produce a differentiated A_s daughter that divides to form a pair of interconnected spermatogonial cells called A_{pair}. The A_{pair} spermatogonial cells can divide synchronously to form a chain of interconnected spermatogonial cells that subsequently become differentiating spermatogonia, spermatocytes, spermatids, and sperm cells.[18] The balance of self-renewal and differentiation of SSCs must be regulated strictly to maintain normal spermatogenesis; however, the mechanisms governing the fate decision – self-renewal or differentiation – are largely unknown.

Sertoli cells, the somatic cells in the seminiferous tubules that physically interact with SSCs, likely constitute a functional SSC niche by providing growth factors that control the balance of self-renewal and differentiation of SSCs. Previous studies showed that Sertoli cells produce glial cell line-derived neurotrophic factor (GDNF) that controls SSC maintenance in a dosage-dependent

manner.[38] GDNF binds two heterologous receptors, Ret and GFRα1, which are expressed in spermatogonial cells. *gdnf*+/−mice lose their SSCs prematurely in testes, indicating that GDNF is essential for SSC self-renewal.[38] In addition to GDNF signaling, BMP signaling also has a role in SSC maintenance.[39,40] Multiple BMPs, BMP4, BMP7, and BMP8, are expressed in male germ cells, while BMP4 is also expressed in Sertoli cells. Intriguingly, targeted disruption of these genes has revealed that they all play important but redundant roles in maintaining the viability of germ cells, including SSCs.[39,40] It remains unclear whether they are required for SSC self-renewal as well. In addition, Sertoli cells also support spermatogenesis.[41] The SCF produced by Sertoli cells activates c-Kit to promote the differentiation of SSC progeny. Mutations in the c-kit gene cause an arrest in an early step of spermatogonia differentiation, suggesting that the SCF/c-Kit pathway is required for germ cell differentiation after birth. How does the SCF/c-Kit system play different roles during fetal PGC migration and spermatogesis after birth? Indeed, spermatogonia have been shown to express the c-Kit receptor, while Sertoli cells produce its ligand, SCF, in both a soluble and a membrane-bound form. At the start of spermatogenesis, shortly after birth, there is a dramatic shift in the production of soluble to membrane-bound SCF by Sertoli cells, which suggests that the membrane-bound SCF is more important in spermatogenesis. The interaction between the c-Kit receptor and membrane-bound SCF appears to be responsible for the adhesion of spermatogonia to Sertoli cells.[41]

Taken together, Sertoli cells are essential for both SSC self-renewal and maintaining spermatogenesis, but it is still not clear whether and how Sertoli cells alone can constitute the SSC niche. Several lines of evidence demonstrate that hormonal factors also play a role in SSC self-renewal and regulation of spermatogenesis through the surrounding testicular somatic cells. Sertoli cells have receptors for follicle-stimulating hormone and testosterone, which are the main hormonal regulators of spermatogenesis.

In the mouse culture experiments, two studies showed that germline stem cells (or SSCs) from neonatal mouse testis can be cultured and expanded indefinitely in vitro in the presence of GDNF and can reconstitute long-term spermatogenesis and restore fertility when transplanted to sterile recipient mice.[2,4] In addition, the cultured SSCs (or germline stem cells) expressed molecular markers similar to undifferentiated ESCs and PGCs, including *Oct4*, Sox2, Rex-1, Stella, and tissue non-specific alkaline phosphatase; however, expression of the third critical molecule, Nanog, could not be detected.[2,4]

Interestingly, after several passages, embryonic stem (ES)-like cell colonies were detected by appearance and expanded when transferred to cultures using standard ESC culture conditions.[2] These ES-like cells are termed multipotent germline stem cells (mGSCs; Figure 2.3). Although the original testis cells and the cultured SSCs do not express Nanog, the mGSCs derived from the cultured SSCs do express Nanog. In addition, similar to ESCs, they are positive for ALP and SSEA1.[2] This indicates that the germline stem cells (or SSCs) may reacquire pluripotency under in vitro culture conditions. Although the mGSCs formed teratomas when injected into the seminiferous tubules of mice, when injected into blastocysts they contributed to chimeras in 25% of embryos and 35% of newborn animals. The mGSCs contributed to multiple somatic cell lineages and the germline in chimeras. However, derivation of mGSCs occurred at a very low efficiency. The age of the donor testis cells raises interesting questions. The number of SSCs in the testis in the first few days of life is low and the majority of germ cells are considered gonocytes, which are still arrested in G0/G1 phase. They resume proliferation about 2 days after birth (Figure 2.3).

In addition, epigenetic studies show that cultured SSCs have a complete androgenetic imprinting pattern, whereas the genomic imprinting is variable in mGSCs.[42] Because the methylation pattern of stem cells tends to change during in vitro culture, it is necessary to investigate the genomic imprinting pattern in differentiated cells derived from ES-like cells.

We found that SSCs present in the testis of adult mice also appear to maintain the potency to generate somatic cells in addition to contributing to the germline.[1] We used transgenic mice that have the *stra8* promoter directing the expression of green fluorescent protein (GFP). Testis cells in culture positive for GFP were selected by cell sorting and cultured in the presence of GDNF for 2–4 weeks, and then in varying conditions to determine whether these cells would develop into ES-like cells. Inclusion of LIF in the medium and culture with mitotically inactive mouse embryonic fibroblasts (MEFs) resulted in the formation of ES-like cell colonies (Figure 2.4a). Derivation of ES-like cells occurred in 27% of mice. We name these cells multipotent adult germline stem cells (maGSCs; Figure 2.3).[1] Similar to mouse ESCs, maGSCs express the cell surface marker SSEA1 (Figure 2.4b), and transcription factors Oct4 (Figure 2.4c), Sox2 (Figure 2.4d), Nanog, and Rex1. They are also positive for ALP (Figure 2.4e). These cells expressed markers associated with different somatic cell lineages after embryoid body formation. When maGSCs are subcutaneously injected into *SCID-beige* mice, mature teratomas containing derivatives of the three embryonic germ layers are found.[1]

However, it is necessary to study the imprinting status of SSCs and maGSCs as well as differentiated cells from maGSCs during in vitro culture.

Cardiac Differentiation of Male Germline Stem Cells In Vitro

As we know, when removed from feeder layers and cultured as multicellular aggregates of differentiated and undifferentiated cells, termed embryoid bodies (EBs), which resemble early postimplantation embryos, ESCs begin to spontaneously differentiate into derivatives of all three embryonal germ layers including functional cardiomyocytes. Similar to ESCs, EGCs derived from PGCs are also able to differentiate into many cell types including cardiomyocytes.[25,26] Human EGCs in vitro also form EBs containing cells that represent all three germ layers, as well as mixed cell populations of less differentiated progenitors and precursors.[31]

When mGSCs derived from germline stem cells of neonatal mouse testis (0–2 days old) are cultured on OP9 stromal cells, they are able to first differentiate into flk1-positive cells, which

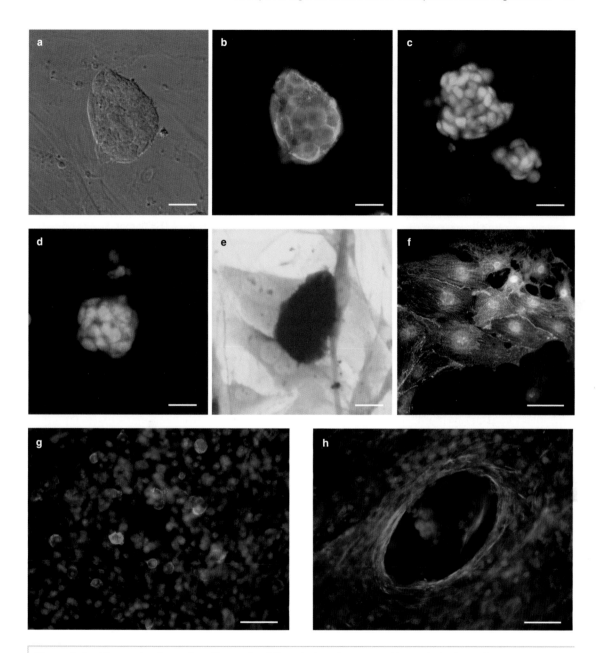

Figure 2.4   *Characterization and cardiovascular differentiation of maGSCs. (a) A typical colony of undifferentiated maGSCs. (b–d) Immunostaining of Stra8-GFP-positive maGSCs with antibodies against GFP (green, b), stage-specific antigen 1 (SSEA1) (red, b), Oct4 (red, c), and Sox2 (red, d). (e) Alkaline phosphatase staining of maGSCs. (f) Connexin 43 staining (green) in a cluster of uninucleate cardiac cells stained for sarcomeric α-actinin (red). (g) von Willebrand factor-positive endothelial cells (red) in embryoid body outgrowths at day 5 + 14. (h) Smooth muscle α-actin-positive cells (red) of tube-like structure in embryoid body outgrowths at day 5 + 14. Nuclei are stained with diamidino-phenylindole (DAPI) (c, d, f, g, and h). Scale bar, 50 μm.*

can further differentiate into beating cardiomyocytes and vascular endothelial and smooth muscle cells.[43]

To induce in vitro differentiation of maGSCs derived from adult mouse testis, we applied the "hanging drop" method used for ESC differentiation.

The differentiation efficiency of beating cardiomyocytes from maGSCs is similar to that from ESCs.[44] Spontaneously and rhythmically contracting cells appeared as clusters and were identified in approximately 80% of the individual EBs at day 5+8 (8 days after plating of 5-day-old EBs on gelatine-coated culture dishes). During EB differentiation, cardiac gene products are expressed in a developmentally controlled manner. The maGSC-derived cardiomyocytes exhibit charac-teristics typical of heart cells in early stages of car-diac development and are functionally viable. They show stable expression of myocytic markers including cardiac-specific L-type Ca^{2+} channels and sarcomeric proteins (Figure 2.4f, and they respond to Ca^{2+} channel modulating drugs. In addition, functional gap junctions are present among cardiomyocytes. Action potential analyses demonstrate that pacemaker-, ventricle-, atrial-, and Purkinje-like cardiomyocytes can be devel-oped from maGSCs. The cardiomyocytes also exhibit the complex functional properties present in native cardiac myocytes, including a positive or negative response to β-adrenergic stimulation, and intact calcium cycling.[44] Besides cardiomy-ocytes, they also give rise to vascular smooth muscle (Figure 2.4g) and endothelial cells (Figure 2.4h). When maGSCs are cultured on OP9 stro-mal cells, they are able to first differentiate into flk1-positive cells (25–55%), which can further differentiate into different cardiovascular lineages including cardiomyocytes and endothelial and smooth muscle cells.

Behavior of maGSCs after Intramyocardial Injection

To test the behavior of maGSCs in vivo within a myocardial environment, undifferentiated maGSCs labeled with Dil (dioctadecylindocarbo-cyanine) were injected into normal mouse hearts. After 1 week, Dil labeled cells could be identified. From histological analysis and expression analy-sis of Oct4 and Ki67, there is considerable evi-dence that proliferation of injected maGSCs occurs.[44] After 4 weeks, Dil labeled cells were still present; however, cardiac differentiation as indi-cated by cardiac troponin T expression did not occur within this short period of observation. Interestingly, no teratoma formation was observed, although we would expect that undifferentiated maGSCs would have the potential for teratoma development.[44] Further studies are needed to evaluate the behavior of maGSCs after injection into infarcted myocardium.

Application of Male Germline Stem Cells in Cardiac Regeneration Therapy

The cardiac differentiation potential of maGSCs opens new possibilities for basic research on car-diac development as well as cardiac regeneration. This includes further studies of the behavior of undifferentiated maGSCs in normal and infarcted myocardium (see above) as well as the behavior of maGSCs predifferentiated into car-diac lineages or differentiated cardiomyocytes derived from maGSCs. The latter would require strategies to select differentiated cells. These selection strategies would require a high level of specification to exclude the use of undifferen-tiated cells with the potential of teratoma development. Particularly the functional car-diomyocytes derived from germline stem cells may be able to be engrafted into the damaged host myocardium and function as cardiomy-ocytes after transplantation into damaged hearts.

The most exciting question now is whether the adult human testis can be a source of ES-like cells. The development of a defined culture system for human SSCs would therefore be of paramount importance. When positive results are obtained, these ES-like cells could be used for autologous regeneration strategies without ethical and immu-nological problems: SSCs and maGSCs could be obtained from testicular biopsies without the use of human embryonic tissue, and the availability of immunocompatible tissue for autotransplantation would circumvent immunological problems asso-ciated with ESC-based therapy. Regeneration strategies using maGSCs may be based on tech-niques that have been developed previously for ESCs. The use of ES-like cell-derived functional cells could potentially offer lifelong treatment.

Before clinical use may be considered, numerous questions have to be answered. Because the population of spontaneously differentiated cells from ES-like cells is always a mixture of different cell types, purifying the cells of interest from the mixed population is essential. Another potential problem is the generation of an adequate number of cells sufficient for active improvement of contractile function. It will be necessary to direct ES-like cells more efficiently to cardiac lineages. Furthermore, an adequate regeneration strategy to substitute for infarcted heart muscle or scar tissue with ES-like cell-derived cardiomyocytes will require that new muscle cells integrate with the existing host muscle and contract in a coordinated and mechanically useful manner. In addition, development of a new blood supply for the transplanted cardiomyocytes is necessary.

Although some male patients could be treated by autologous transplantation of immunocompatible tissue, for allogeneic treatment of multiple patients by the same donor cells, it would be necessary to develop strategies to prevent immune rejection. These strategies to reduce immune rejection may include: (1) the establishment of a human ES-like cell bank, and (2) genetic modulation of ES-like cells to suppress actively the immune response.

In conclusion, germline stem cells may provide a new source of pluripotent cells for regenerative medicine. From mouse studies, we know that germline stem cells can be cultured in vitro for an indefinite period and are able to differentiate into cells from all three germ layers including functional cardiomyocytes. For stem cell-based therapy, a major challenge will be to generate strategies that enable the development of multipotent cells from human adult SSCs and to develop further techniques for their use in organ regeneration.

References

1. Guan K, Nayernia K, Maier LS et al. Pluripotency of spermatogonial stem cells from adult mouse testis. Nature 2006; 440: 1199–203.
2. Kanatsu-Shinohara M, Inoue K, Lee J et al. Generation of pluripotent stem cells from neonatal mouse testis. Cell 2004; 119: 1001–12.
3. Brinster RL, Zimmermann JW. Spermatogenesis following male germ-cell transplantation. Proc Natl Acad Sci USA 1994; 91: 1298–302.
4. Kubota H, Avarbock MR, Brinster RL. Growth factors essential for self-renewal and expansion of mouse spermatogonial stem cells. Proc Natl Acad Sci USA 2004; 101: 16489–94.
5. Kanatsu-Shinohara M, Ikawa M, Takehashi M et al. Production of knockout mice by random or targeted mutagenesis in spermatogonial stem cells. Proc Natl Acad Sci USA 2006; 103: 8018–23.
6. Kubota H, Brinster RL. Technology insight: in vitro culture of spermatogonial stem cells and their potential therapeutic uses. Nat Clin Pract Endocrinol Metab 2006; 2: 99–108.
7. Izadyar F, Creemers LB, van Dissel-Emiliani FM, van Pelt AM, de Rooij DG. Spermatogonial stem cell transplantation. Mol Cell Endocrinol 2000; 169: 21–6.
8. Mahowald AP, Hennen S. Ultrastructure of the "germ plasm" in eggs and embryos of Rana pipiens. Dev Biol 1971; 24: 37–53.
9. Eddy EM, Hahnel AC. Establishment of the germ cell line in mammals. In: McLaren A, Wylie C, eds. Current Problems in Germ Cell Differentiation. Cambridge: Cambridge University Press, 1983: 41–69.
10. McLaren A. Primordial germ cells in the mouse. Dev Biol 2003; 262: 1–15.
11. Saitou M, Barton SC, Surani MA. A molecular programme for the specification of germ cell fate in mice. Nature 2002; 418: 293–300.
12. Sato M, Kimura T, Kurokawa K et al. Identification of PGC7, a new gene expressed specifically in preimplantation embryos and germ cells. Mech Dev 2002; 113: 91–4.
13. Yabuta Y, Kurimoto K, Ohinata Y, Seki Y, Saitou M. Gene expression dynamics during germline specification in mice identified by quantitative single-cell gene expression profiling. Biol Reprod 2006; 75: 705–16.
14. Ohinata Y, Payer B, O'Carroll D et al. Blimp1 is a critical determinant of the germ cell lineage in mice. Nature 2005; 436: 207–13.
15. Monk M, Boubelik M, Lehnert S. Temporal and regional changes in DNA methylation in the embryonic, extraembryonic and germ cell lineages during mouse embryo development. Development 1987; 99: 371–82.
16. Seki Y, Hayashi K, Itoh K et al. Extensive and orderly reprogramming of genome-wide chromatin modifications associated with specification and early development of germ cells in mice. Dev Biol 2005; 278: 440–58.
17. Allegrucci C, Thurston A, Lucas E, Young L. Epigenetics and the germline. Reproduction 2005; 129: 137–49.
18. de Rooij DG. Stem cells in the testis. Int J Exp Pathol 1998; 79: 67–80.

19. Spradling A, Drummond-Barbosa D, Kai T. Stem cells find their niche. Nature 2001; 414: 98–104.

20. Boyer LA, Lee TI, Cole MF et al. Core transcriptional regulatory circuitry in human embryonic stem cells. Cell 2005; 122: 947–56.

21. Loh YH, Wu Q, Chew JL et al. The Oct4 and Nanog transcription network regulates pluripotency in mouse embryonic stem cells. Nat Genet 2006; 38: 431–40.

22. Wang J, Rao S, Chu J et al. A protein interaction network for pluripotency of embryonic stem cells. Nature 2006; 444: 364–8.

23. Pan G, Thomson JA. Nanog and transcriptional networks in embryonic stem cell pluripotency. Cell Res 2007; 17: 42–9.

24. Takahashi K, Yamanaka S. Induction of pluripotent stem cells from mouse embryonic and adult fibroblast cultures by defined factors. Cell 2006; 126: 633–76.

25. Wernig M, Meissner A, Foreman R et al. In vitro reprogramming of fibroblasts into a pluripotent ES-cell-like state. Nature 2007; 448: 318–24.

26. Okita K, Ichisaka T, Yamanaka S. Generation of germline-competent induced pluripotent stem cells. Nature 2007; 448: 313–7.

27. Maherali N, Sridharan R, Xie W et al. Directly Reprogrammed Fibroblasts Show Global Epigenetic Remodeling and Widespread Tissue Contribution. Cell Stem Cell 2007; 1: 55–70.

28. Seydoux G, Braun RE. Pathway to totipotency: lessons from germ cells. Cell 2006; 127: 891–904.

29. Matsui Y, Zsebo K, Hogan BL. Derivation of pluripotential embryonic stem cells from murine primordial germ cells in culture. Cell 1992; 70: 841–7.

30. Resnick JL, Bixler LS, Cheng L, Donovan PJ. Long-term proliferation of mouse primordial germ cells in culture. Nature 1992; 359: 550–1.

31. Shamblott MJ, Axelman J, Wang S et al. Derivation of pluripotent stem cells from cultured human primordial germ cells. Proc Natl Acad Sci USA 1998; 95: 13726–31.

32. Fleischman RA. From white spots to stem cells: the role of the Kit receptor in mammalian development. Trends Genet 1993; 9: 285–90.

33. Donovan PJ, de Miguel MP. Turning germ cells into stem cells. Curr Opin Genet Dev 2003; 13: 463–71.

34. Labosky PA, Barlow DP, Hogan BL. Embryonic germ cell lines and their derivation from mouse primordial germ cells. Ciba Found Symp 1994; 182: 157–68; discussion 168–78.

35. Dean W, Bowden L, Aitchison A et al. Altered imprinted gene methylation and expression in completely ES cell-derived mouse fetuses: association with aberrant phenotypes. Development 1998; 125: 2273–82.

36. Humpherys D, Eggan K, Akutsu H et al. Epigenetic instability in ES cells and cloned mice. Science 2001; 293: 95–7.

37. Onyango P, Jiang S, Uejima H et al. Monoallelic expression and methylation of imprinted genes in human and mouse embryonic germ cell lineages. Proc Natl Acad Sci USA 2002; 99: 10599–604.

38. de Rooij DG. Proliferation and differentiation of spermatogonial stem cells. Reproduction 2001; 121: 347–54.

39. Puglisi R, Montanari M, Chiarella P, Stefanini M, Boitani C. Regulatory role of BMP2 and BMP7 in spermatogonia and Sertoli cell proliferation in the immature mouse. Eur J Endocrinol 2004; 151: 511–20.

40. Zhao GQ, Chen YX, Liu XM, Xu Z, Qi X. Mutation in Bmp7 exacerbates the phenotype of Bmp8a mutants in spermatogenesis and epididymis. Dev Biol 2001; 240: 212–22.

41. de Rooij DG, Grootegoed JA. Spermatogonial stem cells. Curr Opin Cell Biol 1998; 10: 694–701.

42. Kanatsu-Shinohara M, Ogonuki N, Iwano T et al. Genetic and epigenetic properties of mouse male germline stem cells during long-term culture. Development 2005; 132: 4155–63.

43. Baba S, Heike T, Umeda K et al. Generation of cardiac and endothelial cells from neonatal mouse testis-derived multipotent germline stem cells. Stem Cells 2007; 25: 1375–83.

44. Guan K, Wagner S, Unsold B et al. Generation of functional cardiomyocytes from adult mouse spermatogonial stem cells. Circ Res 2007; 100: 1615–25.

chapter 3

Is There Evidence for Cardiogenic Stem Cells Outside the Heart in Adult Mammals?

Elina Minami, Charles E Murry, and Hans Reinecke

Introduction

The mammalian heart has a very limited capacity to regenerate lost cardiomyocytes. Consequently, extensive cardiomyocyte loss (e.g. due to infarction or myocarditis) typically heals by scar formation, which leaves the patient with a contractile deficit that often progresses to heart failure. Prompted by the clinical need to treat heart failure, scientists in the mid-1990s began exploring cell-based cardiac repair in an attempt to remuscularize damaged hearts. Shortly thereafter, researchers in adult stem cell biology advanced the notion of stem cell plasticity, which suggested that adult stem cells could differentiate into unexpected cell types (transdifferentiate) when placed into a new tissue environment.[1] Since that time, many studies have examined the ability of adult stem cells to form new cardiomyocytes or other myocardial cells, and, encouragingly, physiological studies consistently show improved contractile function following transplantation of adult stem cell derivatives (reviewed below). The goal of this chapter is to provide a critical review of the evidence that extracardiac progenitor cells form new myocardium in vitro and in the mammalian heart in vivo. Due to the large body of literature on this topic, we will spend a significant portion covering bone marrow-derived stem cells in this chapter. We recommend the reader to refer to Chapter 6 by Professor Doevendans and colleagues on resident cardiac progenitor cells and Chapter 5 by Professor Kloner and Dr Dai for a more in-depth analysis of mesenchymal stem cells.

In Vitro Observations with Bone Marrow-Derived Stem Cells

Over the last approximately 8 years a variety of extracardiac cell types from various tissues have been reported to adopt a cardiomyocyte phenotype when placed under certain culture conditions. This, per se, is an encouraging fact, and may suggest that infarct remuscularization using autologous cells may one day be feasible. It should be noted, however, that in nearly all studies the candidate progenitors needed a little help to achieve their cardiac potential, in the form of adding the non-specific DNA methyltransferase inhibitor 5-azacytidine (a demethylating agent), or the potent steroid hormone dexamethasone, or by coculturing the candidate cell type with dead or alive cardiomyocytes. These treatments currently may have reduced clinical applicability due to low efficiency or potentially harmful effects, e.g. random DNA demethylation.

Mesenchymal stem cells

One of the most studied candidate cardiac progenitors is the bone marrow-derived mesenchymal stem cell (MSC). MSCs were originally identified based on their ability to generate skeletal muscle after treatment with 5-azacytidine.[2] Subsequently, MSCs were shown to differentiate into various cell types, including bone,[3,4] fat,[5] tendon fibroblasts, or cartilage.[6] Based on these findings, Makino and colleagues hypothesized that marrow stromal cells might also differentiate into cardiomyocytes.[7] The authors isolated bone marrow from adult C3H/He mice and screened marrow stromal cells that began spontaneously beating after exposure to the demethylating agent 5-azacytidine. Conversion rates were reported at ~30%. Reverse transcriptase polymerase chain reaction (RT-PCR) analysis showed that the beating cells expressed several genes found in cardiomyocytes, e.g. atrial natriuretic peptide (ANP), brain natriuretic peptide (BNP), GATA4, and Nkx2-5/Csx, and low levels of α-myosin heavy chain (MHC) and α-cardiac actin. However, abundant expression of β-MHC and α-skeletal actin, main contractile proteins of murine neonatal cardiomyocytes and skeletal muscle, was also reported. Morphologically, the cells clearly appeared as multinucleated skeletal myotubes up to 3 mm in length with hundreds of nuclei. Unfortunately, the authors did not use conventionally derived skeletal myotubes as a control in their PCR-based analysis, nor did they investigate the expression of skeletal muscle-specific genes such as MyoD or skeletal muscle-specific myosin isoforms.

Balana and colleagues similarly attempted to differentiate cardiomyocytes from human mononuclear cells derived from healthy bone marrow donors.[8] The cultures were exposed to 5-azacytidine followed by 6 weeks of further culture. Drug treatment did not induce expression of the skeletal muscle marker MyoD or cardiac markers Nkx2-5 and GATA4, and did not yield beating cells during follow-up. However, in patch clamp experiments, some treated and untreated cells exhibited L-type calcium currents, and almost all cells showed outwardly rectifying potassium currents of rapid or slow activation kinetics. These currents would be expected in cardiomyocytes, but their presence is not specific to cardiomyocytes. Taken together, these data indicate that MSCs can form skeletal muscle in some circumstances after the induction of DNA demethylation (likely by demethylating MyoD family members), but this protocol does not robustly induce cardiac differentiation in vitro.

Other protocols have been used in attempts to induce cardiogenesis from MSCs. Shim et al[9] reported non-contractile cardiomyocyte-like cells derived from bone marrow collected from patients undergoing coronary artery bypass surgery. These authors used insulin, dexamethasone, and ascorbic acid in their differentiation medium and observed the expression of α/β-MHC and GATA4 together with a lack of skeletal MHC and MyoD expression, and an absence of multinucleated myotube formation. Approximately 15–20% of the cardiomyogenic-like cells were found to show cross-striations characterized by α-actinin-positive Z bands. However, the limited number of cells with cross-striations and lack of spontaneous beating in culture suggested that the cells had not fully differentiated into mature cardiomyocytes.[9]

A recent study by Bartunek et al sought to differentiate canine MSCs into a cardiac lineage.[10] These authors attempted to recapitulate signals from embryonic development, where bone morphogenetic protein (BMP)2/4, fibroblast growth factor (FGF), and insulin-like growth factor (IGF), as well as direct cell–cell interactions through specific extracellular matrix (ECM), are required for the specification and stabilization of the mesoderm to form a cardiac field.[11,12] Hence, their cardiac differentiation media contained the cardiomyogenic growth factors basic FGF, BMP2, and IGF1. They found that the treated MSCs showed a uniform expression of the cardiac transcription factors myocyte enhancer factor 2 (MEF2), GATA4, and Nkx2-5. However, treated MSCs did not differentiate into contracting cardiomyocytes, nor did they express sarcomeric myosin heavy chains.

Interestingly, a very recent study by Shiota and colleagues added a sphere formation step to the MSC to cardiomyocyte differentiation protocol.[13] Sphere formation has been utilized as a way to isolate multipotent stem/progenitor cells from various tissues. In this study, multipotent marrow cell populations were isolated using adherent and non-adherent conditions, finally resulting in sphere formation. Under appropriate conditions the sphere-derived cells acquired the phenotype of neurons, adipocytes, osteoblasts, chondrocytes and, most importantly in this context, beating cells. However, morphologically sphere-derived contracting cells resembled skeletal myotubes, and expressed MyoD but not Nkx2-5. Cardiac differentiation with these cells was only reported after grafting into a mouse infarct model. Here, the frequency of the cells engrafted as cardiomyocytes was extremely low at less than 0.001%,[13] i.e. in the range of rare fusion events.

Based on a partial activation of the cardiac gene expression profile, the authors of the above studies interpreted that their findings to indicate that their treatment of MSCs induced cardiac differentiation. However, another interpretation may be that, depending on the growth factor cocktail offered, some cardiac genes may be unchained in vitro, but the full cardiomyogenic program never unfolds. In contrast, if one uses embryonic stem cells as the benchmark, one sees that these cells consistently form beating cardiomyocytes with full activation of the cardiac gene expression profile and expected electrophysiological properties. In differentiating embryonic stem cell cultures, the occurrence of beating is the first marker to gauge the quality of cardiac differentiation and precedes any further evaluation. Should we not use the same stringency for other candidate cell types? Furthermore, given the large number of excellent reagents available to distinguish between skeletal and cardiac muscle, there is no scientific justification for not determining which striated muscle population the cells have formed, yet many papers continue to be published using ambiguous striated muscle markers.

Multipotent adult progenitor cells

In 2002, Verfaillie's group published the derivation of a multipotent adult progenitor cell (MAPC) that copurified with mesenchymal stem cells from bone marrow.[14,15] These MAPCs were then found to reside in normal human, rodent, and possibly other mammalian postnatal tissues. When injected into an early blastocyst, single MAPCs contributed to most, if not all, somatic cell types of the developing embryo including the heart. In vitro differentiation studies showed that MAPCs can be cultured for at least 70 cell doublings, have long telomeres that do not shorten in culture, and have multilineage differentiation potential. Indeed, MAPCs under specific culture conditions differentiated to mesenchymal cell types, i.e. cartilage, bone, fibroblasts, and adipocytes, as well as to cells of almost all other mesodermal cell lineages, namely skeletal, smooth, and cardiac myoblasts and von Willebrand factor-positive endothelial cells.[16] In addition, MAPCs could be induced to differentiate to cells of the neuroectodermal lineage, including neurons expressing β-tubulin III, neurofilament, neuron-specific enolase and glutamate receptor, astrocytes expressing glial fibrillar acidic protein, and oligodendrocytes expressing myelinbasic protein and galactocerebroside. However, cardiogenic differentiation was never shown convincingly, for example MAPCs were never shown to contract in vitro and to express a variety of cardiac-specific markers. Problematic is also the extreme rarity of the cells (1 MAPC in 10–100 million bone marrow cells[16]), and with that the difficult isolation/purification of MAPCs. However, once purified and under proper cell culture conditions, MAPCs appear to be expandable and maintainable in the undifferentiated state.

Endothelium and endothelial progenitor cells

In 2003, Dimmeler's group published the derivation of CD34+ human endothelial progenitor cells (EPCs) obtained from peripheral blood

as Flk1 and CD34 were used to isolate putative angioblasts from the mononuclear cell fraction of peripheral blood.[58] Subsequently, EPCs were also isolated from human umbilical cord blood, bone marrow-derived mononuclear cells, and CD34+ or CD133+ hematopoietic stem cells,[59,61–63] and these cells were shown to differentiate into endothelial cells. Kawamoto and colleagues investigated the effect of direct repopulation of EPCs in a rat model of myocardial infarction.[64] They obtained peripheral blood mononuclear cells from healthy human adults, expanded these in EPC medium, and injected the cells intravenously 3 hours after the induction of myocardial ischemia. The results showed that transplanted EPCs accumulated in the ischemic area and incorporated into foci of myocardial neovascularization. Echocardiography at 4 weeks showed smaller ventricular dimensions, increased fractional shortening, and better regional wall motion in the EPC group. In addition, morphometric analyses revealed greater capillary density in the EPC group.[64] The promising results from initial experimental studies promoted the initiation of clinical pilot studies.

In addition to these studies, Kocher et al mobilized human hematopoietic (CD34+, CD117+) and mesenchymal stem cells (CD34–/CD117–) following treatment of granulocyte colony stimulating factor, labeled them with the fluorescent membrane marker DiI (dioctadecylindocarbocyanine), and injected them intravenously in the rat following myocardial infarction.[65] The cells were detected in the infarct region 2 weeks after infarction, but only the hematopoietic lineage showed increased vascularity and improved ejection fraction, which existed even at 15 weeks. The exact mechanism of how these cells induce angiogenesis is unclear, but potentially these cells trigger proangiogenesis by way of the paracrine effect to alter the milieu of the infarct region and to enhance the restoration of blood flow.[66,67]

Concluding remarks: animal studies

A critical evaluation of the literature reveals that skeletal myoblasts, hematopoietic stem cells, mesenchymal stem cells, and endothelial progenitors, originally postulated to have cardiogenic potential, do not significantly give rise to cardiomyocytes either spontaneously or after in vivo transplantation. While fusion of either circulating cells or those directly injected into the heart results in occasional hybrid cardiomyocytes, these events are so rare that they cannot have an effect on contractile function (although they could potentially influence electrophysiological properties). The report by Yoon et al[25] that non-hematopoietic, non-mesenchymal bone marrow progenitors extensively regenerate the heart has not, to our knowledge, been reproduced. Given that no other investigators had previously isolated such a cell, caution is indicated until these findings are reproduced by an independent group.

There is, however, no doubt that Orlic's provocative study[39] spurred a flurry of bone marrow-based cell transplantation studies in humans (refer to Chapter 10 by Dr Perin and Dr Silva). A clinical implication of the animal studies is that human trials of bone marrow for cardiac repair are unlikely to generate significant numbers of new cardiomyocytes. Nonetheless, it appears that bone marrow-derived cells benefit ventricular remodeling by improving the connective tissue framework, promoting angiogenesis, and enhancing the survival of host cardiomyocytes in chronically ischemic regions through paracrine mechanisms.

Evidence for Extracardiac Progenitors in Humans

Patients with heart transplants or bone marrow transplants offer unique insights into the ability of circulating cells to enter the heart and differentiate into components of myocardium. Most of these studies have used gender-mismatched transplants, where sex chromosomes can identify cells that are not native to the heart. Many reports indicate that extracardiac progenitors can give rise to components of cardiac tissue (Table 3.1).[68–70,72,74] Our group investigated five autopsy specimens from male recipients who received a female donor heart and lived 1–10 years

Table 3.1   Studies of extracardiac progenitor cells in humans

Reference	Donor → recipient	Type of transplant	Method of identification	Percentage of recipient cells
Quaini et al (2002)[68]	Female → male	Heart TX	Fluorescent Y-probe in situ hybridization with smooth muscle α-actin, endothelial, and cardiac markers	Arterioles with Y+ VSMCs 20% Capillaries with Y+ endothelial cells 14% Cardiomyocytes 18%
Laflamme et al (2002)[69]	Female → male	Heart TX	Y-probe in situ hybridization with myosin heavy chain	Cardiomyocytes 0.04%
Glaser et al (2002)[70]	Female → male	Heart TX	Fluorescent Y-probe in situ hybridization with smooth muscle α-actin	VSMCs 5–10%
Muller et al (2002)[71]	Female → male	Heart TX	Fluorescent Y-probe in situ hybridization with sarcomeric actin, smooth muscle actin, von Willebrand factor	Cardiomyocytes 0.16% VSMCs NA Endothelial cells NA
Deb et al (2003)[72]	Male → female	Bone marrow TX	Fluorescent Y-probe in situ hybridization with smooth muscle actin, myosin heavy chain	Cardiomyocytes 0.23%
Simper et al (2003)[73]	Female → male	Heart TX	Fluorescent Y-probe in situ hybridization with CD31	Endothelial cells 1–24%
Hocht-Zeisberg et al (2004)[74]	Female → male	Heart TX	Fluorescent Y-probe in situ hybridization with CD45/CD68, von Willebrand factor Cardiomyocytes detected by autofluorescence	Cardiomyocytes 0.21% (infarct), 0.04% (non-infarct) Endothelial cells 0.56% (infarct), 0.01% (non-infarct)
Minami et al (2005)[75]	Female → male	Heart TX	Y-probe in situ hybridization with smooth muscle actin, endothelial cell and peripheral nerve markers	VSMCs 3.4% Endothelial cells 24% Schwann cells 11%

TX, transplant; VSMCs, vascular smooth muscle cells; NA, not available.

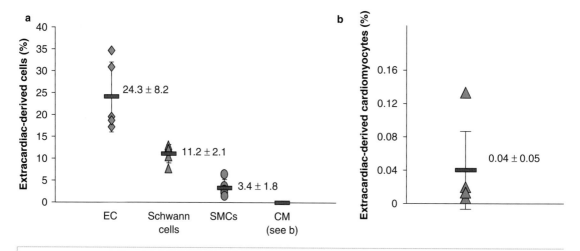

Figure 3.3   *Quantitative analysis of extracardiac-derived endothelial cells (EC), Schwann cells, vascular smooth muscle cells (SMCs), and cardiomyocytes (CM) in autopsy specimens from five patients. Each symbol represents the mean data from a single patient obtained for each cell type. (a) The frequency of extracardiac-derived cells was: endothelial cells 24.3%, Schwann cells 11.2%, vascular smooth muscle cells 3.4%, and cardiomyocytes 0.04%. (b) Expanded scale of the extent of recipient-derived cardiomyocytes. (Modified with permission from reference 75.)*

post-transplantation. While all patients were found to have Y chromosome-positive cardiomyocytes, these averaged only 0.04% of total cardiomyocytes (Figure 3.3). This small number of cells may have arisen via fusion of circulating cells with cardiomyocytes, and would not be expected to have any beneficial impact on myocardial function. In a subsequent study, we found that 3.4% of smooth muscle cells, 24% of endothelial cells, and 11% of Schwann cells were recipient-derived[75] (Figure 3.3). These studies indicate that, while most components of myocardium can be derived from extracardiac progenitors, the frequency varies widely by cell type. The functional significance of these extracardiac-derived cells and their origin still need to be determined. Because endothelial cells are highly immunogenic, we hypothesize that repopulating the coronary circulation with host endothelium may reduce the allograft's immunogenicity by way of tolerance.

Another group studied eight sex-mismatched heart transplant specimens to detect the extent of recipient-derived cells to repopulate endothelial, smooth muscle cells, and cardiomyocytes in transplanted hearts.[68] In this study, the percentage

of Y chromosome-positive microvessels was used rather than the percentage of Y-positive cells, which makes their results not directly comparable for endothelium and smooth muscle cells. Nevertheless, they found that 20% of arterioles had Y-positive smooth muscle cells, 14% of capillaries had Y-positive endothelial cells, and 18% of cardiomyocytes were recipient-derived. While their vascular cell counts are reasonably comparable to ours, their percentage of detected recipient-derived cardiomyocytes is 450-fold greater than our own study.[68,69] As mentioned in Quaini's sudy, heart specimens that were obtained early post-transplantation had higher levels of chimerism, suggesting that many of the Y-positive nuclei could belong to leukocytes, which happen to reside precisely on top of the cell type of interest, giving the false impression of a positive cell. Based on these findings, it is important to exclude false positives by meticulous histological analysis (including confocal microscopy to visualize the tissue in three dimensions (Figure 3.4)) and immunological staining to exclude leukocytes.

Other studies addressed specific forms of injury in the transplanted heart to point out extracardiac

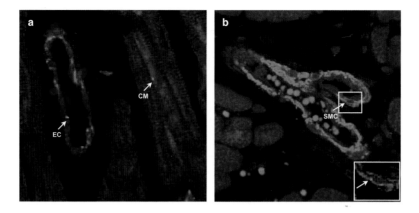

Figure 3.4   *Chimerism in human sex-mismatched heart transplants. Confocal microscopy demonstrates chimerism of an endothelial cell (a: EC, Ulex lectin staining in red), a cardiomyocyte (a: CM, green autofluorescence reveals cross-striations), and a smooth muscle cell (b: SMC, smooth muscle α-actin staining in red), respectively. The inset in panel (b) shows a higher magnification of the boxed area. Arrows indicate the Y-chromosome. (Reproduced with permission from references 75 and 76.)*

stem cells in the reparative process. Simper et al focused on five post-transplant patients who had either transplant arteriopathy or normal arteries and investigated differences in the degree of recipient-derived cells. They also obtained peripheral blood specimens to determine endothelial colonies in these patients. In diseased vessels, the luminal surface had a range of 1–24% recipient-derived endothelial cells, compared to only 0.2% in non-diseased segments.[77] The exact origin of these cells is still undefined, but work from Deb et al suggested a possible bone marrow origin.[72] These investigators studied four autopsy specimens of patients who received sex-mismatched bone marrow transplantation and demonstrated 0.23% of cardiomyocytes as recipient-derived. The study stained for laminin to show the endothelial–basement membrane boundary to minimize false-positive counting. Hocht-Zeisberg et al looked at five autopsy specimens from sex-mismatched heart transplant candidates who had a myocardial infarction of the transplanted heart.[74] They found that the majority of the Y-positive cells were inflammatory cells detected by a pan-leukocyte and macrophage marker (CD45 and CD68, respectively). Only ~0.2% of recipient-derived cardiomyocytes were seen in the infarcted heart, compared to only 0.04% in the non-infarcted heart. In a study by Muller and

colleagues, 21 cardiac biopsy specimens from 13 male heart transplant recipients, who received a female donor heart, were studied to detect the degree of recipient-derived cardiomyocytes in the biopsy specimens.[71] Only 0.16% recipient-derived cardiomyocytes were detected, suggesting that recipient-derived cells do exist, but not sufficient for full reparative capacity.

Concluding remarks: human studies

All of the studies presently discussed and mentioned show that there is evidence for extracardiac progenitor cells that are capable of repopulating the injured heart, but so far, the degree of cardiomyocyte repopulation is too small to make these cell types the ideal cell source for rebuilding the heart. Although animal studies indicate that marrow-derived cells improve cardiac function postinfarction, these cells have not been shown to transdifferentiate into cardiomyocytes efficiently, and likely benefit the heart via paracrine mechanisms. Uncovering the molecules responsible for the paracrine effect may provide new treatment options to patients that bypass the need for cells. As the quest to find sources of stem cells that are unequivocally cardiogenic continues, our group and others are exploring embryonic stem cells for cardiac regeneration. Current work focuses on guided differentiation of embryonic stem cells into a cardiomyogenic phenotype with the goal to use these cells as an efficient source for myocardial repair following injury.[78–83]

References

1. Vieyra DS, Jackson KA, Goodell MA. Plasticity and tissue regenerative potential of bone marrow-derived cells. Stem Cell Rev 2005; 1: 65–9.
2. Wakitani S, Saito T, Caplan AI. Myogenic cells derived from rat bone marrow mesenchymal stem cells exposed to 5-azacytidine. Muscle Nerve 1995; 18: 1417–26.
3. Rickard DJ, Sullivan TA, Shenker BJ et al. Induction of rapid osteoblast differentiation in rat bone marrow stromal cell cultures by dexamethasone and BMP-2. Dev Biol 1994; 161: 218–28.
4. Friedenstein AJ, Chailakhyan RK, Gerasimov UV. Bone marrow osteogenic stem cells: in vitro cultivation and transplantation in diffusion chambers. Cell Tissue Kinet 1987; 20: 263–72.
5. Umezawa A, Maruyama T, Segawa K et al. Multipotent marrow stromal cell line is able to induce hematopoiesis in vivo. J Cell Physiol 1992; 151: 197–205.
6. Ashton BA, Allen TD, Howlett CR et al. Formation of bone and cartilage by marrow stromal cells in diffusion chambers in vivo. Clin Orthop Relat Res 1980; 151: 294–307.
7. Makino S, Fukuda K, Miyoshi S et al. Cardiomyocytes can be generated from marrow stromal cells in vitro. J Clin Invest 1999; 103: 697–705.
8. Balana B, Nicoletti C, Zahanich I et al. 5-Azacytidine induces changes in electrophysiological properties of human mesenchymal stem cells. Cell Res 2006; 16: 949–60.
9. Shim WS, Jiang S, Wong P et al. Ex vivo differentiation of human adult bone marrow stem cells into cardiomyocyte-like cells. Biochem Biophys Res Commun 2004; 324: 481–8.
10. Bartunek J, Croissant JD, Wijns W et al. Pretreatment of adult bone marrow mesenchymal stem cells with cardiomyogenic growth factors and repair of the chronically infarcted myocardium. Am J Physiol Heart Circ Physiol 2007; 292: H1095–104.
11. Arai A, Yamamoto K, Toyama J. Murine cardiac progenitor cells require visceral embryonic endoderm and primitive streak for terminal differentiation. Dev Dyn 1997; 210: 344–53.
12. Auda-Boucher G, Bernard B, Fontaine-Perus J et al. Staging of the commitment of murine cardiac cell progenitors. Dev Biol 2000; 225: 214–25.
13. Shiota M, Heike T, Haruyama M et al. Isolation and characterization of bone marrow-derived mesenchymal progenitor cells with myogenic and neuronal properties. Exp Cell Res 2007; 313: 1008–23.
14. Jiang Y, Jahagirdar BN, Reinhardt RL et al. Pluripotency of mesenchymal stem cells derived from adult marrow. Nature 2002; 418: 41–9.
15. Jiang Y, Vaessen B, Lenvik T et al. Multipotent progenitor cells can be isolated from postnatal murine bone marrow, muscle, and brain. Exp Hematol 2002; 30: 896–904.
16. Reyes M, Lund T, Lenvik T et al. Purification and ex vivo expansion of postnatal human marrow mesodermal progenitor cells. Blood 2001; 98: 2615–25.
17. Dimmeler S, Aicher A, Vasa M et al. HMG-CoA reductase inhibitors (statins) increase endothelial progenitor cells via the PI 3-kinase/Akt pathway. J Clin Invest 2001; 108: 391–7.
18. Badorff C, Brandes RP, Popp R et al. Transdifferentiation of blood-derived human adult endothelial progenitor cells into functionally active cardiomyocytes. Circulation 2003; 107: 1024–32.
19. Koyanagi M, Urbich C, Chavakis E et al. Differentiation of circulating endothelial progenitor cells to a cardiomyogenic phenotype depends on E-cadherin. FEBS Lett 2005; 579: 6060–6.
20. Gruh I, Beilner J, Blomer U et al. No evidence of transdifferentiation of human endothelial progenitor cells into cardiomyocytes after coculture with neonatal rat cardiomyocytes. Circulation 2006; 113: 1326–34.
21. Condorelli G, Borello U, De Angelis L et al. Cardiomyocytes induce endothelial cells to transdifferentiate into cardiac muscle: implications for myocardium regeneration. Proc Natl Acad Sci USA 2001; 98: 10733–8.
22. Welikson RE, Kaestner S, Reinecke H et al. Human umbilical vein endothelial cells fuse with cardiomyocytes but do not activate cardiac gene expression. J Mol Cell Cardiol 2006; 40: 520–8.
23. Terada N, Hamazaki T, Oka M et al. Bone marrow cells adopt the phenotype of other cells by spontaneous cell fusion. Nature 2002; 416: 542–5.
24. Alvarez-Dolado M, Pardal R, Garcia-Verdugo JM et al. Fusion of bone-marrow-derived cells with Purkinje neurons, cardiomyocytes and hepatocytes. Nature 2003; 425: 968–73.
25. Yoon YS, Wecker A, Heyd L et al. Clonally expanded novel multipotent stem cells from human bone marrow regenerate myocardium after myocardial infarction. J Clin Invest 2005; 115: 326–38.
26. Zuk PA, Zhu M, Mizuno H et al. Multilineage cells from human adipose tissue: implications for cell-based therapies. Tissue Eng 2001; 7: 211–28.
27. Erickson GR, Gimble JM, Franklin DM et al. Chondrogenic potential of adipose tissue-derived stromal cells in vitro and in vivo. Biochem Biophys Res Commun 2002; 290: 763–9.

28. Safford KM, Hicok KC, Safford SD et al. Neurogenic differentiation of murine and human adipose-derived stromal cells. Biochem Biophys Res Commun 2002; 294: 371–9.

29. Cousin B, Andre M, Arnaud E et al. Reconstitution of lethally irradiated mice by cells isolated from adipose tissue. Biochem Biophys Res Commun 2003; 301: 1016–22.

30. Planat-Benard V, Menard C, Andre M et al. Spontaneous cardiomyocyte differentiation from adipose tissue stroma cells. Circ Res 2004; 94: 223–9.

31. Yamada Y, Wang XD, Yokoyama S et al. Cardiac progenitor cells in brown adipose tissue repaired damaged myocardium. Biochem Biophys Res Commun 2006; 342: 662–70.

32. Yamada Y, Yokoyama SI, Wang XD et al. Cardiac stem cells in brown adipose tissue express CD133 and induce bone marrow non-hematopoietic cells to differentiate into cardiomyocytes. Stem Cells 2007; 25: 1326–33.

33. Iijima Y, Nagai T, Mizukami M et al. Beating is necessary for transdifferentiation of skeletal muscle-derived cells into cardiomyocytes. FASEB J 2003; 17: 1361–3.

34. Reinecke H, Minami E, Poppa V et al. Evidence for fusion between cardiac and skeletal muscle cells. Circ Res 2004; 94: e56–60.

35. Winitsky SO, Gopal TV, Hassanzadeh S et al. Adult murine skeletal muscle contains cells that can differentiate into beating cardiomyocytes in vitro. PLoS Biol 2005; 3: e87.

36. Deasy BM, Jankowski RJ, Huard J. Muscle-derived stem cells: characterization and potential for cell-mediated therapy. Blood Cells Mol Dis 2001; 27: 924–33.

37. Nussbaum J, Minami E, Laflamme MA et al. Transplantation of undifferentiated murine embryonic stem cells in the heart: teratoma formation and immune response. FASEB J 2007; 21: 1345–57.

38. Swijnenburg RJ, Tanaka M, Vogel H et al. Embryonic stem cell immunogenicity increases upon differentiation after transplantation into ischemic myocardium. Circulation 2005; 112 (9 Suppl): I166–72.

39. Orlic D, Kajstura J, Chimenti S et al. Bone marrow cells regenerate infarcted myocardium. Nature 2001; 410: 701–5.

40. Murry CE, Soonpaa MH, Reinecke H et al. Haematopoietic stem cells do not transdifferentiate into cardiac myocytes in myocardial infarcts. Nature 2004; 428: 664–8.

41. Balsam LB, Wagers AJ, Christensen JL et al. Haematopoietic stem cells adopt mature haematopoietic fates in ischaemic myocardium. Nature 2004; 428: 668–73.

42. Nygren JM, Jovinge S, Breitbach M et al. Bone marrow-derived hematopoietic cells generate cardiomyocytes at a low frequency through cell fusion, but not transdifferentiation. Nat Med 2004; 10: 494–501.

43. Ishikawa F, Shimazu H, Shultz LD et al. Purified human hematopoietic stem cells contribute to the generation of cardiomyocytes through cell fusion. FASEB J 2006; 20: 950–2.

44. Mirotsou M, Zhang Z, Deb A et al. Secreted frizzled related protein 2 (Sfrp2) is the key *Akt*-mesenchymal stem cell-released paracrine factor mediating myocardial survival and repair. Proc Natl Acad Sci USA 2007; 104: 1643–8.

45. Yeh ET, Zhang S, Wu HD et al. Transdifferentiation of human peripheral blood CD34+-enriched cell population into cardiomyocytes, endothelial cells, and smooth muscle cells in vivo. Circulation 2003; 108: 2070–3.

46. Chen SL, Fang WW, Ye F et al. Effect on left ventricular function of intracoronary transplantation of autologous bone marrow mesenchymal stem cell in patients with acute myocardial infarction. Am J Cardiol 2004; 94: 92–5.

47. Zhang S, Shpall E, Willerson JT et al. Fusion of human hematopoietic progenitor cells and murine cardiomyocytes is mediated by alpha 4 beta 1 integrin/vascular cell adhesion molecule-1 interaction. Circ Res 2007; 100: 693–702.

48. Pittenger MF, Martin BJ. Mesenchymal stem cells and their potential as cardiac therapeutics. Circ Res 2004; 95: 9–20.

49. Caplan AI, Bruder SP. Mesenchymal stem cells: building blocks for molecular medicine in the 21st century. Trends Mol Med 2001; 7: 259–64.

50. Bittira B, Kuang JQ, Al-Khaldi A et al. In vitro pre-programming of marrow stromal cells for myocardial regeneration. Ann Thorac Surg 2002; 74: 1154–9; discussion 1159–60.

51. Pittenger MF, Mackay AM, Beck SC et al. Multilineage potential of adult human mesenchymal stem cells. Science 1999; 284: 143–7.

52. Askari AT, Unzek S, Popovic ZB et al. Effect of stromal-cell-derived factor 1 on stem-cell homing and tissue regeneration in ischaemic cardiomyopathy. Lancet 2003; 362: 697–703.

53. Ma J, Ge J, Zhang S et al. Time course of myocardial stromal cell-derived factor 1 expression and beneficial effects of intravenously administered bone marrow stem cells in rats with experimental myocardial infarction. Basic Res Cardiol 2005; 100: 217–23.

54. Mangi AA, Noiseux N, Kong D et al. Mesenchymal stem cells modified with Akt prevent remodeling and restore performance of infarcted hearts. Nat Med 2003; 9: 1195–201.

55. Noiseux N, Gnecchi M, Lopez-Ilasaca M et al. Mesenchymal stem cells overexpressing Akt dramatically repair infarcted myocardium and improve cardiac function despite infrequent cellular fusion or differentiation. Mol Ther 2006; 14: 840–50.

56. Gnecchi M, He H, Liang OD et al. Paracrine action accounts for marked protection of ischemic heart by Akt-modified mesenchymal stem cells. Nat Med 2005; 11: 367–8.

57. Stump MM, Jordan GL Jr, Debakey ME et al. Endothelium grown from circulating blood on isolated intravascular Dacron hub. Am J Pathol 1963; 43: 361–7.

58. Asahara T, Murohara T, Sullivan A et al. Isolation of putative progenitor endothelial cells for angiogenesis. Science 1997; 275: 964–7.

59. Asahara T, Takahashi T, Masuda H et al. VEGF contributes to postnatal neovascularization by mobilizing bone marrow-derived endothelial progenitor cells. EMBO J 1999; 18: 3964–72.

60. Takahashi T, Kalka C, Masuda H et al. Ischemia- and cytokine-induced mobilization of bone marrow-derived endothelial progenitor cells for neovascularization. Nat Med 1999; 5: 434–8.

61. Shi Q, Rafii S, Wu MH et al. Evidence for circulating bone marrow-derived endothelial cells. Blood 1998; 92: 362–7.

62. Murohara T, Ikeda H, Duan J et al. Transplanted cord blood-derived endothelial precursor cells augment postnatal neovascularization. J Clin Invest 2000; 105: 1527–36.

63. Rafii S. Circulating endothelial precursors: mystery, reality, and promise. J Clin Invest 2000; 105: 17–19.

64. Kawamoto A, Gwon HC, Iwaguro H et al. Therapeutic potential of ex vivo expanded endothelial progenitor cells for myocardial ischemia. Circulation 2001; 103: 634–7.

65. Kocher AA, Schuster MD, Szabolcs MJ et al. Neovascularization of ischemic myocardium by human bone-marrow-derived angioblasts prevents cardiomyocyte apoptosis, reduces remodeling and improves cardiac function. Nat Med 2001; 7: 430–6.

66. Rehman J, Li J, Orschell CM et al. Peripheral blood "endothelial progenitor cells" are derived from monocyte/macrophages and secrete angiogenic growth factors. Circulation 2003; 107: 1164–9.

67. Kinnaird T, Stabile E, Burnett MS et al. Bone-marrow-derived cells for enhancing collateral development: mechanisms, animal data, and initial clinical experiences. Circ Res 2004; 95: 354–63.

68. Quaini F, Urbanek K, Beltrami AP et al. Chimerism of the transplanted heart. N Engl J Med 2002; 346: 5–15.

69. Laflamme MA, Myerson D, Saffitz JE et al. Evidence for cardiomyocyte repopulation by extracardiac progenitors in transplanted human hearts. Circ Res 2002; 90: 634–40.

70. Glaser R, Lu MM, Narula N et al. Smooth muscle cells, but not myocytes, of host origin in transplanted human hearts. Circulation 2002; 106: 17–19.

71. Muller P, Pfeiffer P, Koglin J et al. Cardiomyocytes of noncardiac origin in myocardial biopsies of human transplanted hearts. Circulation 2002; 106: 31–5.

72. Deb A, Wang S, Skelding KA et al. Bone marrow-derived cardiomyocytes are present in adult human heart: a study of gender-mismatched bone marrow transplantation patients. Circulation 2003; 107: 1247–9.

73. Simper D, Wang S, Deb A et al. Endothelial progenitor cells are decreased in blood of cardiac allograft patients with vasculopathy and endothelial cells of noncardiac origin are enriched in transplant atherosclerosis. Circulation 2003; 108: 143–9.

74. Hocht-Zeisberg E, Kahnert H, Guan K et al. Cellular repopulation of myocardial infarction in patients with sex-mismatched heart transplantation. Eur Heart J 2004; 25: 749–58.

75. Minami E, Laflamme MA, Saffitz JE et al. Extracardiac progenitor cells repopulate most major cell types in the transplanted human heart. Circulation 2005; 112: 2951–8.

76. Laflamme MA, Murry CE. Regenerating the heart. Nat Biotechnol 2005; 23: 845–56.

77. Caplice NM, Bunch TJ, Stalboerger PG et al. Smooth muscle cells in human coronary atherosclerosis can originate from cells administered at marrow transplantation. Proc Natl Acad Sci USA 2003; 100: 4754–9.

78. Kehat I, Kenyagin-Karsenti D, Snir M et al. Human embryonic stem cells can differentiate into myocytes with structural and functional properties of cardiomyocytes. J Clin Invest 2001; 108: 407–14.

79. Xu C, Police S, Rao N et al. Characterization and enrichment of cardiomyocytes derived from human embryonic stem cells. Circ Res 2002; 91: 501–8.

80. Kehat I, Khimovich L, Caspi O et al. Electromechanical integration of cardiomyocytes derived from human embryonic stem cells. Nat Biotechnol 2004; 22: 1282–9.

81. Laflamme MA, Gold J, Xu C et al. Formation of human myocardium in the rat heart from human embryonic stem cells. Am J Pathol 2005; 167: 663–71.

82. Kofidis T, Lebl DR, Swijnenburg RJ et al. Allopurinol/uricase and ibuprofen enhance engraftment of cardiomyocyte-enriched human embryonic stem cells and improve cardiac function following myocardial injury. Eur J Cardiothorac Surg 2006; 29: 50–5.

83. Rubart M, Field LJ. Cardiac repair by embryonic stem-derived cells. Handb Exp Pharmacol 2006; 174: 73–100.

chapter 4

Myocardial Regeneration via Cell Cycle Activation

Pascal J LaFontant and Loren J Field

Introduction

During development, increases in heart size results as a consequence of the differentiation and proliferation of cardiomyocytes, neurons, interstitial cells, and components of the vasculature. At birth, cardiomyocytes undergo a gradual transition from hyperplastic to hypertrophic growth, such that subsequent increases in myocardial mass result largely from increased myocyte size rather than increased number. In contrast, the other cell types present in the heart retain the ability to proliferate. Consequently, in adults, although cardiomyocytes constitute approximately 90% of the mass of the heart, they constitute less than 20% of the total number of cells present.

The proliferative capacity of adult cardiomyocytes is quite limited, although the exact level of cardiomyocyte cell cycle activity in the adult is the subject of debate.[1,2] Consequently, injured myocardium typically is replaced by the more rapidly proliferating cell types rather than by functional cardiomyocytes. While some data support the notion of the presence of cardiac resident and/or peripheral stem cells with cardiomyogenic activity,[3] the extent to which this occurs is subject to debate.[4] Regardless of the absolute levels of cardiomyocyte cell cycle and/or cardiomyogenic stem cell activity in the adult heart, they are insufficient to reverse the progression to heart failure following severe injury.

The absence of robust regeneration has prompted a number of approaches to attempt to increase cardiomyocyte numbers in diseased hearts. Clearly, interventions aimed at salvaging at-risk myocardium during the acute or chronic phases of injury can have a pronounced impact on cardiac function post-injury, and such cardioprotective activities are likely to underlie at least some of the beneficial effects seen with cell transplantation.[5,6] True regenerative growth, however, requires the replacement of lost cardiomyocytes with new cells able to participate in a functional syncytium with the surviving myocardium. Several approaches have emerged to attempt to accomplish this, including the direct transplantation of cardiomyocytes or cardiomyogenic stem cells,[7] mobilization of cardiac-resident or peripheral stem cells,[8] and induction of cell cycle activity in surviving cardiomyocytes.[9]

This chapter will discuss the potential utility of cell cycle activation as a means to induce regenerative growth of the heart. Initial discussions will focus on studies in several non-mammalian species which exhibit relatively robust myocardial regeneration following experimental injury to the heart. Experiments examining cardiomyocyte cell cycle activity in non-human mammalian species will then be reviewed. Finally, analyses examining cardiomyocyte cell cycle activity in human hearts will be reviewed.

Lessons from Non-Mammalian Species

Frogs, newts, and axolotls

The marked ability of many non-mammalian vertebrates to regenerate organs such as limbs, livers, and fins has fascinated researchers for centuries. Studies establishing a robust ability of many non-mammalian vertebrates including frogs, newts, axolotls, and reptiles to regenerate their hearts have also been reported. For example, the ability of adult frogs to regenerate a significant portion of a severed heart was reported more than four decades ago.[10] These studies, which utilized electron microscopy to identify cardiomyocytes and tritiated thymidine uptake coupled with autoradiography to identify cells undergoing DNA synthesis, provided evidence that myofiber-containing cardiomyocytes in the injured frog heart were able to re-enter the cell cycle. The marked degree of regenerative growth seen in these studies suggested that cardiomyocyte DNA synthesis culminated with mitosis and cytokinesis.

Robust heart regeneration was also observed in the adult newt and axolotl. In the newt, mitotic bodies within cells containing myofibers were observed at the border zone of injuries.[11] Once again, thymidine incorporation coupled with ultrastructural analysis revealed that cardiomyocytes at the border zone actively entered S-phase.[12-14] In vitro studies further supported the notion that subpopulations of newt cardiomyocytes are able to progress through the cell cycle.[15] Similar results were observed in the axolotl. Collectively these studies established that, in frogs, newts, and axolotls, differentiated adult cardiomyocytes have the ability to progress through the cell cycle and form regenerated myocardium following experimental injury.

Zebrafish

The amenability of zebrafish to genetic manipulations (including mutagenesis, transgenesis, and gene silencing using morpholinos)[16-19] makes them an ideal model system to study developmental processes. It is therefore not surprising that numerous studies examining heart patterning and cell fate mapping have emerged. Zebrafish also exhibit regenerative cardiac growth following experimental injury. In one study, adult zebrafish hearts were completely regenerated 60 days following resection of 20% of the myocardium.[20] Thirty percent of the cardiomyocytes adjacent to the area of injury

exhibited bromodeoxyuridine (BrdU) immune reactivity at 14 days post-resection (BrdU was injected daily for 7 days prior to analysis). Phosphorylated histone H3 immune reactivity (a marker of mitotic cells)[21] was also observed. In contrast to the results reported for frogs, newts, and axolotls, regeneration in the zebrafish was not accompanied by the development of persistent fibrosis.

Similar results were obtained following myocardial resection in zebrafish with a cardiomyocyte-restricted enhanced green fluorescent protein (EGFP) reporter transgene.[22] A quasi-complete regeneration and repatterning of the amputated myocardium was evident 30 days post-injury. Once again, high levels of cardiomyocyte BrdU incorporation were observed following 7 days of nucleotide injection. Interestingly, in situ analyses indicated that *Nkx2-5* expression was not upregulated in the regenerating myocardium (*Nkx2-5* is expressed in cardiac progenitors during zebrafish development). Additional studies were performed in transgenic fish expressing a CARP-promoted EGFP reporter transgene. CARP (cardiac ankyrin repeat protein) is a downstream target of *Nkx2-5*, and the reporter transgene is actively expressed during cardiac development but not in adult hearts. The reporter transgene was not induced in the regenerating cells following myocardial resection, consistent with the observed absence of *Nkx2-5* expression via in situ analysis. Moreover, the msxB and msxC transcription factors (which are induced in regenerating zebrafish tissues) were observed to be induced during heart regeneration, but not during cardiac development.[22] These observations led the investigators to conclude that the observed regenerative growth is not a simple recapitulation of events that occur during normal cardiac development.

Although the studies mentioned above documented the proliferation of differentiated cardiomyocytes following injury in adult zebrafish hearts, they did not rule out the potential role of stem cells in the regenerative process. To address this issue, myocardial regeneration was monitored in transgenic fish which expressed a nuclear localized red fluorescent protein (nRFP) reporter and a cytoplasmic EGFP reporter, both driven by the cardiomyocyte-restricted *cmlc2* promoter.[23] This system takes advantage of the observation that newly synthesized EGFP rapidly assumes a correct tertiary structure and exhibits epifluorescence, whereas the appropriate folding, nuclear transport, and epifluorescence of newly formed nRFP occurs much more slowly. Using this system, cardiomyocytes with cytoplasmic EGPF epifluorescence but lacking nRFP epifluorescence were observed at early stages of regeneration, suggesting that these cells arose from de novo differentiation as opposed to proliferation of pre-existing cardiomyocytes. It is, however, noteworthy that induction of *Nkx2-5* (as well as a number of other transcription factors associated with normal cardiac development) was detected in regions of active myocardial regeneration;[23] this result is in marked contrast to those observed previously.[22] Given this discrepancy, the conclusion that the observed myocardial regeneration is stem cell-mediated becomes highly dependent upon the reporter transgene system's ability to accurately discriminate between newly born versus proliferating cardiomyocytes. Nonetheless, these studies collectively demonstrate that zebrafish have a remarkable capacity to regenerate cardiac tissue following injury, and that cardiomyocyte cell cycle progression is a major component of that process.

Lessons from Non-human Mammals

Surveys of cardiomyocyte cell cycle activity in normal and injured hearts

Quantitation of cardiomyocyte proliferation entails assessment of some aspect of cell cycle activity. Although this is a relatively straightforward exercise in instances where the proliferation index is high (as in the examples presented above), there are several factors that complicate such analyses in mammalian hearts where adult cardiomyocyte activity is much lower. First, the method used to distinguish cardiomyocytes (and in particular, cardiomyocyte nuclei) from other cells is critical. Given the prevalence of non-cardiomyocyte nuclei in a typical histological section (>80%, see argument in the Introduction), a certain degree of subjectivity can be encountered when assigning a nucleus to a given cell type. Other difficulties are encountered when choosing a marker with which to score cell cycle activity. As indicated above, scoring DNA synthesis directly (i.e. by monitoring incorporation of modified nucleotides such as tritiated thymidine or BrdU) can clearly mark cells in S-phase. However, care must be exercised in studies which utilize long-term nucleotide delivery in light of the relative high rates of DNA turnover in non-proliferating cells (including adult cardiomyocytes).[24] Biochemical markers (i.e. Ki67 and proliferating cell nuclear antigen (PCNA) immune reactivity) are more tenuous because they provide only an indirect read-out of DNA synthesis, and their expression is known to occur in non-cycling cells.[25]

The difficulties encountered in scoring cardiomyocyte DNA synthesis are perhaps best illustrated by a simple survey of the literature for the values in uninjured adult hearts. In contrast to analysis of infarcted hearts, potential complications arising from varying degrees of myocardial injury and misidentification of infiltrating cells during wound healing would not confound the results. Nonetheless, even under these seemingly benign conditions, the reported rates of cardiomyocyte DNA synthesis in uninjured adult mice and rats ranged from as low as 0.0006% to as high as 3%.[1] The published values for cardiomyocyte cell cycle activity following injury are even more disparate, and undoubtedly reflect at least in part the nature of the different cell cycle assays employed and in part the fidelity of cardiomyocyte nucleus identification.[1,26]

Analysis of cell cycle progression is further complicated due to the presence of extensive multinucleation, which is thought to arise from acytokinetic mitoses. In agreement with this, anillin (a protein required for cleavage furrow formation and cytokinesis) fails to concentrate at the midbody during the formation of binucleated cardiomyocytes;[27] however, it is not clear whether this is causal for multinucleation. In mice, any amount from 3 to 13% of the cardiomyocytes in the adult ventricle are mononucleated (depending on genetic background), with the vast majority of the remaining cells being binucleated (although tri- and tetranucleated cells can be detected).[28] Similar levels of multinucleation occur in other species.[29]

Cardiomyocyte nuclei can also exhibit various levels of polyploidy. Although the majority of cardiomyocyte nuclei in adult mouse hearts contain a normal diploid DNA content, rare nuclei with as high as 16C DNA content have been detected.[30] Cardiomyocyte polyploidy is more prevalent in higher species. Endomitosis is thought to contribute to cardiomyocyte polyploidization,[31] although the potential contribution of cell fusion events[32,33] cannot be ruled out. The functional consequences of cardiomyocyte polyploidization in the adult heart are not clear, although a recent study suggested that it may reflect an adaptive response to aerobic energy deficiency.[34]

In the mouse, reporter transgenes have been used in conjunction with nucleotide incorporation assays to track cardiomyocyte DNA synthesis. For example, a reporter transgene utilizing the cardiomyocyte-restricted α-myosin heavy chain (MHC) promoter[35] to target expression of nuclear-localized β-galactosidase permits unambiguous identification of cardiomyocyte nuclei in tissue sections.[36,37] Cardiomyocyte nuclei can easily be identified in mice carrying the transgene with simple X-GAL (5-bromo-4-chloro-3-indolyl-β-D-galactoside) staining. X-GAL is a chromogenic substrate of β-galactosidase, and gives rise to a blue signal in the presence of the enzyme. To monitor cardiomyocyte DNA synthesis, the transgenic mice are given labeled deoxyribonucleotide (i.e. tritiated thymidine or BrdU), and sections prepared from the hearts are stained with X-GAL and processed to image for the presence of the labeled nucleotide (i.e. autoradiography or anti-BrdU immune reactivity, see Figure 4.1). The transgene reporter system can also be used to assist in the identification of cardiomyocyte-restricted phosphorylated histone H3 immune reactivity.[38]

Using this approach, cardiomyocyte DNA synthesis rates were monitored in adult hearts in the absence or presence of injury in DBA/2J inbred background. In uninjured hearts, DNA synthesis was observed in only 0.0006% of the ventricular cardiomyocytes (more than 180 000 nuclei were screened).[36] Focal necrotic damage (via application of a cautery iron to the epicardial surface of the left ventricle) increased the level of ventricular cardiomyocyte DNA synthesis to 0.008% at the injury border zone, while no cardiomyocyte DNA synthesis was observed in regions remote from the injury (assayed 7 days post-injury).[36] A similar induction in peri-injury cell cycle activity was observed following myocardial infarction, with DNA synthesis in 0.004% and 0.008% of the cardiomyocytes at 7 and 28 days post-infarction, respectively.[39] The main potential caveat of transgenic reporter approaches is that they require that the reporter transgene remains active in the proliferating cells.

Use of genetically modified animals to identify cardiomyocyte cell cycle regulators

The use of permanent (i.e. transgenesis, gene targeting) or transient (i.e. viral transduction) genetic modification approaches have in many cases demonstrated a direct correlation between the presence or absence of a given gene product and cardiomyocyte cell cycle activity.[9] In most instances, these studies focused on cardiomyocyte cell cycle activity during development, and did not examine proliferation in adults.

The number of studies wherein genetic manipulation impacted upon cardiomyocyte proliferation in adult hearts is rather limited. In most cases, the genetic modification was present throughout ontogeny (and thus was in place during the temporal window when cardiomyocyte terminal differentiation occurs). Thus, it remains possible that in some instances the introduction of the same genetic modification in genetically naive, terminally differentiated adult cardiomyocytes may not yield the same effect. However, given that cardiomyocyte cell cycle activity is apparent in genetically naive adult hearts (albeit at low levels), this caveat is less of a concern. It is also possible that cardiomyocyte cell cycle activity

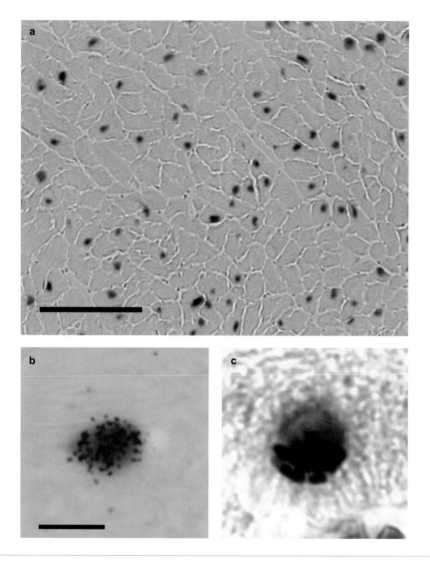

Figure 4.1 *Use of a reporter transgene to identify cardiomyocyte nuclei.[38] (a) An X-GAL-stained section from a mouse expressing a nuclear-localized β-galactosidase reporter under the regulation of the MHC promoter. Cardiomyocyte nuclei are readily identified by the robust blue signal. Bar, 100 μm. (b) An autoradiograph of an X-GAL-stained section from a mouse heart expressing the nuclear β-galactosidase reporter. The mouse received a single injection of tritiated thymidine prior to sacrifice. Silver grains are apparent over a blue nucleus, indicative of cardiomyocyte DNA synthesis. Bar, 10 μm. (c) An X-GAL-stained section from a mouse heart expressing the nuclear β-galactosidase reporter which was also processed for phosphorylated histone H3 immune reactivity (signal was developed with a horseradish peroxidase-conjugated secondary antibody and diaminobenzidine (DAB) reaction). The dark brown signal over a blue nucleus is indicative of cardiomyocyte mitosis or endomitosis. Magnification is the same as in (b).*

in genetically modified animals may be due in part to proliferation of de novo myocytes arising from cardiomyogenic stem cells[32] or alternatively from fusion events between cardiomyocytes and non-myocytes with proliferative potential.[40] However, in most instances both the kinetics and magnitude of the proliferative response are indicative of a direct effect of the genetic manipulation on pre-existing cardiomyocytes. Thus the available data strongly support the notion that genetic manipulation can directly induce cardiomyocyte cell cycle activity. Several of these studies are considered below.

D-type cyclins   Restriction point transit requires the induction of D-type cyclin family members (cyclin D1, D2, and D3), which, when bound to cyclin dependent kinase (CDK) 4, catalyze the phosphorylation of retinoblastoma protein family members. In cultured cells, restriction point transit commits the cell to a new round of division. Transgenic mice expressing cyclin D1, D2, or D3 under the transcriptional regulation of the MHC promoter exhibited robust accumulation of nuclear-localized cyclin D.[39,41] Interestingly, transgene expression resulted in concomitant induction and nuclear localization of the endogenous CDK4 protein in these animals. Nuclear cyclin D accumulation was associated with cell cycle activity: 0.09–0.3% of the cardiomyocytes in adult transgenic hearts were observed to be in S-phase (as evidenced by tritiated thymidine incorporation following a single injection of isotope).[39,41] In contrast, cardiomyocyte thymidine incorporation in mice lacking a D-type cyclin transgene never exceeded 0.0006%. Thus, expression of cyclin D1, D2, or D3 was sufficient to enhance cardiomyocyte DNA synthesis under baseline conditions in adult mice. Similar results were obtained with adenoviral delivery of cyclin D1 carrying a nuclear localization motif in rats,[42] indicating that genetically naive adult cardiomyocytes are also responsive.

To determine whether cyclin D-induced cardiomyocyte cell cycle activity could promote regenerative growth, the transgenic models were subjected to myocardial injury. Surprisingly, injury resulted in cytoplasmic accumulation of transgene-encoded cyclin D1 and D3, whereas cyclin D2 was retained in the nucleus. A concomitant marked reduction in cardiomyocyte DNA synthesis was observed in the cyclin D1 and cyclin D3 transgenic mice.[39] In contrast, injury resulted in enhanced levels of cardiomyocyte DNA synthesis,

as well as cardiomyocyte phosphorylated-histone H3 immune reactivity, in cyclin D2 transgenic mice. Histological analyses revealed a progressive increase in the number of cardiomyocytes in infarcted transgenic hearts, but not in infarcted non-transgenic hearts, providing additional proof of cyclin D2-induced proliferation. Cardiomyocyte proliferation led to a 50% reduction in infarct size at 150 days post-injury as compared to that observed in non-transgenic littermates at the same time point (Figure 4.2). In other experiments, cardiac function (as measured by intraventricular pressure/volume catheters) increased concomitantly with structural improvement following myocardial infarction.[43]

Cyclin D2-induced cardiomyocyte cell cycle activity appears to be beneficial in other injury models. For example, expression of a transgene encoding constitutively active transforming growth factor β1 (TGFβ1) results in atrial fibrosis. Cyclin D2-induced cardiomyocyte cell cycle activation antagonized atrial fibrosis in double transgenic animals (Figure 4.3).[44] Collectively these data indicate that targeted expression of D-type cyclins is sufficient to promote restriction point transit and cardiomyocyte DNA synthesis in the adult heart. Furthermore, in the case of cyclin D2, transgene-induced cell cycle activity is sufficient to promote regenerative growth of the heart following infarction.

p38 MAP kinase   The p38 mitogen activated protein (MAP) kinase signaling cascade has been implicated in the pathogenesis of heart failure, and in vitro studies have suggested that this pathway can play a role in hypertrophic growth of the myocardium.[45] In other studies, pharmacologic[46] or transgenic[47] inhibition of the pathway was associated with protection against reperfusion injury-induced cardiomyocyte apoptosis in mice. Recent studies have examined the role of p38 MAP kinase in the regulation of cardiomyocyte proliferation. Pharmacologic inhibition of p38 MAP kinase resulted in a 2–3-fold increase in the levels of fibroblast growth factor 1 (FGF1)-stimulated DNA synthesis (3 day treatment, BrdU labeling during the last 24 hours)

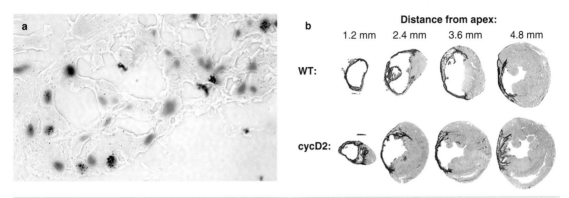

Figure 4.2   *Cyclin D2-induced cardiomyocyte proliferation results in infarct regression.[39] (a) A section from the heart of a mouse expressing the nuclear β-galactosidase reporter and cyclin D2 which was subjected to permanent coronary artery occlusion. The animal received a single injection of tritiated thymidine 7 days post-injury. The heart was then harvested and sectioned. Sections were then stained with X-GAL and subjected to autoradiography. Relatively high levels of cardiomyocyte DNA synthesis, as evidenced by the presence of silver grains over blue nuclei, were apparent at the infarct border zone. Bar, 50 μm. (b) Sections from wild type (WT) or cyclin D2 (cycD2) transgenic mice which were subjected to permanent coronary artery occlusion. Hearts were harvested 150 days post-injury and fixed, and transverse sections were prepared. The image shows sections sampled at 1.2-mm intervals from the apex to the base of the heart. Sections were stained with Sirius red (stains collagen red) and fast green (stains viable myocardium green). The infarct in mice expressing cyclin D2 is markedly reduced as compared to the wild type animals. In contrast, infarct size was similar in both groups at 7 days post-injury.[39] Thus, cardiomyocyte cell cycle activation resulted in infarct regression.*

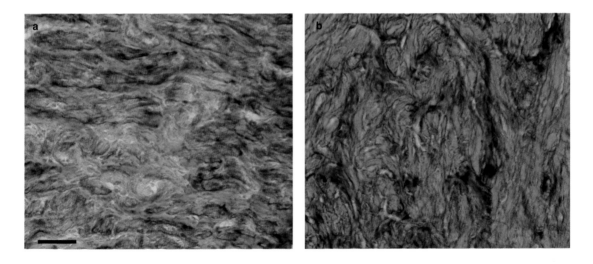

Figure 4.3   *Cyclin D2-induced cardiomyocyte proliferation antagonizes transforming growth factor β1 (TGFβ1)-induced atrial fibrosis.[44] (a) A section from the left atrium of a mouse carrying a transgene encoding mutant TGFβ1 which is constitutively active. The section was stained with Sirius red (stains collagen red) and fast green (stains viable myocardium green). Constitutive TGFβ1 activity induced marked atrial fibrosis, as indicated by the intense and widespread Sirius red staining. (b) A section of the left atrium of a mouse carrying both a TGFβ1 transgene and a cyclin D2 transgene. The level of atrial fibrosis is markedly reduced, as indicated by the reduction in Sirius red staining. Thus, cardiomyocyte cell cycle activation antagonized atrial fibrosis. Bar, 20 μm.*

and phosphorylated histone H3 immune reactivity in cultured neonatal rat cardiomyocytes.[48] An increase in total cell number was also noted. Interestingly, adult cardiomyocytes are also responsive to this signaling pathway. For example, cardiomyocyte restricted deletion of the p38 MAP kinase gene resulted in a 20-fold increase in cardiomyocyte BrdU incorporation in vivo in adult mice. In agreement with this, pharmacologic inhibition of p38 MAP kinase, in conjunction with FGF1 treatment, induced DNA synthesis and cytokinesis in cultured adult rat cardiomyocytes.[48] Although previous studies clearly demonstrated growth factor-induced DNA synthesis in cultured adult cardiomyocytes, cytokinesis was not observed.[49]

In a subsequent study, adult rats with myocardial infarction were treated with FGF1 (delivered via self-assembling peptide nanofibers) and p38 MAP kinase inhibitor.[50] Although no difference in the level of cardiomyocyte S-phase entry was noted at 2 weeks post-injury (as estimated by the level of cyclin D2 immune reactivity), a 2–3-fold increase in cyclin A2 and phosphorylated histone H3 immune reactivity was seen as compared to infarcted animals without pharmacologic treatment. At 3 months post-injury, echocardiography and histology analyses indicated that this intervention resulted in both functional and structural improvement (despite the fact that the duration of p38 MAP kinase inhibition was limited to 1 month due to the cardiotoxic effects of the drug). Collectively, these data clearly indicate that inhibition of p38 MAP kinase renders neonatal and adult cardiomyocytes more responsive to mitogenic stimuli in vitro and in vivo. The mechanistic basis of combinatorial p38 MAP kinase inhibition/FGF1 treatment on regenerative growth and functional improvement following myocardial infarction is more difficult to interpret due to the acute cardioprotective activity of p38 MAP kinase inhibition,[46,47] the necessity of using only short-term inhibitor treatment, and the proangiogenic activity of FGF1.

Cyclin A2

Cyclin A2 regulates multiple points of the cell cycle: when bound to CDK2 it facilitates restriction point transit, and when bound to CDK1 it facilitates mitosis entry.[51,52] This dual activity makes cyclin A2 an interesting candidate to promote cardiomyocyte proliferation. Western blot analyses of transgenic mice carrying an MHC-promoted cyclin A2 transgene revealed cyclin A2 accumulation predominantly in the nucleus at postnatal day 7, but predominantly in the cytoplasm by postnatal day 14.[53] In agreement with this, elevated levels of PCNA and phosphorylated histone H3 immune reactivity were noted during late embryonic and early neonatal life. However, at 6 months of age, phosphorylated histone H3 immune reactivity was detected in only a few scattered cardiomyocytes. Nonetheless, transgene-induced proliferation resulted in an increase in total cardiomyocyte number at 6 months of age, as determined by morphometric analyses based on estimates of whole heart volume and calculated values of average myocyte volume.[53]

Based on these results, an additional study was performed wherein adenoviruses with a cytomegalovirus-promoted cyclin A2 transgene was delivered to the infarct border zone of adult rats following permanent coronary artery ligation.[54] Viral transduction was associated with an increase in cyclin A2 expression as assessed by Western blot analysis, although immune histology to monitor transgene expression was not performed. Increased levels of PCNA, Ki67, and BrdU immune reactivity were observed in treated animals receiving viral therapy as compared to the untreated controls. Viral treatment was associated with an improvement in cardiac geometry and function, as measured by histologic and hemodynamic analyses, respectively.[54] Collectively, these studies indicate that targeted expression of cyclin A2 can increase cardiomyocyte cell cycle activity during early neonatal life, giving rise to an increase in cardiomyocyte number in adult animals. Viral delivery of cyclin A2 following infarction was associated with increased cell cycle activity as well as improved cardiac function; however, histochemical analyses to demonstrate that functional improvement correlated with increased cardiomyocyte number (as opposed to potential impact from cyclin

A2-induced proliferation of non-myocytes) were not performed.

Other genetic models

A number of other genetic models exhibiting cell cycle activity in adult hearts have been reported. For example, expression of the SV40 large T antigen oncoprotein under the regulation of atrial natriuretic factor, MHC, or protamine promoters resulted in overt cardiomyocyte proliferation in the atria[55,56] or ventricles.[57] Efforts aimed at establishing the mechanism of cardiomyocyte proliferation in these models identified a prominent T antigen-binding protein, designated p193,[58,59] which was subsequently shown to be a new member of the cullin protein family.[60] Expression of a mutant p193 molecule with apparent dominant interfering activity potentiates cardiomyocyte cell cycle activity following E1A-transduction in cultured embryonic stem cell-derived cardiomyocytes,[61] as well as following myocardial infarction in transgenic mice.[38] In the latter study, the magnitude of cardiomyocyte cell cycle activity (as measured by tritiated thymidine incorporation) was roughly similar to the level of cardiomyocyte apoptosis (as measured by activated caspase 3 immune reactivity), and was associated with a reduction of injury-induced cardiomyocyte hypertrophy. These observations raise the possibility that cell cycle induction abated post-injury hypertrophic growth by replacing cardiomyocytes which were lost due to apoptosis.

Given the impact of D-type cyclin expression noted above, it is likely that modulation of the expression of retinoblastoma (RB) protein family members would also impact on cardiomyocyte cell cycle activity. Although cardiomyocyte-restricted deletion of the *RB* gene had no overt phenotype, crossing these animals into a p130 deficient background resulted in a profound increase in heart mass[62] (p130 is an RB family member). The increase in heart size appeared to result from a combination of cardiomyocyte hypertrophy and cell division, as a marked increase in the level of cardiomyocyte DNA synthesis (as evidenced by BrdU incorporation) and karyo- or cytokinesis (as evidenced by phosphorylated histone H3 immune activity) was

apparent in the genetically modified animals as compared to the controls.

Transgenic animals expressing other fundamental cell cycle regulatory genes have been studied. For example, although targeted expression of the c-*myc* proto-oncogene during development led to a two-fold increase in cardiomyocyte number, overt cell cycle activity was not observed in adult transgenic hearts.[63] In contrast, activation of a tamoxifen-inducible c-*myc* transgene in adult cardiomyocytes led to hypertrophic growth which was accompanied by cardiomyocyte DNA synthesis, phosphorylated histone H3 immune reactivity, and an increase in ploidy.[64] In other studies, transgenic mice expressing dominant interfering versions of the tuberous sclerosis complex 2[65] or the p53[38] tumor suppressor proteins under the regulation of the MHC promoter exhibited enhanced cardiomyocyte DNA synthesis following isoproterenol-induced hypertrophy and myocardial infarction, respectively (using tritiated thymidine incorporation as the experimental read-out); however, the level of cell cycle activity was too small to impact upon cardiac structure. Targeted expression of the prosurvival protein Bcl-2 resulted in a two-fold increase in cardiomyocyte DNA synthesis (measured via BrdU incorporation in vivo),[66] while expression of insulin-like growth factor I resulted in a 16-fold increase (measured in acutely isolated adult cardiomyocyte cultures).[67] Finally, targeted expression of CDK2[68] resulted in a modest increase in cardiomyocyte DNA synthesis in adult transgenic mice. Collectively, these studies indicate that genetic manipulation can induce cell cycle activity in adult cardiomyocytes, and that in some cases this can result in cardiomyocyte proliferation.

Studies in Human Hearts

Although no efforts to therapeutically induce cardiomyocyte proliferation have been attempted, there are numerous studies examining cell cycle activity in the normal, and in particular the injured, adult human heart. The level of cardiomyocyte multinucleation reported for human hearts ranges from 10 to 75%.[69] Moreover, exceedingly high levels of polyploidization are observed in primate cardiomyocyte nuclei (including humans).[29] In one study, roughly 50% of adult human cardiomyocytes were observed to have a $4C \times 2$ nuclear content (that is, binucleate cells with each nucleus containing a 4C DNA content), while roughly 15% had a $2C \times 2$ nuclear content. The remaining cells had variable nuclear content, and some nuclei exhibited as high as a 32C DNA content.[30] Differences in the reported values for polyploidization are likely attributable to differences in the assay systems employed, potential tissue degradation in instances where autopsy materials were analyzed, the nature and severity of the disease process, and finally natural variations in the population.

Given these considerations, it is not surprising that a survey of the literature revealed differences with regard to cardiomyocyte cell cycle activity in diseased human hearts. For example, fluorescent immune histologic examination of hearts from patients who died between 4 and 12 days post-infarction revealed that roughly 4% of the border zone cardiomyocytes exhibited Ki67 immune reactivity.[70] This was accompanied by cardiomyocyte mitotic indices of roughly 0.08% (although the presence or absence of nuclear membranes was not ascertained in this study). Light microscopic analysis of a similar group of hearts (harvested between 1 and 21 days post-infarction) revealed a similar level of Ki67 immune reactivity in the infarct border zone (4.84%).[31] However, in all but three of the cells examined, an intact nuclear membrane was observed, leading these investigators to conclude that cell cycle activation led to endomitosis rather than cytokinesis. The level of polyploidy resulting from endomitosis in this study was in good agreement with previously published values.[71,72] Of note, cell cycle induction was limited to two or three rows of surviving cardiomyocytes at the infarct border. Similarly, polyploidy cardiomyocytes in the absence of mitosis were also observed in left ventricular myectomy samples from patients with pressure overload-induced heart failure.[73]

Summary

The studies cited above provide compelling support of the notion that cell cycle activation can give rise to myocardial repair following injury. This process occurs spontaneously in lower species. Although the level of spontaneous cell cycle activation in mammalian hearts is much lower, genetic manipulation can readily increase rates to the point that proliferation based regenerative growth can be achieved, with a positive impact on cardiac structure and function. As indicated above, it remains possible that some of the observed effects are mediated via cardiomyogenic stem cells. Regardless of the origin of the proliferating cells (i.e. cardiomyocyte-autonomous or progenitor-derived), it is clear that enhancing the capacity of cardiomyocyte proliferation is beneficial in injured hearts. Thus, continued study of the molecular regulation of cardiomyocyte proliferation is warranted.

References

1. Soonpaa MH, Field LJ. Survey of studies examining mammalian cardiomyocyte DNA synthesis. Circ Res 1998; 83: 15–26.
2. Anversa P, Kajstura J. Ventricular myocytes are not terminally differentiated in the adult mammalian heart. Circ Res 1998; 83: 1–14.
3. Dimmeler S, Zeiher AM, Schneider MD. Unchain my heart: the scientific foundations of cardiac repair. J Clin Invest 2005; 115: 572–83.
4. Chien KR. Stem cells: lost in translation. Nature 2004; 428: 607–8.
5. Field LJ. Unraveling the mechanistic basis of mesenchymal stem cell activity in the heart. Mol Ther 2006; 14: 755–6.
6. Reinlib L, Field L. Cell transplantation as future therapy for cardiovascular disease?: A workshop of the National Heart, Lung, and Blood Institute. Circulation 2000; 101: E182–7.
7. Dowell JD, Rubart M, Pasumarthi KB, Soonpaa MH, Field LJ. Myocyte and myogenic stem cell transplantation in the heart. Cardiovasc Res 2003; 58: 336–50.
8. Kovacic JC, Muller DW, Graham RM. Actions and therapeutic potential of G-CSF and GM-CSF in cardiovascular disease. J Mol Cell Cardiol 2007; 42: 19–33.
9. Pasumarthi KB, Field LJ. Cardiomyocyte cell cycle regulation. Circ Res 2002; 90: 1044–54.

10. Rumyantsev PP. Interrelations of the proliferation and differentiation processes during cardiac myogenesis and regeneration. Int Rev Cytol 1977; 51: 186–273.

11. Oberpriller J, Oberpriller JC. Cell division in adult newt cardiac myocytes. In: Oberpriller J, Oberpriller JC, Maruro A, eds. The Development and Regenerative Potential of Cardiac Muscle. Chur: Harwood Academic Publishers, 1991: 293–312.

12. Oberpriller JO, Oberpriller JC. Response of the adult newt ventricle to injury. J Exp Zool 1974; 187: 249–53.

13. Bader D, Oberpriller JO. Repair and reorganization of minced cardiac muscle in the adult newt (Notophthalmus viridescens). J Morphol 1978; 155: 349–57.

14. Bader D, Oberpriller J. Autoradiographic and electron microscopic studies of minced cardiac muscle regeneration in the adult newt, notophthalmus viridescens. J Exp Zool 1979; 208: 177–93.

15. Bettencourt-Dias M, Mittnacht S, Brockes JP. Heterogeneous proliferative potential in regenerative adult newt cardiomyocytes. J Cell Sci 2003; 116: 4001–9.

16. Huang CJ, Jou TS, Ho YL et al. Conditional expression of a myocardium-specific transgene in zebrafish transgenic lines. Dev Dyn 2005; 233: 1294–303.

17. Mably JD, Chuang LP, Serluca FC et al. santa and valentine pattern concentric growth of cardiac myocardium in the zebrafish. Development 2006; 133: 3139–46.

18. Lien CL, Schebesta M, Makino S, Weber GJ, Keating MT. Gene expression analysis of zebrafish heart regeneration. PLoS Biol 2006; 4: e260.

19. Wang WD, Huang CJ, Lu YF et al. Heart-targeted overexpression of Nip3a in zebrafish embryos causes abnormal heart development and cardiac dysfunction. Biochem Biophys Res Commun 2006; 347: 979–87.

20. Poss KD, Wilson LG, Keating MT. Heart regeneration in zebrafish. Science 2002; 298: 2188–90.

21. Wei Y, Mizzen CA, Cook RG, Gorovsky MA, Allis CD. Phosphorylation of histone H3 at serine 10 is correlated with chromosome condensation during mitosis and meiosis in Tetrahymena. Proc Natl Acad Sci USA 1998; 95: 7480–4.

22. Raya A, Koth CM, Buscher D et al. Activation of Notch signaling pathway precedes heart regeneration in zebrafish. Proc Natl Acad Sci USA 2003; 100 (Suppl 1): 11889–95.

23. Lepilina A, Coon AN, Kikuchi K et al. A dynamic epicardial injury response supports progenitor cell activity during zebrafish heart regeneration. Cell 2006; 127: 607–19.

24. Pelc SR. Labelling of DNA and cell division in so called non-dividing tissues. J Cell Biol 1964; 22: 21–8.

25. van Oijen MG, Medema RH, Slootweg PJ, Rijksen G. Positivity of the proliferation marker Ki-67 in noncycling cells. Am J Clin Pathol 1998; 110: 24–31.

26. Field LJ. Modulation of the cardiomyocyte cell cycle in genetically altered animals. Ann NY Acad Sci 2004; 1015: 160–70.

27. Engel FB, Schebesta M, Keating MT. Anillin localization defect in cardiomyocyte binucleation. J Mol Cell Cardiol 2006; 41: 601–12.

28. Soonpaa MH, Field LJ. Assessment of cardiomyocyte DNA synthesis during hypertrophy in adult mice. Am J Physiol 1994; 266: H1439–45.

29. Rumiantsev PP. Growth and Hyperplasia of Cardiac Muscle Cells. London: Harwood Academic Publishers, 1991.

30. Brodsky V. Cell ploidy in the mammalian heart. In: Oberpriller J, Oberpriller JC, Mauro A, eds. The Development and Regenerative Potential of Cardiac Muscle. Chur: Harwood Academic Publishers, 1991: 253–87.

31. Meckert PC, Rivello HG, Vigliano C et al. Endomitosis and polyploidization of myocardial cells in the periphery of human acute myocardial infarction. Cardiovasc Res 2005; 67: 116–23.

32. Oh H, Bradfute SB, Gallardo TD et al. Cardiac progenitor cells from adult myocardium: homing, differentiation, and fusion after infarction. Proc Natl Acad Sci USA 2003; 100: 12313–18.

33. Alvarez-Dolado M, Pardal R, Garcia-Verdugo JM et al. Fusion of bone-marrow-derived cells with Purkinje neurons, cardiomyocytes and hepatocytes. Nature 2003; 425: 968–73.

34. Anatskaya OV, Vinogradov AE. Paradoxical relationship between protein content and nucleolar activity in mammalian cardiomyocytes. Genome 2004; 47: 565–78.

35. Gulick J, Subramaniam A, Neumann J, Robbins J. Isolation and characterization of the mouse cardiac myosin heavy chain genes. J Biol Chem 1991; 266: 9180–5.

36. Soonpaa MH, Field LJ. Assessment of cardiomyocyte DNA synthesis in normal and injured adult mouse hearts. Am J Physiol 1997; 272: H220–6.

37. Soonpaa MH, Koh GY, Klug MG, Field LJ. Formation of nascent intercalated disks between grafted fetal cardiomyocytes and host myocardium. Science 1994; 264: 98–101.

38. Nakajima H, Nakajima HO, Tsai SC, Field LJ. Expression of mutant p193 and p53 permits cardiomyocyte cell cycle reentry after myocardial infarction in transgenic mice. Circ Res 2004; 94: 1606–14.

39. Pasumarthi KB, Nakajima H, Nakajima HO, Soonpaa MH, Field LJ. Targeted expression of cyclin D2 results in cardiomyocyte DNA synthesis and infarct regression in transgenic mice. Circ Res 2005; 96: 110–18.

40. Matsuura K, Wada H, Nagai T et al. Cardiomyocytes fuse with surrounding noncardiomyocytes and reenter the cell cycle. J Cell Biol 2004; 167: 351–63.

41. Soonpaa MH, Koh GY, Pajak L et al. Cyclin D1 overexpression promotes cardiomyocyte DNA synthesis and multinucleation in transgenic mice. J Clin Invest 1997; 99: 2644–54.

42. Tamamori-Adachi M, Ito H, Sumrejkanchanakij P et al. Critical role of cyclin D1 nuclear import in cardiomyocyte proliferation. Circ Res 2003; 92: e12–19.

43. Hassink RJ, Pasumarthi KB, Nakajima H et al. Cardiomyocyte cell cycle activation improves cardiac function after myocardial infarction. Submitted.

44. Nakajima H, Nakajima HO, Dembowsky K, Pasumarthi KB, Field LJ. Cardiomyocyte cell cycle activation ameliorates fibrosis in the atrium. Circ Res 2006; 98: 141–8.

45. Petrich BG, Wang Y. Stress-activated MAP kinases in cardiac remodeling and heart failure; new insights from transgenic studies. Trends Cardiovasc Med 2004; 14: 50–5.

46. Kaiser RA, Lyons JM, Duffy JY et al. Inhibition of p38 reduces myocardial infarction injury in the mouse but not pig after ischemia-reperfusion. Am J Physiol Heart Circ Physiol 2005; 289: H2747–51.

47. Kaiser RA, Bueno OF, Lips DJ et al. Targeted inhibition of p38 mitogen-activated protein kinase antagonizes cardiac injury and cell death following ischemia-reperfusion in vivo. J Biol Chem 2004; 279: 15524–30.

48. Engel FB, Schebesta M, Duong MT et al. p38 MAP kinase inhibition enables proliferation of adult mammalian cardiomyocytes. Genes Dev 2005; 19: 1175–87.

49. Claycomb WC, Moses RL. Growth factors and TPA stimulate DNA synthesis and alter the morphology of cultured terminally differentiated adult rat cardiac muscle cells. Dev Biol 1988; 127: 257–65.

50. Engel FB, Hsieh PC, Lee RT, Keating MT. FGF1/p38 MAP kinase inhibitor therapy induces cardiomyocyte mitosis, reduces scarring, and rescues function after myocardial infarction. Proc Natl Acad Sci USA 2006; 103: 15546–51.

51. Sherr CJ, Roberts JM. Inhibitors of mammalian G1 cyclin-dependent kinases. Genes Dev 1995; 9: 1149–63.

52. Pagano M, Pepperkok R, Verde F, Ansorge W, Draetta G. Cyclin A is required at two points in the human cell cycle. EMBO J 1992; 11: 961–71.

53. Chaudhry HW, Dashoush NH, Tang H et al. Cyclin A2 mediates cardiomyocyte mitosis in the postmitotic myocardium. J Biol Chem 2004; 279: 35858–66.

54. Woo YJ, Panlilio CM, Cheng RK et al. Therapeutic delivery of cyclin A2 induces myocardial regeneration and enhances cardiac function in ischemic heart failure. Circulation 2006; 114: I206–13.

55. Field LJ. Atrial natriuretic factor-SV40 T antigen transgenes produce tumors and cardiac arrhythmias in mice. Science 1988; 239: 1029–33.

56. Behringer RR, Peschon JJ, Messing A et al. Heart and bone tumors in transgenic mice. Proc Natl Acad Sci USA 1988; 85: 2648–52.

57. Katz EB, Steinhelper ME, Delcarpio JB et al. Cardiomyocyte proliferation in mice expressing alpha-cardiac myosin heavy chain-SV40 T-antigen transgenes. Am J Physiol 1992; 262: H1867–76.

58. Daud AI, Lanson NA Jr, Claycomb WC, Field LJ. Identification of SV40 large T-antigen-associated proteins in cardiomyocytes from transgenic mice. Am J Physiol 1993; 264: H1693–700.

59. Tsai SC, Pasumarthi KB, Pajak L et al. Simian virus 40 large T antigen binds a novel Bcl-2 homology domain 3-containing proapoptosis protein in the cytoplasm. J Biol Chem 2000; 275: 3239–46.

60. Dias DC, Dolios G, Wang R, Pan ZQ. CUL7: a DOC domain-containing cullin selectively binds Skp1.Fbx29 to form an SCF-like complex. Proc Natl Acad Sci USA 2002; 99: 16601–6.

61. Pasumarthi KB, Tsai SC, Field LJ. Coexpression of mutant p53 and p193 renders embryonic stem cell-derived cardiomyocytes responsive to the growth-promoting activities of adenoviral E1A. Circ Res 2001; 88: 1004–11.

62. MacLellan WR, Garcia A, Oh H et al. Overlapping roles of pocket proteins in the myocardium are unmasked by germ line deletion of p130 plus heart-specific deletion of Rb. Mol Cell Biol 2005; 25: 2486–97.

63. Jackson T, Allard MF, Sreenan CM et al. The c-myc proto-oncogene regulates cardiac development in transgenic mice. Mol Cell Biol 1990; 10: 3709–16.

64. Xiao G, Mao S, Baumgarten G et al. Inducible activation of c-Myc in adult myocardium in vivo provokes cardiac myocyte hypertrophy and reactivation of DNA synthesis. Circ Res 2001; 89: 1122–9.

65. Pasumarthi KB, Nakajima H, Nakajima HO, Jing S, Field LJ. Enhanced cardiomyocyte DNA synthesis during myocardial hypertrophy in mice expressing a modified TSC2 transgene. Circ Res 2000; 86: 1069–77.

66. Limana F, Urbanek K, Chimenti S et al. bcl-2 overexpression promotes myocyte proliferation. Proc Natl Acad Sci USA 2002; 99: 6257–62.

67. Reiss K, Cheng W, Ferber A et al. Overexpression of insulin-like growth factor-1 in the heart is coupled with myocyte proliferation in transgenic mice. Proc Natl Acad Sci USA 1996; 93: 8630–5.

68. Liao HS, Kang PM, Nagashima H et al. Cardiac-specific overexpression of cyclin-dependent kinase 2 increases smaller mononuclear cardiomyocytes. Circ Res 2001; 88: 443–50.

69. Brodsky V, Sarkisov DS, Arefyeva AM, Panova NW, Gvasava IG. Polyploidy in cardiac myocytes of normal and hypertrophic human hearts; range of values. Virchows Arch 1994; 424: 429–35.

70. Beltrami AP, Urbanek K, Kajstura J et al. Evidence that human cardiac myocytes divide after myocardial infarction. N Engl J Med 2001; 344: 1750–7.

71. Ebert L, Pfitzer P. Nuclear DNA of myocardial cells in the periphery of infarctions and scars. Virchows Arch B Cell Pathol 1977; 24: 209–17.

72. Herget GW, Neuburger M, Plagwitz R, Adler CP. DNA content, ploidy level and number of nuclei in the human heart after myocardial infarction. Cardiovasc Res 1997; 36: 45–51.

73. Hein S, Arnon E, Kostin S et al. Progression from compensated hypertrophy to failure in the pressure-overloaded human heart: structural deterioration and compensatory mechanisms. Circulation 2003; 107: 984–91.

chapter 5

Mesenchymal Stem Cell Therapy for the Injured Heart

Wangde Dai and Robert A Kloner

Introduction

A variety of cell types, such as fetal or neonatal cardiomyocytes, skeletal muscle myoblasts, mesenchymal stem cells (MSCs), hematopoietic stem cells, adult cardiac resident stem cells, embryonic stem cells, and others, are potential cell sources for cell transplantation therapy in the heart (for review, see references 1 and 2). This chapter will focus on the bone marrow-derived MSCs in cardiac regeneration.

Definition and Characteristics of Bone Marrow-Derived Mesenchymal Stem Cells

Bone marrow-derived MSCs are clonogenic non-hematopoietic stem cells within the bone marrow, and have the capacity to differentiate into mesoderm-type lineages, such as chondrocytes, osteoblasts, and endothelial cells. MSCs are able to adhere to plastic and expand in tissue culture with a finite lifespan of 15–50 cell doublings. They are a relatively rare cell population in the bone marrow. Assessed by colony forming unit fibroblasts, there is about 1 MSC in 34 000 bone marrow nucleated cell population in humans,[3] and 1 MSC in 11 300–27 000 bone marrow nucleated cells in mice.[4] Due to the low frequency in bone marrow and lack of information with respect to specific surface markers, relatively little is known about the characteristics of MSCs

in vivo. Most of the information about their characteristics is derived from in vitro studies.

As a stem cell, one of the defining characteristics of MSCs is their self-renewal potential. The self-renewal potential of MSCs during in vitro serial propagation is highly variable due to the different methods employed to derive populations and culture conditions, such as serum growth factors, the addition of specific growth factors,[5] and the cell seeding density.[6] Another characteristic is that MSCs have multilineage differentiation potential. MSCs have been demonstrated to differentiate into a variety of cell types, including bone, cartilage, tendon, muscle, adipose tissue, endothelial cells, and possibly cardiomyocytes.

The characteristics of MSCs, including morphology and surface markers, have been extensively analyzed in culture. There are two types of morphology: one is characterized by large, flat cells, another by elongated, fibroblastoid cells. The functional significance of these differing morphologies remains unknown. MSCs are generally negative for the hematopoietic markers CD34 and CD45. MSCs exhibit some heterogeneity during long-term culture, but similar immunophenotypic profiles are observed in functionally different cultures. Currently there are no characteristic surface markers that can be used to definitively identify MSCs, although a series of antibodies to surface markers have been employed by several investigators.[7–10] For example, Pittenger and Martin[11] have listed a number of surface molecules on human MSCs in Figure

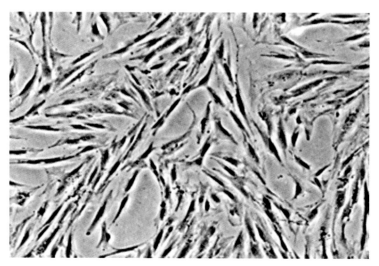

hMSC surface markers

Positive	Negative
CD13, CD29, CD44, CD49a, b, c, d, e, f, CD51, CD54, CD58, CD71, CD73, CD90, CD102, CD105, CD106, CDw119, CD120a, CD120b, CD123, CD124, CD126, CD127, CD140a, CD166, P75, TGFβ1R, TGFβ2R, HLAA,B,C, SSEA3, SSEA4, D7	CD3, CD4, CD6, CD9, CD10 CD11a, CD14, CD15, CD18, CD21, CD25, CD31, CD34, CD36, CD38, CD45*, CD49d, CD50, CD62E,L,S, CD80, CD86, CD95, CD117, CD133, SSEA1

Figure 5.1   Human mesenchymal stem cells (hMSCs) in culture appear fibroblastic and homogeneous in size and morphology by second passage. Flow cytometry applying fluoresceinated antibodies was used to determine surface molecules present in the expanded cell population, and both positive and negative surface molecules are listed. (Reproduced with permission from reference 11.)

5.1, but these are still incomplete. Most of the surface markers are not adequate to identify stem cells, because they may only express on a stem cell at a certain stage or under certain conditions, or also express on non-stem cells. Table 5.1 demonstrates surface antigen comparison among MSC-like cells cultured in different conditions from several laboratories. Thus, searching specific surface markers for purifying MSCs is a challenge for MSC therapy in cardiac regeneration.

Isolation and Culture of Mesenchymal Stem Cells

In general, isolation of adult stem cells requires detailed characterization based on their immunophenotypic or functional traits. Since MSCs lack clearly defined surface markers, their isolation relies on their ability to adhere to plastic surfaces. There are adherent and non-adherent cells within the total population of bone marrow cells. After plating the total cells onto tissue culture dishes, the non-adherent cells are removed by changing the culture medium. The remaining adherent cells will be relatively homogeneous in morphology and immunophenotype after maintenance with medium change, removal of non-adherent cells, and periodic passages. In order to enrich the frequency of MSCs in this initial cell population, various methods have been developed. MSCs can expand rapidly if plated at very low density (approximately 100–500 cells per cm²), and form single-cell-derived colonies.

Table 5.1   Surface antigen comparison among mesenchymal stem cell (MSC)-like cells

Surface antigen	MSCs[12]	MAPCs[13]	RS1[14]	PLAs[15]	APCs[16]
CD9					+
CD10		−	−		+
CD11a, b	−		−		−
CD13	+	+		+	+
CD14	−		−	−	−
CD18 integrin β2	−				−
CD29	+			+	+
CD31 PECAM	−	−	+/−	−	
CD34	−	−	−	−	+
CD44	+		+	+	+
CD45	−a	−	−	−	−
CD49b integrin α2	+	+			
CD49d integrin α4	−			+	+
CD49e integrin α5	+		+		+
CD50 ICAM3	−	−			−
CD54 ICAM1	+				+
CD56 NCAM				−	−
CD62E E-selectin	−	−		−	−
CD71 transferrin rec	+		+	+	
CD73 SH3	+			+	
CD90 Thy1	+	+	+/−	+	
CD105 endoglin, SH2	+			+	+
CD106 VCAM	+	−		−	+
CD117	−	−			
CD133	−	(+)	−	−	
CD166 ALCAM	+				+
Others					
β2 microglobulin	+	+			
nestin	+			+	
p75	+			+	
HLA ABC	+		+/−		+
HLA DR	− induc	−	−		−
SSEA4	+	+			
TRK (A, B, C)	+		+		
Differentiation in vitro					
osteo	+	+	+	+	+
adipo	+	+	+	+	+
chondro	+	+	+	+	
neural	(+)			(+)	
stromal	+	+			
myoblast Sk	(+)	+		+	
endothelial	(+)	+			

(+) indicates detection varied; aositive upon isolation:[17] MAPCs, multipotent adult progenitor cells; RS1, recycling stem cells; PLAs, processed liposuction aspirates; APCs, adipose progenitor cells; PECAM, platelet endothelial cell adhesion molecule; ALCAM, activated leukocyte cell adhesion molecule; ICAM, intercellular adhesion molecule; NCAM, neural cell adhesion molecule; VCAM, vascular cell adhesion molecule; HLA, human leukocyte antigen (Reproduced with permission from Reference 11).

Eslaminejad et al[18] plated mouse bone marrow mononuclear cells at about 500 cells per well of 24-well plates, and observed that fibroblastic clones formed at 7 days after culture. The fibroblastic clones were pooled together and expanded through several subcultures. These isolated cells were able to differentiate into the osteoblastic, chondrocytic, and adipocytic lineages. Thus, MSCs can be isolated by a low density primary culture system.

Density centrifugation can isolate a mononuclear cell fraction from bone marrow.[19] MSCs can be sieved out from other bone marrow cells by a culture device that is a 10-cm plastic culture dish comprising a plate with 3-μm pores.[20] Unwanted cells, such as hematopoietic contaminants, can be eliminated by immunodepletion using antibodies against CD34, CD45, and CD11b.[21,22] Other methods, such as magnetic activated cell sorting,[23] fibrin microbeads,[24] and fluorescence automated cell sorting,[25] are also used for MSC isolation. Because none of these approaches are efficient to establish homogeneous cell cultures, the isolation and expansion of homogeneous MSCs with specific criteria remains a challenge in this research field, which depends on a better understanding of the nature of MSCs.

Another challenge is how to expand MSCs ex vivo without affecting their differentiation potential, because the multipotent MSCs decrease in number during long-term culture. Therefore, strategies are needed to enhance and maintain the multilineage differentiation potential of MSCs during in vitro culture expansion.

Cardiomyogenic Lineage Differentiation of Mesenchymal Stem Cells

In vitro studies suggest that MSCs can be induced to differentiate into cell types such as osteoblasts, chondrocytes, endothelial cells, neuron-like cells, and, in several studies, cardiomyocytes. In vitro cultured MSCs have great heterogeneity in their differentiation potential. There are a minority of cells that seem to be pluripotent within established cultures, whereas most may be committed to more differentiated phenotypes which have bi- or only unilineage differentiation capacity.[26] Pittenger et al[12] showed that only one-third of the MSC clones derived from established cultures are pluripotent. The phenotype of differentiated cells is determined by morphological, immunophenotypic, and functional criteria. For instance, the identification of cardiac myocytes is determined by immunocytochemistry with antibodies specific for cardiomyocyte-specific markers, and by functional assessment such as observation of spontaneous beating and electrocardiography (ECG).

Numerous experiments have been performed to elucidate the factors and techniques needed to induce adult stem cells to differentiate into cardiomyocytes.[27] Shim et al[28] demonstrated that MSCs differentiated into cardiomyocyte-like cells in a cardiomyogenic differentiation medium containing insulin, dexamethasone, and ascorbic acid. The agent 5-azacytidine has induced MSCs, which are isolated from murine,[29] rat,[30] rabbit,[31] and human[32] to differentiate into cardiomyocytes in cell culturing experiments. Hakuno et al[29] demonstrated that murine MSC-derived cardiomyocytes induced by 5-azacytidine spontaneously beat in vitro and expressed functional adrenergic and muscarinic receptors. Platelet-derived growth factor (PDGF)-A and -B has also been used to induce the differentiation of cardiac myocytes from bone marrow cells both in vitro and in vivo.[33] Another approach is to coculture MSCs with adult cardiomyocytes. Cultured adult cardiomyocytes may provide an environment that stimulates the induction of cardiomyocyte differentiation of MSCs by cell–cell interaction, electrical and/or mechanical stimulation, and/or undetermined growth factors. Fukuhara et al[34] cocultured mice bone marrow stromal cells with rat cardiomyocytes. The bone marrow stromal cells incorporated in parallel with cardiomyocytes and revealed myotube-like formation; expressed myosin heavy chain, cardiac-specific troponin I, and connexin 43; and contracted synchronously with cardiomyocytes. Xie et al[17] demonstrated that conditioned medium of cultured cardiomyocytes under hypoxic conditions induced MSC differentiation into myocardial-like cells. However, Wang et al[35] cultured rat MSCs with adult rat cardiomyocytes in direct coculture, indirect coculture, and conditioned culture, respectively. Only direct coculture with direct cell-to-cell contact between MSC and adult cardiomyocyte resulted in the differentiation of MSCs into cardiomyocytes, while the soluble signaling molecules in the indirect coculture group and conditioned culture group did not. These results suggested that cardiac environmental factors are powerful inducers of cardiomyogenic differentiation of bone marrow stromal cells. However, future studies are needed to investigate whether cell fusion between the MSCs and cocultured cardiomyocytes explain some of the results of the coculture experiments described above. Cultured bone marrow cells may have adopted the phenotype of the cocultured cells by spontaneous cell fusion.[36]

The ability of MSCs to differentiate into cardiomyocytes in in vitro studies theoretically makes them ideal candidates for the restoration of injured cardiac muscle. Many factors can affect this differentiation process. For example, Zhang et al[14] observed that 5-azacytidine induced passage 4, but not passages 1 and 8 of rat bone marrow MSCs to form myotubes and express cardiomyocyte-associated markers, because passage 4 rat MSCs had a growth-arrest appearance, while passages 1 and 8 rat MSCs displayed an exponential growth pattern. These results suggest that the passage and proliferative ability of rat MSCs influence their potential to differentiate into cardiomyocytes. The underlying mechanism of cardiomyogenic transdifferentiation from MSCs is still unknown. Thus, better understanding of the regulation of the transdifferentiation of MSCs is needed for exploiting the therapeutic potential of MSCs.

Immunobiology of Mesenchymal Stem Cells

MSCs are thought to be able to avoid allogeneic rejection, because they lack human leukocyte antigen (HLA) class II antigens, prevent T cell response, and induce a suppressive local microenvironment through the production of prostaglandins and interleukin 10 as well as by the expression of indoleamine 2,3,-dioxygenase.[37] Adult MSCs express intermediate levels of HLA class I, but not HLA class II antigens on the cell surface.[38] This pattern of HLA expression does not change even after differentiation into bone, cartilage, or adipose tissue.[38] In vitro studies show that MSCs seem to escape the immune system. Undifferentiated MSCs suppress allogeneic T-cell proliferation in vitro.[39] These data suggest that MSCs can be transplantable across allogeneic barriers without being rejected.

Aging of Mesenchymal Stem Cells

The low frequency of MSCs in bone marrow (BM) necessitates their in vitro expansion for the generation of large numbers of MSCs. The differentiation potential and proliferation rate decline in aged MSCs. The replicative senescence of MSCs in culture is different between species. Murine MSCs can be passaged for more than 100 population doublings,[4] whereas human MSCs can only be passaged around 40–50 population doublings.[40] MSCs isolated from donors with increasing age are associated with decreased proliferation and multipotentiality of differentiation. Human MSCs that were derived from old donors exhibited accelerated senescence and a decreased maximal lifespan compared with cells from young donors. The increase in proliferative response to serum stimulation was significantly lower in MSCs from the older donors than from the younger donors.[40] Besides these intrinsic factors, some other extrinsic factors, such as the bone marrow microenvironment, may contribute to the reduced function of aged MSCs (for review, see reference 13).

By morphologic assessment, young donor-derived MSCs exhibit a spindle-type shape, whereas MSCs from older donors show a larger and flatter morphology, with no spindle-type morphology observed even at primary passage in culture.[41] Expansion in vitro can age the MSCs derived from young donors, with a progressive change in cell morphology from a spindle-type shape to a wider and flatter shape. Bonab et al[42] observed that cultured MSCs showed abnormalities after a long period of normal growth. On average, granules were noted in the cytoplasm at 84 days after primary culture, and the cells with granules began to become vacuolated, rounded, and finally detached from the base of the flasks at around day 120.

There is a correlation between telomere length and proliferative capacity of the human MSC. In order to bring about regenerative capacity and ability to differentiate, the MSC must express at least some telomerase activity. Telomerase deficiency (telomerase is a crucial enzyme for the synthesis of telomeres) impairs differentiation of mesenchymal stem cells in vitro.[43] Cells stop dividing and enter senescence when telomeres reach a certain length. Human MSC lines show erosion of telomeres at each cell division until they reach a threshold around 10 kb, where cells stop dividing.[41] Overexpression of telomerase can result in long telomeres, and maintain proliferative ability.[16] In addition to the importance of the telomere, other molecular changes, such as changes in growth factors and inflammatory cytokines, may be associated with MSC aging (for review, see reference 13). Understanding the molecular mechanisms underlying the phenomenon of in vitro aging of MSCs will help to establish methods to expand MSCs without affecting their proliferative ability and differentiation potential.

Therapeutic Application

Repair of damaged myocardium

MSCs might theoretically be used for cardiac regeneration due to their self-renewal and differentiation into cardiomyocytes. MSCs can be induced to differentiate into cardiomyocytes in vitro, and then be transplanted into the heart. Yoon et al[15] demonstrated that bone morphogenetic protein 2 (BMP2) and fibroblast growth factor 4 (FGF4) induced myogenic differentiation of MSCs in vitro. BMP2/FGF4-pretreated MSCs had better myogenic differentiation within the

infarcted myocardium, and significantly prevented dilatation of the infarcted region and improved heart function compared with MSCs untreated with BMP2/FGF4 in a rat myocardial infarct model. Hattan et al[44] transfected murine MSCs with a recombinant plasmid containing enhanced green fluorescent protein cDNA under the control of the myosin light chain 2v promoter, and induced the MSCs to differentiate into cardiomyocytes by 5-azacytidine. Differentiated cardiomyocytes expressed green fluorescent protein, and were purified by fluorescence activated cell sorting. The authors transplanted purified cardiomyocytes from bone marrow mesenchymal stem cells into the left ventricle of adult mouse hearts, and observed that the grafted cells survived and oriented in parallel to the cardiomyocytes of the recipient heart at 3 months after transplantation.

Undifferentiated MSCs can also be used for cell therapy, and might differentiate depending on the local milieu and signals generated by the microenvironment of the heart. Shake et al[45] injected autologous MSCs directly into the infarct of a swine myocardial infarction model. Grafted MSCs expressed muscle-specific proteins as early as 2 weeks, and significantly attenuated contractile dysfunction and pathologic thinning. Piao et al[46] injected allogeneic MSCs or media into the center and the border area of the infarct scar in a rat myocardial infarction model. At 4 weeks after transplantation, the transplanted MSCs formed islands of cell clusters on the border of the infarct scar, and the cells expressed cardiac muscle proteins α-actinin and cardiac troponin T. The regional and global left ventricular function was significantly improved in the cell-treated group compared with the media control group.

However, whether MSCs can transdifferentiate into cardiomyocytes in vivo within the recipient heart remains controversial. Fazel et al[47] demonstrated that the transplanted MSCs from β-galactosidase transgenic mice were not induced to transdifferentiate into cardiomyocytes in the host cardiomyocytes in vivo. Berry et al[48] directly injected human MSCs into acutely ischemic myocardium in Lewis rats. After 8 weeks, the grafted cells expressed a cardiomyocyte protein, but stopped short of full differentiation. Although the MSC injection did not regenerate contracting cardiomyocytes in the myocardial infarction, it preserved some cardiac function by reducing the stiffness of the subsequent scar and attenuated postinfarction remodeling.

Improvement of cardiac function by MSC transplantation may involve a paracrine mechanism. Our group[49] has previously demonstrated that allogeneic MSCs did not express muscle-specific markers α-actinin, myosin heavy chain, phospholamban, and tropomyosin at 2 weeks after transplantation into rat myocardial infarction. Although the engrafted MSCs expressed the above muscle-specific markers at 6 months after transplantation (Figures 5.2–5.5), they did not fully evolve into an adult cardiac phenotype (Figure 5.6). MSC transplantation significantly improved left ventricular function at 4 weeks, while this benefit was lost at 6 months. These results suggest a possible early paracrine effect of engrafted MSCs on cardiac functional improvement. Recently, Gnecchi et al[50] collected the conditioned medium from hypoxic *Akt*-MSC, and observed that the conditioned medium markedly inhibited hypoxia-induced apoptosis and triggered vigorous spontaneous contraction of adult rat cardiomyocytes in vitro. *Akt*-MSC-conditioned medium also significantly limited infarct size and improved ventricular function when injected into infarcted hearts. These data provide evidence that transplanted MSCs protected the myocardium and improved cardiac function through paracrine mechanisms, rather than true transdifferentiation of the MSCs into new functioning phenotypic cardiac myocytes.

Therapeutic neovascularization

Restoration of the supply of oxygen and nutriment through the regrowth of functional blood vessels to the ischemic myocardium is important to decrease apoptosis of hypertrophied myocytes in the peri-infarct region, improve long-term salvage and survival of viable myocardium, reduce collagen deposition, and sustain improvement in cardiac function.[51] Recent studies have suggested that transplantation of MSCs enhances therapeutic angiogenesis after myocardial infarction in animal models.[52–55] The mechanism whereby engrafted MSCs stimulate angiogenesis in the ischemic heart remains controversial.[56] Paracrine action of MSCs might play a crucial role in the induction of neovascularization. Tang et al[52] injected autologous MSCs or culture medium intramyocardially into the peri-infarct zone in a rat myocardial infarction model. Two weeks later, the angiogenic factors basic fibroblast growth factor, vascular endothelial growth factor, and stem cell homing factor (stromal cell derived factor 1α) increased significantly in the MSC-treated hearts compared with medium-treated hearts. At 8 weeks after implantation, capillary density increased about 40% and left ventricular function improved significantly in MSC-treated hearts compared with medium-treated hearts. The results suggested that the major mechanism of increasing angiogenesis appears to be a paracrine action of the engrafted cells. Zhang et al[53] also showed that transplanted human MSCs upregulated vascular endothelial growth factor (VEGF) expression, enhanced angiogenesis, and improved the functional recovery in a rat myocardial infarction model. Recently, Shyu et al[54] compared the effects of MSC therapy and angiogenic growth factor gene therapy in a model of acute myocardial infarction in mice. Human MSCs or angiogenic growth factor genes (angiopoietin 1 or VEGF) were injected intramuscularly at the left anterior ventricular free wall. Human MSC transplantation markedly increased capillary density compared with angiogenic growth factor gene therapy. MSCs were superior to angiogenic growth factor genes for improving myocardial performance in this study.

MSCs might contribute to collateral vessel formation through cell incorporation into new or remodeling vessels. Oswald et al[55] cultured human MSCs in the presence of 2% fetal calf serum and 50 ng/ml VEGF, and observed that these MSCs were induced to differentiate into endothelial-like cells, which expressed endothelial-specific marker von Willebrand factor. The differentiated cells formed characteristic capillary-like structures when cultured with an in vitro angiogenesis test kit. This study showed that human

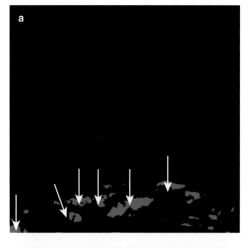

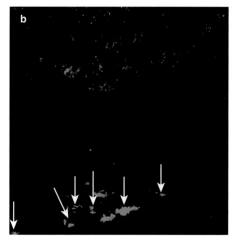

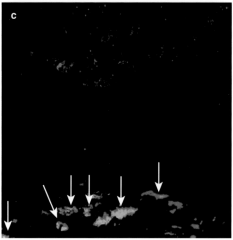

Figure 5.2 *Confocal microscopy of fluorescent immunohistochemical staining of DiI-labeled (DIL is dioctadecylindocarbocyanine) cells in infarcted myocardium for α-actinin at 6 months. (a) DiI-labeled MSCs appear red (white arrows). (b) Sections stained with antibody to muscle marker α-actinin appear green. White arrows point to MSC transplant. (c) Merged image of (a) and (b) shows that DiI-labeled MSCs express α-actinin (yellow cells; white arrows). Original magnification x 400. (Reproduced with permission from reference 49.)*

MSCs differentiated into cells with phenotypic and functional features of endothelial cells. In vivo study also demonstrated that the engrafted MSCs formed vascular structures and were positive for von Willebrand factor or smooth muscle actin in myocardium.[57] Our recently published data[49] also demonstrated that engrafted MSCs expressed von Willebrand factor and incorporated as endothelial cells into the vasculature at 6 months after transplantation into the myocardial infarction in rats (Figure 5.7). The total blood vessel density that stained positive for von Willebrand factor (including capillaries) in the scar area was significantly greater in the MSC group than in the saline group at 6 months after MSC or saline treatment. However, the density of arterioles and small arteries in the scar area was similar in the two groups.

Prevention of arrhythmias

MSC transplantation could be a possible biological alternative for the treatment of abnormalities of the pacemaker function of the heart, or abnormalities of cardiac impulse conduction. MSCs may be used as platforms for delivery of pacemaker genes to the myocardium to create biologic cardiac pacemakers. Potapova et al[58] transfected human MSCs with a cardiac pacemaker gene, *mHCN2*, by electroporation. The genetically modified human MSCs were able to express functional HCN2 (hyperpolarization-activated cyclic nucleotide-gated cation) channels

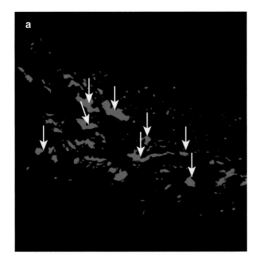

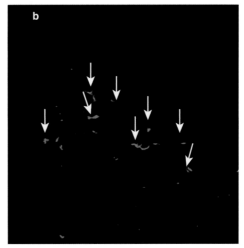

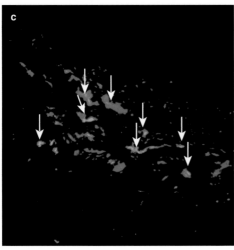

Figure 5.3   *Confocal microscopy of fluorescent immunohistochemical staining of DiI-labeled cells in infarcted myocardium for MF20 at 6 months. (a) DiI-labeled MSCs appear red (white arrows). (b) Sections stained with antibody to muscle marker MF20 appear green. White arrows point to MSC transplant. (c) Merged image of (a) and (b) shows that DiI-labeled MSCs express MF20 (yellow cells; white arrows). Original magnification × 400. (Reproduced with permission from reference 49.)*

in vitro and in vivo, mimicking overexpression of HCN2 genes in cardiac myocytes. Transfected hMSCs influenced the in vitro beating rate of neonatal rat ventricular myocytes in culture. After subepicardial transplantation of transfected hMSCs in the canine left ventricular wall, animals developed spontaneous rhythms of left-sided origin during sinus arrest, and engrafted MSCs formed gap junctions with adjacent myocytes within the injected regions. These findings demonstrate that genetically modified human MSCs that express a cardiac pacemaker gene represent a novel delivery system for this type of gene.

MSCs can contribute to the formation of a conduction system in the heart. Airey et al[59] injected human MSCs intraperitoneally into sheep fetuses in utero. The engrafted MSCs formed segments of Purkinje fibers during late fetal development. Beeres et al[60] cultured neonatal rat cardiomyocytes on multielectrode arrays. At 48 hours after culturing, conduction block was induced by abrasion of a 200–450-μm-wide channel to cause several asynchronously beating fields of cardiomyocytes. Application of human MSCs into the culture restored synchronization of the cardiomyocytes. Immunostaining for connexins and intercellular dye transfer (calcein)

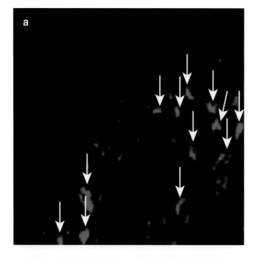

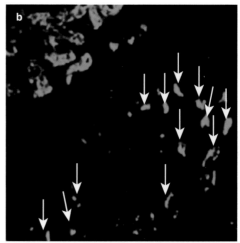

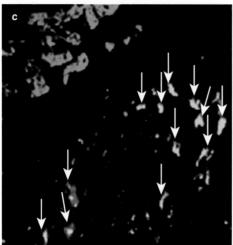

Figure 5.4 *Confocal microscopy of fluorescent immunohistochemical staining of DiI-labeled cells in infarcted myocardium for phospholamban at 6 months. (a) DiI-labeled MSCs appear red (white arrows). (b) Sections stained with antibody to muscle marker phospholamban appear green. White arrows point to MSC transplant. (c) Merged image of (a) and (b) shows that DiI-labeled MSCs express phospholamban (yellow cells; white arrows). Original magnification x 400. (Reproduced with permission from reference 49.)*

showed the presence of functional gap junctions between human MSCs and cardiomyocytes. Intracellular action potential recordings indicated cross-channel electrical conduction. Human MSCs appear to have the potential to repair conduction block, although this field is still in its infancy. There are complex problems concerning safety and efficacy that need to be resolved before clinical evaluation.

Combination of cell and gene therapy

MSCs can be used as a vehicle for delivery of therapeutic target genes in vivo. Matsumoto et al[61] transfected a human VEGF165 gene to cultured

MSCs of Lewis rats, and then injected the VEGF-transfected MSCs into myocardial infarction of syngeneic rats. High expression of VEGF was detected in the VEGF-transfected MSC-treated group at 1 week. Infarct size, left ventricular dimensions, ejection fraction, and capillary density of the infarcted region were significantly improved in the VEGF group at 4 weeks after myocardial infarction, compared with the non-VEGF-transfected MSC or medium group. This study suggests that a combined strategy of MSC transplantation with gene therapy could be useful for the treatment of myocardial infarction. The combined strategy may represent a

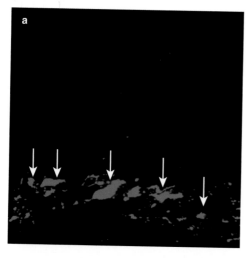
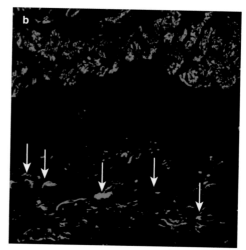
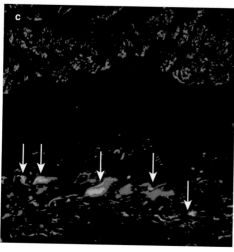

Figure 5.5 *Confocal microscopy of fluorescent immunohistochemical staining of DiI-labeled cells in infarcted myocardium for tropomyosin at 6 months. (a) DiI-labeled MSCs appear red (white arrows). (b) Sections stained with antibody to muscle marker tropomyosin appear green. White arrows point to MSC transplant. (c) Merged image of (a) and (b) shows that DiI-labeled MSCs express tropomyosin (yellow cells; white arrows). Original magnification x 400. (Reproduced with permission from reference 49.)*

reversible and safe gene delivery approach, because the gene expression could be stopped by combined transfection with a suicide gene in the event of an unexpected adverse reaction or when expression of the protein of interest is no longer required.[62]

Genetic manipulation can increase the survival rate of transplanted MSCs within myocardial infarction. Lim et al[63] transduced MSCs with myristoylated (myr)-*Akt* and transplanted the cells into porcine hearts after experimental myocardial infarction. MSCs transduced with myr-*Akt* were more resistant to apoptosis compared with MSCs without myr-*Akt*. Other genes, such as hypoxia-regulated heme oxygenase 1 gene,[64] fibroblast growth factor 2 (FGF2) gene,[65] VEGF, and insulin-like growth factor I gene,[66] have also been used to improve the survival of transplanted stem cells during myocardial hypoxia or ischemia.

Homing of MSCs to the Injured Myocardium

In response to ischemic injury, cardiac muscle activates signaling cascades that can attract circulating stem cells. These stem cells migrate to the site of damage through the peripheral blood, adhere to the endothelium of the vasculature, and

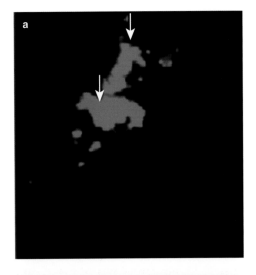

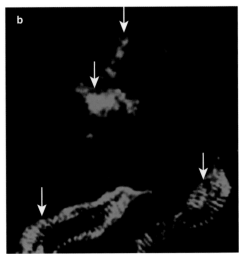

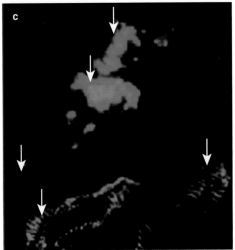

Figure 5.6   *Higher-power magnification (x 600) confocal microscopy of fluorescent immunohistochemical staining of DiI-labeled cells in infarcted myocardium for α-actinin at 6 months. (a) DiI-labeled MSCs appear red (white arrows). (b) Sections stained with antibody to muscle marker α-actinin appear green. White arrows point to MSC transplant without typical cross-striation. Red arrows point to host cardiac cells with cross-striations. (c) Merged image of (a) and (b) shows that DiI-labeled MSCs express α-actinin without typical cross-striation (yellow cells; white arrows). (Reproduced with permission from reference 49.)*

transmigrate across the physical endothelium and extracellular matrix barrier to the damaged host tissues. This process is termed "homing". "Homing" of circulating MSCs may contribute to the repair process of the injured myocardium. Wang et al[67] observed that circulating MSCs spontaneously increased within 3 days after the onset of an acute myocardial infarction in patients; then the cell counts decreased and normalized at 1 month. Segers et al[68] demonstrated that circulating MSCs adhered to the cardiac microvascular endothelium in rat ischemia reperfusion injured hearts in vivo. Cardiac homing of MSCs was

significantly enhanced by the activation of MSCs with tumor necrosis factor α (TNFα) before injection. Schmidt et al[69] detected tight cell–cell contacts between MSCs and endothelial cells at the capillary vessel, and demonstrated MSCs transmigrating across the endothelial barrier in an isolated heart perfusion model. Jiang et al[70] injected MSCs intravenously through the tail vein in a rat myocardial infarction model. The injected MSCs homed to the ischemic myocardium, and expressed cardiac muscle proteins troponin and desmin, the smooth muscle cell marker α-actin, and endothelial cell marker CD31 at 4 and 8

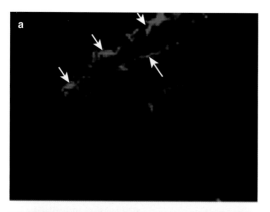

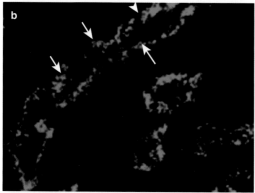

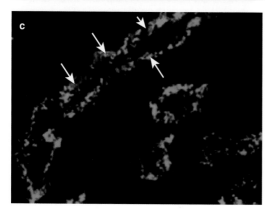

Figure 5.7 *Confocal microscopy of fluorescent immunohistochemical staining of DiI-labeled cells in infarcted myocardium for von Willebrand factor at 6 months. (a) DiI-labeled MSCs appear red (white arrows). (b) Sections stained with antibody to endothelium marker von Willebrand factor appear green and define endothelium of several blood vessels. White arrows point to MSC transplant. (c) Merged image of (a) and (b) shows that DiI-labeled MSCs express von Willebrand factor (yellow cells; white arrows). Original magnification x 400. (Reproduced with permission from reference 49.)*

weeks after transplantation. The cardiac function was significantly improved in the MSC group compared with the medium control group. Although homing of MSCs is a promising approach for cardiac repair, many factors can influence this homing process. In the heart, the specific signals for stem cell homing are only expressed for a short time following injury.[71] Therefore, deciphering these specific homing signals and reestablishing their expression at a time remote from injury may allow for the development of better strategies to repair damaged myocardium. In vitro propagation of BM-derived MSCs may decrease the homing ability of MSCs.[72] The molecular signals regulating MSC trafficking to sites of injury remain unclear.[73] More basic research is needed before MSC homing therapy for myocardial infarction becomes part of routine clinical practice.

In contrast, our research group[74] recently labeled rat MSCs with isotopic colloidal nanoparticles (europium) and injected them either directly into an experimental myocardial infarction, or intravenously via the tail vein of a rat after acute myocardial infarction. There were 25% of labeled cells remaining in the heart at day 4 after injection; however, no labeled cells were detected in the heart when cells were administered intravenously. Our data suggest that "homing" of intravenous injected MSCs may not be an appropriate route of delivery as a treatment immediately after myocardial infarction.

Clinical Trials

Because autologous bone marrow-derived stem cells are easy to isolate and expand in culture, and have great plasticity, they are the most ideal cell source currently selected for cell therapy of myocardial infarction in clinical trials. Because there are no specific surface markers that are reliable parameters for MSC purity, only unselected bone marrow stem cells containing MSCs have been used in patients. Recently, several groups reported their randomized clinical trial data. Schachinger et al[75] enriched bone marrow-derived progenitor cells with Ficoll–Hypaque centrifugation to obtain a cell suspension which consisted of hematopoietic, mesenchymal, and other mononuclear cells. The cell suspension was infused into the infarct coronary artery at 3–7 days after successful reperfusion therapy in 101 patients with acute myocardial infarction. The randomized control group ($n=98$) received an intracoronary infusion of placebo medium. At 4 months, the absolute improvement in global left ventricular ejection fraction was significantly greater in the cell group ($5.5\pm7.3\%$) compared with the control group ($3.0\pm6.5\%$; $p=0.01$). At 1 year, adverse clinical events including death, recurrence of myocardial infarction, and any revascularization procedure were significantly reduced in the cell group (2%, $n=101$) compared with the placebo control group (12%, $n=103$). Assmus et al[76] isolated progenitor cells from bone marrow by Ficoll density-gradient centrifugation. The progenitor cells contained fewer than 1% hematopoietic progenitor cells. Intracoronary infusion of bone marrow-derived progenitor cells resulted in moderate but significant improvements in left ventricular ejection fraction in patients with ischemic heart disease ($n=24$) at 3 months after treatment, compared with those patients who received intracoronary infusion of circulating blood progenitor cells ($n=24$) or no cell infusion ($n=23$). However, other groups reported negative results. Lunde et al[77] prepared mononuclear cells from bone marrow by Ficoll density gradient. At day 3–5 after myocardial infarction patients were treated with acute percutaneous coronary intervention; they received intracoronary infusion of bone marrow-derived mononuclear cells ($n=47$) or no cell infusion ($n=50$). There was no significant difference in global left ventricular function between the two groups at 6 months after treatment. Meyer et al[78] processed bone marrow with gelatin polysuccinate density-gradient sedimentation and obtained cell suspensions containing nucleated cells, CD34+ cells, and hematopoietic colony-forming cells. The patients who received intracoronary cell infusion ($n=30$) had a significant increase of left ventricular ejection fraction compared with those who received no cell infusion ($n=30$) at 6 months, but the benefit was lost at 18 months. These findings were similar to the findings in our experimental study in which adult

bone marrow-derived MSCs resulted in a transient improvement in left ventricular function that was lost long term.[49] The available clinical trial data are mixed, and are not sufficient to decide whether stem cell therapy for myocardial infarction is ready for general clinical practice.

Concerns Regarding Mesenchymal Stem Cell Therapy

Because mesenchymal stem cells maintain their multipotential capacity after transplantation, they may form unexpected tissue. For example, Grinnemo et al[79] demonstrated that transplanted human MSCs differentiate into fibroblasts, not cardiomyocytes, in a rat myocardial infarction model. How to induce and enhance the cardiomyocyte differentiation of MSCs remains a major issue in the field of myocardial regeneration.

Another challenge to MSC therapy is the issue of how to increase the survival rate of transplanted MSCs in the ischemic myocardium. Transplanted MSCs can be washed out through the blood vessels,[80] or die due to lack of blood supply. Strategies are needed to keep the cells at the desired site after transplantation, and to increase their capacity to resist a hostile environment such as local ischemia.

Although no serious ventricular arrhythmias have been reported after MSC transplantation into hearts in both animal experiments and clinical trials, Chang et al[81] demonstrated the proarrhythmic potential of MSCs in an in vitro coculture model, in which human MSCs were cocultured with neonatal rat ventricular myocytes. Compared with myocyte-only culture, cocultures decreased conduction velocity and induced re-entrant arrhythmias. The results suggested that cocultures of MSCs and ventricular myocytes can produce an arrhythmogenic substrate. Thus, local transplantation of MSCs may predispose the heart to re-entrant arrhythmias.

There are still concerns over whether transplanted MSCs express cardiac cell markers through transdifferentiation or cell fusion. Bae et al[82] demonstrated that there was cell fusion of transplanted MSCs with Purkinje neurons in Niemann–Pick type C mice.

Whether MSCs are "immune privileged" remains controversial. Grinnemo et al[83] injected human MSCs into the myocardium of Sprague–Dawley rats. In a mixed lymphocyte reaction test, human MSCs induced significant proliferation of rat peripheral blood lymphocytes. Hematoxylin and eosin staining and immunohistochemistry demonstrated a significant infiltration of round cells, mostly macrophages, into the area of injection of MSCs in rat hearts. This study suggests that MSCs may cause immunoreactivity in a xenogenic model.

Summary

Current cumulative evidence demonstrates that MSC transplantation may be a novel therapy for the repair of damaged myocardium due to the ability of MSCs to self-renew and, in some but not all studies, to differentiate into cardiomyocytes in vitro and in vivo. Some studies suggest that the benefit of these cells is not due to true transdifferentiation into cardiomyocytes with replacement of heart muscle but due to a paracrine effect. MSCs are generally identified through a combination of poorly defined physical, phenotypic, and functional properties because their properties are poorly understood. In order to compare the data on MSC therapy in heart disease from different laboratories, there is an urgent need for a more comprehensive view of how to identify characteristics, and standardize the MSCs that will be utilized in trials. Other questions, such as which approach, intravenous or intramyocardial, is better for cell delivery; how many cells should be used; when is the best time for cell transplantation after myocardial infarction; and what kind of patient can benefit from cell therapy, will require further investigation.

References

1. Wold LE, Dai W, Sesti C et al. Stem cell therapy for the heart. Congest Heart Fail 2004; 10: 293–301.
2. Dai W, Hale SL, Kloner RA. Stem cell transplantation for the treatment of myocardial infarction. Transpl Immunol 2005; 15: 91–7.
3. Wexler SA, Donaldson C, Denning-Kendall P et al. Adult bone marrow is a rich source of human mesenchymal "stem" cells but umbilical cord and mobilized adult blood are not. Br J Haematol 2003; 121: 368–74.
4. Meirelles Lda S, Nardi NB. Murine marrow-derived mesenchymal stem cell: isolation, in vitro expansion, and characterization. Br J Haematol 2003; 123: 702–11.
5. Bianchi G, Banfi A, Mastrogiacomo M et al. Ex vivo enrichment of mesenchymal cell progenitors by fibroblast growth factor 2. Exp Cell Res 2003; 287: 98–105.
6. Colter DC, Class R, DiGirolamo CM, Prockop DJ. Rapid expansion of recycling stem cells in cultures of plastic-adherent cells from human bone marrow. Proc Natl Acad Sci USA 2000; 97: 3213–18.
7. Bianco P, Riminucci M, Gronthos S et al. Bone marrow stromal stem cells: nature, biology, and potential applications. Stem Cells 2001; 19: 180–92.
8. Barry FP, Boynton RE, Haynesworth S et al. The monoclonal antibody SH-2, raised against human mesenchymal stem cells, recognizes an epitope on endoglin (CD105). Biochem Biophys Res Commun 1999; 265: 134–9.
9. Barry F, Boynton R, Murphy M et al. The SH-3 and SH-4 antibodies recognize distinct epitopes on CD73 from human mesenchymal stem cells. Biochem Biophys Res Commun 2001; 289: 519–24.
10. Gronthos S, Simmons PJ, Graves SE et al. Integrin-mediated interactions between human bone marrow stromal precursor cells and the extracellular matrix. Bone 2001; 28: 174–81.
11. Pittenger MF, Martin BJ. Mesenchymal stem cells and their potential as cardiac therapeutics. Circ Res 2004; 95: 9–20.
12. Pittenger MF, Mackay AM, Beck SC et al. Multilineage potential of adult human mesenchymal stem cells. Science 1999; 284: 143–7.
13. Sethe S, Scutt A, Stolzing A. Aging of mesenchymal stem cells. Ageing Res Rev 2006; 5: 91–116.
14. Zhang FB, Li L, Fang B et al. Passage-restricted differentiation potential of mesenchymal stem cells into cardiomyocyte-like cells. Biochem Biophys Res Commun 2005; 336: 784–92.
15. Yoon J, Min BG, Kim YH et al. Differentiation, engraftment and functional effects of pre-treated mesenchymal stem cells in a rat myocardial infarct model. Acta Cardiol 2005; 60: 277–84.
16. Simonsen JL, Rosada C, Serakinci N et al. Telomerase expression extends the proliferative life-span and maintains the osteogenic potential of human bone marrow stromal cells. Nat Biotechnol 2002; 20: 592–6.
17. Xie XJ, Wang JA, Cao J, Zhang X, Xu HZ. Differentiation of bone marrow mesenchymal stem cells induced by myocardial medium under hypoxic conditions. Acta Pharmacol Sin 2006; 27: 1153–8.

18. Eslaminejad MB, Nikmahzar A, Taghiyar L, Nadri S, Massumi M. Murine mesenchymal stem cells isolated by low density primary culture system. Dev Growth Differ 2006; 48: 361–70.

19. Sekiya I, Larson BL, Smith JR et al. Expansion of human adult stem cells from bone marrow stroma: conditions that maximize the yields of early progenitors and evaluate their quality. Stem Cells 2002; 20: 530–41.

20. Hung SC, Chen NJ, Hsieh SL et al. Isolation and characterization of size-sieved stem cells from human bone marrow. Stem Cells 2002; 20: 249–58.

21. Baddoo M, Hill K, Wilkinson R et al. Characterization of mesenchymal stem cells isolated from murine bone marrow by negative selection. J Cell Biochem 2003; 89: 1235–49.

22. Ortiz LA, Gambelli F, McBride C et al. Mesenchymal stem cell engraftment in lung is enhanced in response to bleomycin exposure and ameliorates its fibrotic effects. Proc Natl Acad Sci USA 2003; 100: 8407–11.

23. Stenderup K, Justesen J, Eriksen EF, Rattan SI, Kassem M. Number and proliferative capacity of osteogenic stem cells are maintained during aging and in patients with osteoporosis. J Bone Miner Res 2001; 16: 1120–9.

24. Zangi L, Rivkin R, Kassis I et al. High-yield isolation, expansion, and differentiation of rat bone marrow-derived mesenchymal stem cells with fibrin microbeads. Tissue Eng 2006; 12: 2343–54.

25. Fickert S, Fiedler J, Brenner RE. Identification, quantification and isolation of mesenchymal progenitor cells from osteoarthritic synovium by fluorescence automated cell sorting. Osteoarthritis Cartilage 2003; 11: 790–800.

26. Digirolamo CM, Stokes D, Colter D et al. Propagation and senescence of human marrow stromal cells in culture: a simple colony-forming assay identifies samples with the greatest potential to propagate and differentiate. Br J Haematol 1999; 107: 275–81.

27. Heng BC, Haider HKh, Sim EK, Cao T, Ng SC. Strategies for directing the differentiation of stem cells into the cardiomyogenic lineage in vitro. Cardiovasc Res 2004; 62: 34–42.

28. Shim WS, Jiang S, Wong P et al. Ex vivo differentiation of human adult bone marrow stem cells into cardiomyocyte-like cells. Biochem Biophys Res Commun 2004; 324: 481–8.

29. Hakuno D, Fukuda K, Makino S et al. Bone marrow-derived regenerated cardiomyocytes (CMG Cells) express functional adrenergic and muscarinic receptors. Circulation 2002; 105: 380–6.

30. Wakitani S, Saito T, Caplan AI. Myogenic cells derived from rat bone marrow mesenchymal stem cells exposed to 5-azacytidine. Muscle Nerve 1995; 18: 1417–26.

31. Rangappa S, Fen C, Lee EH, Bongso A, Sim EK. Transformation of adult mesenchymal stem cells isolated from the fatty tissue into cardiomyocytes. Ann Thorac Surg 2003; 75: 775–9.

32. Xu W, Zhang X, Qian H et al. Mesenchymal stem cells from adult human bone marrow differentiate into a cardiomyocyte phenotype in vitro. Exp Biol Med (Maywood) 2004; 229: 623–31.

33. Xaymardan M, Tang L, Zagreda L et al. Platelet-derived growth factor-AB promotes the generation of adult bone marrow-derived cardiac myocytes. Circ Res 2004; 94: E39–45.

34. Fukuhara S, Tomita S, Yamashiro S et al. Direct cell-cell interaction of cardiomyocytes is key for bone marrow stromal cells to go into cardiac lineage in vitro. J Thorac Cardiovasc Surg 2003; 125: 1470–80.

35. Wang T, Xu Z, Jiang W, Ma A. Cell-to-cell contact induces mesenchymal stem cell to differentiate into cardiomyocyte and smooth muscle cell. Int J Cardiol 2006; 109: 74–81.

36. Terada N, Hamazaki T, Oka M et al. Bone marrow cells adopt the phenotype of other cells by spontaneous cell fusion. Nature 2002; 416: 542–5.

37. Ryan JM, Barry FP, Murphy JM, Mahon BP. Mesenchymal stem cells avoid allogeneic rejection. J Inflamm (Lond) 2005; 2: 8.

38. Le Blanc K, Tammik C, Rosendahl K, Zetterberg E, Ringden O. HLA expression and immunologic properties of differentiated and undifferentiated mesenchymal stem cells. Exp Hematol 2003; 31: 890–6.

39. Tse WT, Pendleton JD, Beyer WM, Egalka MC, Guinan EC. Suppression of allogeneic T–cell proliferation by human marrow stromal cells: implications in transplantation. Transplantation 2003; 75: 389–97.

40. Stenderup K, Justesen J, Clausen C, Kassem M. Aging is associated with decreased maximal life span and accelerated senescence of bone marrow stromal cells. Bone 2003; 33: 919–26.

41. Baxter MA, Wynn RF, Jowitt SN et al. Study of telomere length reveals rapid aging of human marrow stromal cells following in vitro expansion. Stem Cells 2004; 22: 675–82.

42. Bonab MM, Alimoghaddam K, Talebian F et al. Aging of mesenchymal stem cell in vitro. BMC Cell Biol 2006; 7: 14.

43. Liu L, DiGirolamo CM, Navarro PA, Blasco MA, Keefe DL. Telomerase deficiency impairs differentiation of mesenchymal stem cells. Exp Cell Res 2004; 294: 1–8.

44. Hattan N, Kawaguchi H, Ando K et al. Purified cardiomyocytes from bone marrow mesenchymal stem cells produce stable intracardiac grafts in mice. Cardiovasc Res 2005; 65: 334–44.

45. Shake JG, Gruber PJ, Baumgartner WA et al. Mesenchymal stem cell implantation in a swine

myocardial infarct model: engraftment and functional effects. Ann Thorac Surg 2002; 73: 1919–25.

46. Piao H, Youn TJ, Kwon JS et al. Effects of bone marrow derived mesenchymal stem cells transplantation in acutely infarcting myocardium. Eur J Heart Fail 2005; 7: 730–8.

47. Fazel S, Chen L, Weisel RD et al. Cell transplantation preserves cardiac function after infarction by infarct stabilization: augmentation by stem cell factor. J Thorac Cardiovasc Surg 2005; 130: 1310.

48. Berry MF, Engler AJ, Woo YJ et al. Mesenchymal stem cell injection after myocardial infarction improves myocardial compliance. Am J Physiol Heart Circ Physiol 2006; 290: H2196–203.

49. Dai W, Hale SL, Martin BJ et al. Allogeneic mesenchymal stem cell transplantation in postinfarcted rat myocardium: short- and long-term effects. Circulation 2005; 112: 214–23.

50. Gnecchi M, He H, Noiseux N et al. Evidence supporting paracrine hypothesis for Akt-modified mesenchymal stem cell-mediated cardiac protection and functional improvement. FASEB J 2006; 20: 661–9.

51. Itescu S, Kocher AA, Schuster MD. Myocardial neovascularization by adult bone marrow-derived angioblasts: strategies for improvement of cardiomyocyte function. Heart Fail Rev 2003; 8: 253–8.

52. Tang YL, Zhao Q, Qin X et al. Paracrine action enhances the effects of autologous mesenchymal stem cell transplantation on vascular regeneration in rat model of myocardial infarction. Ann Thorac Surg 2005; 80: 229–36.

53. Zhang S, Jia Z, Ge J et al. Purified human bone marrow multipotent mesenchymal stem cells regenerate infarcted myocardium in experimental rats. Cell Transplant 2005; 14: 787–98.

54. Shyu KG, Wang BW, Hung HF, Chang CC, Shih DT. Mesenchymal stem cells are superior to angiogenic growth factor genes for improving myocardial performance in the mouse model of acute myocardial infarction. J Biomed Sci 2006; 13: 47–58.

55. Oswald J, Boxberger S, Jorgensen B et al. Mesenchymal stem cells can be differentiated into endothelial cells in vitro. Stem Cells 2004; 22: 377–84.

56. Heil M, Ziegelhoeffer T, Mees B, Schaper W. A different outlook on the role of bone marrow stem cells in vascular growth: bone marrow delivers software not hardware. Circ Res 2004; 94: 573–4.

57. Nagaya N, Kangawa K, Itoh T et al. Transplantation of mesenchymal stem cells improves cardiac function in a rat model of dilated cardiomyopathy. Circulation 2005; 112: 1128–35.

58. Potapova I, Plotnikov A, Lu Z et al. Human mesenchymal stem cells as a gene delivery system to create cardiac pacemakers. Circ Res 2004; 94: 952–9.

59. Airey JA, Almeida-Porada G, Colletti EJ et al. Human mesenchymal stem cells form Purkinje fibers in fetal sheep heart. Circulation 2004; 109: 1401–7.

60. Beeres SL, Atsma DE, van der Laarse A et al. Human adult bone marrow mesenchymal stem cells repair experimental conduction block in rat cardiomyocyte cultures. J Am Coll Cardiol 2005; 46: 1943–52.

61. Matsumoto R, Omura T, Yoshiyama M et al. Vascular endothelial growth factor-expressing mesenchymal stem cell transplantation for the treatment of acute myocardial infarction. Arterioscler Thromb Vasc Biol 2005; 25: 1168–73.

62. Miyagawa S, Sawa Y, Fukuda K et al. Angiogenic gene cell therapy using suicide gene system regulates the effect of angiogenesis in infarcted rat heart. Transplantation 2006; 81: 902–7.

63. Lim SY, Kim YS, Ahn Y et al. The effects of mesenchymal stem cells transduced with Akt in a porcine myocardial infarction model. Cardiovasc Res 2006; 70: 530–42.

64. Tang YL, Tang Y, Zhang YC et al. Improved graft mesenchymal stem cell survival in ischemic heart with a hypoxia-regulated heme oxygenase-1 vector. J Am Coll Cardiol 2005; 46: 1339–50.

65. Song H, Kwon K, Lim S et al. Transfection of mesenchymal stem cells with the FGF-2 gene improves their survival under hypoxic conditions. Mol Cells 2005; 19: 402–7.

66. Yau TM, Kim C, Li G et al. Maximizing ventricular function with multimodal cell-based gene therapy. Circulation 2005; 112 (9 Suppl): I123–8.

67. Wang Y, Johnsen HE, Mortensen S et al. Changes in circulating mesenchymal stem cells, stem cell homing factor, and vascular growth factors in patients with acute ST elevation myocardial infarction treated with primary percutaneous coronary intervention. Heart 2006; 92: 768–74.

68. Segers VF, Van Riet I, Andries LJ et al. Mesenchymal stem cell adhesion to cardiac microvascular endothelium: activators and mechanisms. Am J Physiol Heart Circ Physiol 2006; 290: H1370–7.

69. Schmidt A, Ladage D, Steingen C et al. Mesenchymal stem cells transmigrate over the endothelial barrier. Eur J Cell Biol 2006; 85: 1179–88.

70. Jiang W, Ma A, Wang T et al. Homing and differentiation of mesenchymal stem cells delivered intravenously to ischemic myocardium in vivo: a time-series study. Pflugers Arch 2006; 453: 43–52.

71. Penn MS, Zhang M, Deglurkar I, Topol EJ. Role of stem cell homing in myocardial regeneration. Int J Cardiol 2004; 95 (Suppl 1): S23–5.

72. Rombouts WJ, Ploemacher RE. Primary murine MSC show highly efficient homing to the bone marrow but lose homing ability following culture. Leukemia 2003; 17: 160–70.

73. Schenk S, Mal N, Finan A et al. MCP-3 is a myocardial mesenchymal stem cell homing factor. Stem Cells 2007; 25: 245–51.

74. Hale SL, Dow JS, Dai W, Kloner RA. Homing of mesenchymal stem cells following intravenous injection: the wrong approach for cell delivery to infarcted myocardium? A quantitative assessment using nanoparticle labeling [Abstract]. Circulation 2006; 114 (Suppl): II79.

75. Schachinger V, Erbs S, Elsasser A et al. Intracoronary bone marrow-derived progenitor cells in acute myocardial infarction. N Engl J Med 2006; 355: 1210–21.

76. Assmus B, Honold J, Schachinger V et al. Transcoronary transplantation of progenitor cells after myocardial infarction. N Engl J Med 2006; 355: 1222–32.

77. Lunde K, Solheim S, Aakhus S et al. Intracoronary injection of mononuclear bone marrow cells in acute myocardial infarction. N Engl J Med 2006; 355: 1199–209.

78. Meyer GP, Wollert KC, Lotz J et al. Intracoronary bone marrow cell transfer after myocardial infarction: eighteen months' follow-up data from the randomized, controlled BOOST (BOne marrOw transfer to enhance ST-elevation infarct regeneration) trial. Circulation 2006; 113: 1287–94.

79. Grinnemo KH, Mansson-Broberg A, Leblanc K et al. Human mesenchymal stem cells do not differentiate into cardiomyocytes in a cardiac ischemic xenomodel. Ann Med 2006; 38: 144–53.

80. Dow J, Simkhovich BZ, Kedes L, Kloner RA. Washout of transplanted cells from the heart: a potential new hurdle for cell transplantation therapy. Cardiovasc Res 2005; 67: 301–7.

81. Chang MG, Tung L, Sekar RB et al. Proarrhythmic potential of mesenchymal stem cell transplantation revealed in an in vitro coculture model. Circulation 2006; 113: 1832–41.

82. Bae JS, Furuya S, Shinoda Y et al. Neurodegeneration augments the ability of bone marrow-derived mesenchymal stem cells to fuse with Purkinje neurons in Niemann-Pick type C mice. Hum Gene Ther 2005; 16: 1006–11.

83. Grinnemo KH, Mansson A, Dellgren G et al. Xenoreactivity and engraftment of human mesenchymal stem cells transplanted into infarcted rat myocardium. J Thorac Cardiovasc Surg 2004; 127: 1293–300.

chapter 6

Myocardial Regeneration via Intracardiac Stem Cells

Sophie Bekkers, Rian Nijmeijer, Patrick van Vliet, Sander Smits, Marie-José Goumans, and Pieter A Doevendans

Introduction

Ischemic heart disease is the leading cause of mortality in the Western world. Myocardial infarction (MI) is frequently complicated by maladaptive left ventricular (LV) remodeling, which is characterized by ventricular dilatation and diminished cardiac performance. This may contribute to the progression into congestive heart failure. The current treatment option to reduce ischemic cardiovascular damage is to provide reperfusion of the infarct-related coronary artery by, for example, percutaneous transluminal coronary angioplasty (PTCA) or thrombolysis. The other option is to revascularize the ischemic area by coronary artery bypass grafting (CABG). These therapies have successfully reduced MI size and decreased the mortality of acute MI. However, when patients present late (> 12 hours after MI) or fail to respond to therapy, a transmural MI will develop, characterized by cell death (Figure 6.1). The prevalence of congestive heart failure continues to increase and remains associated with a more than 10-fold elevated risk of death, despite the introduction of multiple treatment strategies to reduce the infarct size and LV remodeling. The search for alternative therapies remains necessary. At present, cell transplantation appears a promising treatment to repair the damaged myocardium and restore cardiac function, augmenting the inadequate intrinsic repair mechanisms within the diseased heart. Cell transplantation therapy might enhance the formation of vascular structures and serve as a source of new cardiomyocytes to restore ventricular wall thickness and improve the contractile function of the heart. Additionally, transplanted cells may activate resident progenitor cells in the heart via a paracrine pathway.

The success of stem cell therapy stands or falls with the quality and potential of the cell population used. Theoretically, different types of cells can be used for this purpose, namely embryonic stem cells (ESCs) or (adult) somatic stem cells derived from several sources (for an overview see references 1 and 2). In vitro ESCs can differentiate into rhythmically contracting cardiomyocytes coupled by gap junctions, but with a fetal electrophysiological phenotype.[3,4] Transplantation of differentiated ESCs has shown the most promising results in preclinical studies to date; however, ethical controversy, tumorgenicity, and immunity issues limit their use. Somatic stem cells harvested from the bone marrow are at present the most frequently used adult stem cell population for cardiac repair in clinical trials. To date, differentiation of bone marrow cells into cardiomyocytes in vivo is under debate. Even in experimental studies using different types of bone marrow-derived stem cells, differentiation into myocytes occurs rarely.[5] Additionally, clinical trials have been performed using skeletal myoblasts. Since skeletal muscle cells have a greater tolerance to ischemia than cardiac cells, these cells seem to be well suited for cardiac repair after MI. However, skeletal muscle has different electrical and mechanical properties from cardiac muscle,

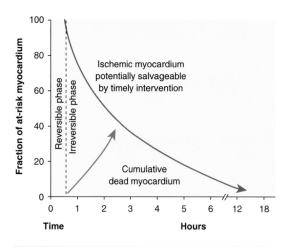

Figure 6.1 *Salvageable period after acute myocardial infarction. In the first hours after acute myocardial infarction (MI), reperfusion therapy can rescue cardiomyocytes from irreversible cell death. Thirty minutes after acute coronary occlusion the first cardiomyocytes, located subendocardially, are irreversibly damaged.*

which raises the risk of life-threatening arrhythmias.[6] The quest for the best cell for cardiac replacement therapy continues.[7]

Until recently, the heart was considered to be a terminally differentiated organ with no regenerative capacity. Cardiomyocytes were believed to respond to disease only by hypertrophy. Although in many adult tissues, such as blood, skin, liver, skeletal muscle, and even the central nervous system, stem cells have been isolated, no evidence was found that stem cells could be harvested from the adult heart.[8] However, Anversa and co-workers repeatedly described the existence of mitotic cardiomyocytes in normal and pathological conditions.[9] In 1998, mitotic figures were detected using confocal microscopy in patients with ischemic heart failure, but also in healthy controls.[10] Recent experiments in patients after acute myocardial infarction suggested activation of cell cycle entry by mitotic figures in sarcomeric α-actinin-expressing cells or Ki67 expression in laminin-expressing cells.[11] Patients with aortic stenosis showed increased telomerase activity in myocytes, indicative of DNA synthesis

and nuclear division.[12] The methods used to identify dividing cardiomyocytes are under debate. Observations of DNA synthesis and binucleated cardiomyocytes are essentially different from cell division, especially since cardiomyocytes can be multinucleated. Furthermore, in sex mismatched transplantation studies, XY-cardiomyocytes and vascular cells have been identified within female donor hearts.[13] These studies brought to light a new view on the dogma of the heart being a static postmitotic organ, opening the possibility of myocardial regeneration by either bone marrow-derived cells or resident cardiac stem cells. Several studies showed that indeed certain cardiac cell populations harbor stem cell characteristics with respect to their gene expression profile, growth, and differentiation potential. Furthermore, some of these cardiac stem/progenitor cells also express early cardiac genes and transcription factors essential for differentiation along the cardiomyocyte lineage. These cardiac stem/progenitor cells seem to be ideal for cardiac repair, since they are already committed to the cardiac lineage. So far, different sources of stem cells have been identified within the adult mouse heart. The isolation of different cardiac progenitor cell populations, characterized by their specific expression profile of marker proteins, provides new opportunities to ultimately find the best progenitor cell for cell transplantation-based cardiac regeneration.

Cardiac Stem Cells and Progenitor Cells

All somatic adult tissues with regenerative capacity harbor a resident stem cell or progenitor cell population which functions in the maintenance and regeneration of the respective tissues. Since the heart has always been considered to be a terminally differentiated organ without any regenerative capacity, the existence of a cardiac progenitor cell population was not underscored. However, accumulating evidence suggested the existence of a stem cell population within the heart, initiating the quest for the cardiac stem/progenitor cell. Recently, several groups independently identified and isolated 'different' cell populations present within the mammalian heart based on the expression of several markers for primitive cells.

Side population (SP) cells were the first murine adult cardiac stem cell population isolated from hearts from wild type and reporter mouse strains.[14-16] These cells can be characterized by the capacity for Hoechst dye efflux via multidrug resistance (MDR) channels that are verapamil sensitive, and can be isolated by fluorescence activated cell sorting (FACS), an established protocol for bone marrow stem cell isolation.[17] Cardiac SP cells differ from bone marrow-derived SP cells, lacking CD45 and c-Kit expression. In addition to isolation based on Hoechst dye efflux, SP cells were recently characterized by their expression of the adenosine triphosphate (ATP)-binding cassette (ABC) transporter. When SP cells were cocultured with adult cardiomyocytes, the SP cells differentiated into cardiomyocytes as well.[14,18] Murine cardiac SP cells positive for the hematopoietic stem cell antigen 1 (Sca1, a Ly6 family member[19]) have also been isolated.[18] This cardiac SP subgroup already expressed cardiac, smooth muscle, and endothelial cell markers, and the CD31 negative fraction was shown to have the highest differentiation potential towards the cardiomyocyte lineage, but only after coculture. When cocultured with adult rat cardiomyocytes, improved differentiation of the cardiac SP cells and spontaneous contractions combined with calcium transients was observed. Fusion was ruled out in the majority of differentiated cells based on the absence of Cre–lox recombination and non-colocalization of green-fluorescent SP cells and red-fluorescent cardiomyocytes. Interestingly, in hearts from Mef2c double-negative mice, which is a model for chronic heart failure, FACS analysis revealed that SP cells were substantially reduced with a concurrent increase of cardiomyocytes, suggesting that SP cells differentiated into cardiomyocytes in vivo.[14]

Based on other markers known from bone marrow stem cell isolation, different cell populations were isolated from rodent hearts and tested for their cardiomyogenic potential in vitro. Cardiac stem/progenitor cells expressing Sca1 or the stem cell factor (SCF) receptor c-Kit[20] were isolated from mice[21-23] and rats.[24] The murine adult heart contains Sca1 and CD31 positive, c-Kit, CD34, and CD45 negative cardiac progenitor cells.[22] The Sca1 positive progenitor cells showed expression of early cardiomyogenic transcription factors, and the presence of endogenous telomerase activity revealed their potential for self-renewal. These Sca1+ cells differentiated into cardiomyocytes after stimulation with 5-azacytidine as determined by staining and marker expression. In vitro knockout of the bone morphogenetic protein (BMP) receptor 1A decreased expression of the growth factor BMP2, the cardiac transcription factor *Mef2c*, and the sarcomeric protein α-myosin heavy chain (MHC), confirming the involvement of auto- and/or paracrine growth factor cascade during their differentiation. Similar to the progenitor cells in the study of Oh et al,[22] Sca1 positive cardiac progenitor cells expressing hematopoietic genes were shown to differentiate into spontaneously beating areas after stimulation with oxytocin.[21] Further analysis of the Sca1+ cells revealed a cardiomyocyte-specific gene expression in the differentiated cardiac progenitor cells on both an RNA and a protein level. Calcium current measurements in combination with isoproterenol administration enhanced the beating rate, indicating a functional β-adrenergic signaling pathway in differentiated cells. Remarkably, the Sca1 positive progenitor cells also developed osteocyte- and adipocyte-related characteristics when specifically stimulated with osteogenic inducers or cultured in adipogenic culture medium, respectively, suggesting an even broader differentiation potential.

How Sca1 positive cardiac progenitor cells differ from cardiac SP cells is not clear. FACS analysis suggested that the SP cells described above are in fact a subpopulation of the Sca1 positive cardiac progenitor cells. Therefore, it might be that only the Sca1+/CD31– SP cells are responsible for the observed cardiomyogenic potential of this progenitor cell population.[18] Support for the cardiomyogenic potential of CD31 negative progenitor cells came when Sca1+/CD31– progenitor cells were shown to be able to differentiate into endothelial and cardiomyogenic lineages.[23] In *in vitro* assays, stimulation of Sca1+/CD31– progenitor cells with vascular endothelial growth factor (VEGF) resulted in enhanced network formation and endothelial cell marker expression. Stimulation with 5-azacytidine and several growth factors induced a cardiomyocyte differentiation. As with the Sca1+/CD31– SP cells described by Pfister et al,[18] the differentiation of Sca1+/CD31– progenitor cells was improved when cocultured with rat cardiomyocytes.

A third population of rodent cardiac stem/progenitor cells was identified based on the expression of c-Kit. c-Kit positive cardiac stem cells were found in the interstitia of rats and, like Sca1+cells, expressed cardiomyocyte specific transcription factors such as Nkx2-5, GATA4, and *Mef2c*.[24] In vitro, the c-Kit positive cardiac stem cells differentiated into a mixed population of primitive cardiomyocytes, smooth muscle cells, endothelial cells, and fibroblasts after culture in differentiation medium containing dexamethasone. However, these myocytes appeared to be immature both morphologically as well as functionally, and did not contract spontaneously. The c-Kit positive cells share some similarities with previously described cardiac progenitor populations, but it remains to be determined whether they have been derived from a common ancestor. Recently, the dog heart was used to isolate c-Kit+/Sca1+/MDR+ (MDR is multidrug resistance protein) stem/progenitor cells with cardiomyogenic differentiation potential.[25] Upon differentiation, the c-Kit+ cells acquired a cardiomyocyte, smooth muscle, endothelial, or fibroblast phenotype. Interestingly, the canine cardiac stem cells expressed hepatocyte growth factor (HGF), insulin-like growth factor (IGF), and their specific receptors.

Another recently identified cardiac progenitor cell population in the heart of mice, rats, and humans is the Islet 1 (Isl1)-expressing progenitor cell.[26] Staining and Isl1-based reporter gene expression showed that the Isl1-positive cardiac progenitors could be found in the atria, ventricles, and outflow tract from embryonic and postnatal hearts and that these cells differentiated into cardiomyocytes in vivo. Isl1-positive cells were then isolated from postnatal murine hearts, FACS sorted, and expanded in culture. The Isl+ cells do not express any of the frequently used stem cell markers, such as c-Kit or Sca1, which makes these cells distinct from the cells described before. The cultured cells revealed expression of early cardiac transcription factors Nkx2-5 and GATA4, indicating that these cells are already committed to the cardiac lineage. Furthermore, Isl+ cells could be expanded in vitro without spontaneous differentiation when using a feeder layer. Coculture experiments with viable and non-viable neonatal mouse cardiomyocytes induced adult cardiomyocyte gene expression, suggesting differentiation without fusion. Real-time intracellular calcium imaging and electrical stimulation of the differentiated progenitor cell suggested the presence of a functional β-adrenergic signaling pathway and excitation–contraction coupling. Further electrophysiological evaluation indicated that the differentiated progenitor cells had reached a neonatal cardiomyocyte phenotype.

The last group of cardiac progenitor cells has not been identified on the basis of marker expression, but by culture procedure. Multicellular clusters of fibroblast-like cells termed "cardiospheres" were isolated from postnatal human heart biopsies as well as murine hearts by culturing percutaneous endomyocardial biopsies in primary cultures.[27] Cardiospheres are a mixture of young and adult cells and at the same time a mixture of the three cardiac cell types: myocytes, smooth muscle cells, and endothelial cells. c-Kit+-expressing cells were found in the proliferating core; c-Kit was the only conserved cardiac stem cell marker in the development and maturation of these cardiospheres. Cardiospheres were able to differentiate into cardiomyocyte-like cells when cultured in medium containing endothelial and basic fibroblast growth factors. Upon differentiation, spontaneous beating was observed in both murine and human cell clusters, even though the human equivalent only did this after coculture and cellular coupling with adult rat cardiomyocytes.

Cells from these clusters showed DNA synthesis, suggestive of cell cycling, and were positive for stem cell-, cardiomyocyte-, or endothelial cell-specific markers. Importantly, the grown cardiospheres could be plated to yield cardiosphere-derived cells (CDCs) expressing stem cell-specific antigens as well as proteins vital for cardiac contractile and electrical function.[28] Human and porcine CDCs, when cocultured with neonatal rat ventricular myocytes, exhibited biophysical signatures of myocyte characteristics including calcium transients synchronous with those of neighboring myocytes. These single cells derived from the cardiospheres could form new clusters with similar functional and phenotypic characteristics, including spontaneous beating, indicating the presence of a uniform cardiac progenitor cell with endothelial and cardiomyogenic differentiation potential.

The above-described experiments have shown that embryonic and postnatal hearts contain progenitor cells that can be identified throughout development and be isolated, expanded, and differentiated when cocultured into functional cardiomyocytes.

Preclinical Studies

In this section, we will compare the different preclinical transplantation studies in rodents using cardiac progenitor cells, including Sca1 cells, c-Kit cells, and cardiospheres. Neither SP cells, cardiac progenitor cells identified by their dye efflux, nor the recently identified cardiac progenitor Islet 1+ cells have been used in *in vivo* experiments and will therefore not be discussed. To date, six preclinical transplantation studies have been published using c-Kit+ cells, Sca1+ cells, and cardiospheres (Table 6.1).

To explore the differentiation capacity of Sca1+ cells in vivo, isolated Sca1+ progenitors, from the myocyte depleted fraction, were injected intravenously after left ventricular ischemia–reperfusion injury using a heart-specific Cre–loxP-mediated excision reporter system.[22] Chronically instrumented mice with an implantable occluder were used to exclude the effects of an inflammatory response due to the

open-chest procedure. Only a few of the genetically tagged transplanted cardiac progenitor cells could be found in the left ventricle shortly after MI. Twenty-four hours after transplantation, Sca1+ cells were present in the myocardium, but no cells were present within the infarcted area. Two weeks after cell injection, persistence of the grafted cells was confirmed in 10 out of 14 transplanted mice. The donor cells were mainly located in the infarct border zone, and 60% of the grafted cells expressed the adult cardiac marker sarcomeric α-actinin. By using Cre–lox-mediated heart-specific reporter gene expression in vivo, this is the first study elegantly assessing the occurrence of fusion. Fusion of the Cre expressing progenitor cell with the loxP–lacZ expressing recipient mouse would result in blue cardiomyocytes. Cell fusion with host cells was found in 50% of the transplanted cells, demonstrating that those donor cardiac progenitor cells that formed cardiomyocytes either differentiated into new cardiomyocytes or fused with cardiomyocytes from the recipient. Although Sca1+ cells are able to incorporate and differentiate in the injured heart, their influence on cardiac function was not assessed in this study. Interestingly, FACS analysis of cardiac and circulating cell suspensions following left anterior descending artery (LAD) ligation revealed a relative increase and subsequent decrease of resident, but not circulating, Sca1+/CD31– cells in time.[23] This might suggest local proliferation and differentiation of resident cardiac progenitor cells after cardiac damage, but more research is needed to prove this. Direct intramyocardial Sca1+/CD31– progenitor cell transplantation after MI showed improved cardiac function and enhanced efficiency in cardiac energy metabolism. Despite increased myocardial neovascularization, endothelial cell and cardiomyocyte differentiation remained limited, suggesting a mainly paracrine effect in the peri-infarct region. Altogether, Sca1+ progenitor cells are inclined to migrate to, survive in and integrate with the infarct border zone between 12 hours and 14 days after acute MI in both a fusion dependent and a fusion independent way in a 50:50 ratio.

Table 6.1 Preclinical studies using intracardiac stem cells

Pre-clinical trial	Stem cell markers	Early cardiac markers	Hema/endoth	Species	n	In vitro diff	Number of cells	Route of adm	Model	Follow-up (days)	Genetic tagging	Fusion?	Cardiac markers	Vasc/endoth marker	Results echo
Beltrami, 2003[24]	c-Kit+	Nlx+ Mef2c+ GATA 4/5+	Lin- CD34-,45-	Rat	22	+	1×10^5	IM border	Infarct	20	BrdU	2N DNA	+	ND	EF 45%tr vs 34%untr
Beltrami, 2003[24]	c-Kit+	Nkx Mef2c+ GATA 4/5+	Lin- CD34-,45-	Rat	6	+	2×10^5 (1 clone)	IM border	Infarct	20	EGFP	2N DNA	ND	ND	ND
Dawn, 2005[29]	c-Kit+	ND	ND	Rat	24	ND	1×10^6	Aortic root	Isch-rep	35	EGFP	2N DNA, 2 chrom 12	+	+	FS 29%tr vs 22%untr
Messina, 2004[27]	c-Kit+ Sca1+	Nkx- Mef2c+ GATA4+	Lin+ CD31+ 31+, CD 34+,45+	Human-into-mouse	4	+	60 spheres	IM border	Infarct	18	lacZ/ EGFP	ND	+	+	FS 37%tr vs 18%untr
Oh, 2003[22]	Sca1+	Nkx2-5- Mef2c+ GATA4+	Lin- CD 34, 45- CD 31, 38+	Mouse	14	+	1×10^6	IV	Isch-rep	14	PKH2-GL α-MHC-CreCre-lox	50%	+	ND	ND
Smith, 2007[28]	c-Kit+	Nkx- Mef2c+ GATA4+	CD31+, 34+, 45-, 105+	Human-into-mouse	11	+	1×10^5	IM border	Infarct	20	EGFP	ND	+	+	EF 4%tr vs 25%untr
Wang, 2006[23]	Sca1+ CD31-	Nkx2-5- GATA4-	ND	Mouse	6	+	1×10^6	IM border	Infarct	21	lacZ	ND	+	+	EF 38%tr vs 33%untr

ND, not determined; Hema/endoth, hematological endothelial lineage; In vitro diff, in vitro differentiation; Number of cells, number of transplanted cells; Route of adm, route of administration; IM border, intramyocardial in border zone; IV, intravenous vena jugular vein; Isch-rep, ischemia-reperfusion; BrdU, bromo deoxyuridine; EGFP, enhanced green fluorescent protein; MHC, myosin heavy chain; chrom, chromosome; Vasc/endoth marker, vascular or endothelial markers; Results echo, echocardiographic results; EF, ejection fraction; FS, fractional shortening; tr, treated; untr, untreated.

Beltrami and co-workers identified c-Kit+ cells as possible cardiac stem cells.[24] Whether this pool of putative c-Kit positive stem cells is resident in the heart since fetal life or originates from the bone marrow and homes to the myocardium is still debatable. During myocardial ischemia, stem cell factor (SCF), the ligand of the c-Kit receptor, is upregulated. This source of SCF might function as a homing signal for bone marrow-derived c-Kit+ cells. Beltrami et al determined whether c-Kit+ cells are suitable for myocardial regeneration therapy using an experimental mouse model for acute MI. To be able to track the injected cells in vivo bromodeoxyuridine (BrdU) was added to the culture medium before cell transplantation to label the nuclei of the donor cells. BrdU-expressing c-Kit+ cardiac progenitor cells were injected directly into the hearts of mice shortly after permanent LAD ligation. Immunohistochemical analysis revealed that BrdU positive cardiomyocytes, as well as non-cardiomyocytes, were present within the infarcted area as well as in spared myocardium 20 days after transplantation. The use of genetically labeled enhanced green fluorescent protein (EGFP) positive cardiac c-Kit+ cells supported the finding that transplanted c-Kit+ cells could enter and survive in the infarcted region. An increased density of capillaries and arterioles was reported within the infarcted area, harboring EGFP-expressing donor cells in the vessel wall, suggesting that some of the c-Kit+ cardiac stem cells differentiated into vascular cells. Interestingly, using echocardiography, a significant improvement of functional performance was found in stem cell-treated compared to sham mice,[24] demonstrating that allogenic c-Kit+ cardiac cell transplantation in a mouse MI model, when injected in the border zone, is safe and has cardioprotective capacity. This cardioprotective mechanism remains largely unknown; c-Kit+ cells appear to differentiate into cardiomyocytes and cardiac vascular cells, but cell fusion was not excluded.

Dawn et al also explored the ability of c-Kit+ cardiac stem cells to enhance cardiac repair, but used a different experimental rat model.[29] In this study, experimental ischemia–reperfusion injury

was used as a model for patients who received early reperfusion therapy after acute myocardial infarction. c-Kit+ cells, injected 4 hours after reperfusion into the aortic root, entered the coronary circulation, crossed the vessel wall, and entered the myocardial interstitium within a few hours. In all treated rats subjected to ischemia–reperfusion, EGFP+ cells were found both in the infarcted region and in the non-infarcted myocardium. Two days after transplantation a comparable deterioration of left ventricular systolic function was observed in treated and untreated rats. However, while untreated rats exhibited progressive remodeling 35 days after ischemia–reperfusion injury, this process was inhibited by cell transplantation. In the non-infarcted area, newly formed EGFP+ myocytes were indistinguishable from the adjacent host cardiomyocytes. However, the regenerated myocytes within the infarcted area harbored a strikingly different phenotype and organization. The cells were small, resembled neonatal cells, and were found in small clusters surrounded by scarred tissue. A possible explanation is the necessity of contact with mature myocytes for terminal differentiation. DNA content in EGFP+ nuclei was 2N and the normal two copies of a randomly chosen chromosome were detected, opposing but not excluding cell fusion. Thus, c-Kit+ cardiac cells administered in the aortic root in a rat ischemia–reperfusion model migrate to the infarcted area within a few hours, integrate, and differentiate into cardiomyocytes with a fetal phenotype and vascular cells.

In a different study, Messina et al used the so-called cardiospheres, self-adherent cell clusters obtained by mild digestion of murine and human biopsy specimens, for cell transplantation.[27] Cardiospheres were transduced with a lentiviral vector expressing GFP and transplanted into the viable myocardium adjacent to a recently induced myocardial infarction in mice. Eighteen days after orthotopic transplantation, systolic left ventricular function was better preserved, compared to untreated mice. Throughout the infarcted area, bands of transplanted cells were visualized. This study does not determine which cell types are responsible for this effect, but mainly demonstrates that it is possible to isolate cells from small fragments of human myocardium and expand these cells in vitro without losing their differentiation state. Subcutaneous transplantation of murine cardiospheres expressing the cardiac-specific promoters myosin light chain 3 (MLC3) or cardiac troponin I (cTnI)-promoter coupled to EGFP demonstrated beating areas visible through the mouse skin. Although it took 10 days to evolve, obviously contact with adult cardiomyocytes is not required for differentiation of mouse cardiospheres into rhythmically beating cardiomyocytes. Recently, adenoviral transduced human cardiosphere-derived cells (CDCs), isolated by pre-plating dissociated cardiospheres, were injected into the border zone of SCID (severe combined immune deficient) mice after myocardial infarction.[28] β-Galactosidase-expressing CDCs engrafted and migrated into the infarcted area. Twenty days after transplantation, the percentage of viable myocardium as well as the ejection fraction was higher in the CDC-transplanted mice compared to the fibroblast-injected control group. Immunohistochemical analysis revealed very little differentiation of CDCs into cardiomyocytes, although there were numerous areas of myocardial regeneration, suggesting a paracrine effect.

Study Interpretation

To date, four different cardiac progenitor or stem cells have been described: SP cells, c-Kit+ cells, Sca1+ cells, and Isl1+ cells. Preclinical cell transplantation studies are performed with rodent c-Kit+ cells, Sca1+ cells, and cardiospheres or CDCs, a mixture of human cardiac-derived cell types. Due to incomplete characterization of the different populations and the use of different stem cell markers, it is unclear how one cell type differs from another. Stem cell populations are dynamic and the expression of markers could change in time, depending on the time of isolation and in vitro culture conditions. One of the pitfalls in preclinical studies is, among others, that bone marrow-derived stem cell transplantation is tracking the in vivo fate of transplanted cells within the host. In cardiac regeneration studies that used myoblasts and bone marrow-derived

progenitor cells, identification of transplanted cells by immunohistochemistry was complicated due to the high density of muscle-specific proteins causing non-specific antibody binding in the heart. To be able to identify the transplanted cells once injected into the host, genetic tagging is a powerful tool. The expression of EGFP or *lacZ* facilitated recognition of the stem cells. Furthermore, transplanting cells expressing a reporter gene under the control of a cardiomyocyte-specific promoter will allow indisputable identification of stem cell differentiation into myocytes. However, the high levels of autofluorescence due to the MI and scar tissue complicate immunofluorescent analysis of the GFP signal. Another complication in the interpretation of results from stem cell transplantation studies is that the results can be confusing due to the fusion of transplanted cells with host myocardium. Genetic analysis using two different transgenic mouse lines has successfully been used to identify fusion.[22]

Until now, preclinical transplantation studies for cardiac regeneration have used an acute LAD ligation model with or without reperfusion. The extreme ischemic response in the acute phase of myocardial infarction with a release of cytokines, angiogenic factors, and other growth factors might be needed to stimulate the proliferation and/or differentiation of transplanted cells. Therefore, one should be careful when extrapolating these observed results to chronic ischemic heart failure. The optimal route for administration of progenitor cells has not been assessed yet, which is why different methods, intramyocardial, intra-aortal, or intravenous delivery, are used. In the experimental MI models, cells were injected in the border zone.[24,27] Up to 20 days after cell transplantation, cardioprotective effects were reported. Immunohistochemical analysis showed an increase in neoangiogenesis after transplantation and the transplanted cells migrated into the infarcted area and expressed biochemical markers of adult cardiomyocytes. However, cell fusion was not excluded. Using an ischemia–reperfusion model,[22] Sca1+ cells were injected intravenously and migrated into the infarct border zone, but no cells were seen in the necrotic area during follow-up. However, c-Kit+ cells, injected in the aortic root, did migrate into the infarcted area within a few hours by crossing the vessel wall, most likely due to the method used for administering the cells. Many cells might be lost in the circulation or end up in the spleen when injected intravenously, reducing the number of cells available for the myocardial tissue. The treated rats in the study of Dawn et al showed a reduction of negative remodeling after ischemia–reperfusion damage.[29] In the reperfused area transplanted cells could survive up to 35 days, but the phenotype of EGFP+ myocytes derived from transplanted cells was immature.

Injection of cells in the infarct border zone seems a more efficient way to deliver the cells, although ischemic conditions may decrease cell survival. Moreover, in clinical practice the invasive aspect of intramyocardial injection is undesired, and technically it is difficult to determine where exactly the infarct border zone is located. If the cells are injected intravenously these cells need to migrate to the infarcted area, and many cells will be lost in this process. Furthermore, during the migration process in patients who have systemic vascular disease the cells can adhere to the vessel wall at undesired sites in the coronary or systemic circulation, raising the risk for atherosclerotic plaque progression and (re)stenosis.

It is important to unravel the mechanism responsible for the reported beneficial effects on cardiac performance. It has been suggested that newly formed stem cell-derived myocytes replace the ones that are lost. Clearly this assumption is precocious, since the number of transplanted cells found in the infarcted area seems too low to be able to rebuild the ventricular wall and improve cardiac function. Furthermore, the study performed by Oh et al genetically determined the role of fusion of stem cells with host cells, and showed that there was considerable contribution.[22] The transplanted cells could also exert beneficial effects on angiogenesis, improvement of scar tissue, and cytoprotection in a paracrine way or via the transplanted cells themselves.[30] A recent study by Gnecci et al evaluated the effects of intramyocardial injection of conditioned medium from hypoxic mesenchymal stem cells (MSCs) overexpressing the pro-survival gene *Akt1* after MI in rats.[31] In rats treated with conditioned medium only, improvement of ventricular function was comparable to that in rats treated with the MSC itself. In a canine MI model, positive results for cardiac function were obtained after intramyocardial administration of HGF and IGFI.[25] These studies support the hypothesis that paracrine effects of transplanted stem cells could be one mechanism for functional improvements.

In conclusion, cell transplantation in the acute phase of myocardial infarction in rodents had no adverse effects. In the first 2–5 weeks after transplantation, preclinical studies report a reduction of negative remodeling, transplanted cells integrate and differentiate in vivo, but the efficiency is low. Cell delivery in the infarct border zone seems most efficient, although intra-aortal injection is also effective and less invasive.

From Bench to Bed

With our current knowledge of stem cell biology, the positive effects of stem cell transplantation cannot be explained solely by known mechanisms of stem cells to affect the heart. Furthermore, it remains to be determined whether indeed different populations of resident stem cells exist and what their natural purpose is. The crucial pathways in stem cell activation and differentiation remain to be clarified. Another interesting question is why the repair mechanism in, for example, the liver is far more eligible to replace large defects compared to the heart. From an evolutionary view, an explanation could be that a large defect in the heart is lethal in contrast to the liver where there is just more time to repair the damage.

In preclinical studies, different animal models were used to imitate the patient with MI. The studies of Dawn et al and Oh et al used the ischemia–reperfusion model to translate results to the clinical setting of acute MI followed by primary PTCA, currently the established therapy. In theory, cardiac progenitor cells are able to regenerate myocardium and compensate for the limited loss of cardiomyocytes due to subendocardial infarction and apoptotic damage due to ischemia–reperfusion. But should we aim at these patients that have a relatively low incidence of advanced heart failure in the long term? In the follow-up period after successful early primary PTCA, cardiac function improves without transplantation therapy in the majority of patients, probably due to the recovery of stunned myofibers.[32] Furthermore, it is very difficult to accomplish autologous cardiac progenitor cell transplantation in the acute phase of MI, which is the highest risk period for mortality, since in vitro expansion takes at least several days. To optimize treatment for patients with acute MI, early revascularization and reduction of reperfusion damage will improve recovery of cardiac function instead of cell replacement therapy. Of more importance is to educate the general population to call the emergency services as quickly as possible when there are signs of acute MI.

Patients with MI who present late, when the period of myocardial salvage has passed, could however benefit from cardiac replacement therapy. Patients who received reperfusion therapy between 12 hours and several days after acute MI to minimize ventricular remodeling are still at risk to develop symptoms of heart failure, especially patients with anterior wall infarction. The infarcted area in this group of patients has been reperfused, which creates a beneficial environment for stem cells to survive.

The patients who would gain most from stem or progenitor cell therapy are patients with end-stage ischemic heart disease when therapeutic options are very limited and poor. These patients underwent MI before the fibrinolytic (let alone the PTCA) era, presented late, had reperfusion therapy which was not successful, or have extensive coronary artery disease leading to a substantial reduction of viable cardiomyocytes and pump-function. To reestablish functional myocardium, restoration of blood supply is crucial. Therefore, the main focuses for new treatment strategies to rebuild the infarcted or ischemic myocardium are:

- restoration of vascularization
- cardiomyocyte replacement therapy.

Recently, an embryonic stem cell-derived multipotent cardiovascular progenitor cell has been identified using genetic fate mapping which expresses the transcription factors Isl1, Nkx2-5, and flk1. These cells can spontaneously differentiate into cardiomyocyte, endothelial, and vascular smooth muscle cells in vitro.[33,34] Whether these multipotent cardiovascular progenitor cells exist and can be isolated from somatic tissue is an important question for future research. However, even if multipotential progenitor cells can be obtained for clinical application of cardiac regeneration in the future, it remains to be seen whether preferential routes are taken depending on the cardiac environment. For example, all multipotent progenitors could differentiate into vascular cells in an environment with many angiogenic factors, as in ischemic myocardium, leaving no cells to differentiate into myocytes. Mechanisms to create an environment for successful stem cell transplantation after MI are: capillary formation by sprouting of pre-existing vessels (angiogenesis), or monocyte-aided increase in the caliber of existing arteriolar collaterals (arteriogenesis).[35] Injected endothelial progenitor cells derived from monocytes improve angio- and arteriogenesis of ischemic hind limbs and ischemic hearts in animal models by physical incorporation and by paracrine mechanisms.[36]

Future Perspectives

Evaluating the results from rodent preclinical studies as well as pilot and randomized clinical trials (2002–2006), stem cells still remain a promising therapeutic modality for the large number of patients suffering congestive heart failure who cannot be adequately treated with conventional therapeutic approaches. However, these studies also indicate that stem cell therapy is still in its infancy. The search for the holy grail for cardiac regeneration started with the most primitive stem cell, the embryonic stem cell, and has now progressed to the adult heart itself as a potential source of stem cells.[37,38] The advantages of primitive cells are pluripotency, high plasticity, and high proliferation capacity, but there is a risk for tumor formation. With adult cardiac stem cells, autologous transplantation remains an option, the cells are committed to the cardiac lineage, another advantage is the better functional integration, and tumors will not be formed. The presence of these cells provides new treatment options for cellular replacement as an alternative therapy for heart failure after MI. However, cardiac resident progenitor cells are not easily accessible for use in transplantation studies. Translated to a clinical setting, these cells can only be harvested from cardiac biopsies or resection specimens during heart surgery, or biopsies obtained by cardiac catheterization. To date, five preclinical studies using adult cardiac stem cells have been executed. Unfortunately, it is not yet the right time to translate these results into clinical studies. First, we need to answer the following questions:

- Are Sca1, c-Kit, and *Isl1*+ cells three different cardiac progenitor cell populations, or do they originate from the same founders with the markers indicating successive differentiation stages?
- Are the cardiac progenitor cells developmental remnants, or is there recruitment of cells from the bone marrow during postnatal life? Can we increase the endogenous pool of cardiac stem cells?
- How can we manipulate adult cardiac progenitor cells in vivo?
- What pretreatments give the best results in cell proliferation, survival, and maintenance?

Pilot studies with small numbers of patients using different cells from bone-marrow aspirate, circulating progenitor cells (CPCs), endothelial progenitor cells (EPCs), or skeletal myoblasts have already been executed since 2002 with mixed results. In these studies there was a variety of stem cell types, culture methods, number of transplanted cells, patient categories, routes of administration, and endpoints. In randomized clinical trials of 170 patients with chronic

ischemic heart failure and 210 patients with acute MI, minor beneficial effects were observed.[39] Autologous bone-marrow cell transplantation did not have severe adverse effects. Autologous myoblast transplantation studies in general showed a significant improvement of cardiac function; the cells are less sensitive to oxygen-deprived conditions, but muscle cell progenitors failed to couple electrically to the surrounding cardiomyocytes, leading to arrhythmias in a small number of patients. To overcome this essential problem, skeletal myoblasts are engineered to express gap junctional proteins, e.g. connexin 43, to decrease arrhythmogenicity.[40] Four years after the start of the first clinical studies using somatic progenitor cells for cardiac regeneration, however, the most essential research questions still remain unanswered:

- What is the most suitable somatic stem cell population to use, and when, how, and what number of cells do we need to transplant?
- What do the cells actually do within the injured myocardium, influencing cell survival, neoangiogenesis, and/or muscle regeneration?
- Can we develop effective non-invasive therapies to stimulate somatic progenitor cells in situ?

The answers to these questions can be obtained by adequate preclinical studies and basic research going from bed to bench. At the bench, much work has to be done to understand the scientific underpinnings of migration, maintenance, proliferation, differentiation, and maintenance of cardiac stem or progenitor cells. Stem cell research in regenerative tissues such as the skin and intestine is pioneer in unraveling the mechanisms of differentiation and proliferation of stem cells. Increasing evidence supports a role for BMP, fibroblast growth factor and Wnt signaling in stem cell maintenance and regulation.[41,42] Understanding the scientific underpinnings of the growth factor pathways involved in stem cell regeneration opens a new window for future regenerative medicine. Stem cell transplantation might be circumvented if growth factors and cytokines activate the endogenous cardiac stem cells in situ or enhance cellular protection. However, until now no studies have been published describing the capacity of growth factors to induce the cascade of myocardial regeneration in humans. However, more research is needed to ensure that these growth factors will have a long-term effect. Further developments of factors or cell types that stimulate vascularization in the ischemic and infarcted myocardium are indispensable for cardiac regeneration. A promising technique that combines neovascularization and cardiac regeneration is human cardiac tissue engineering. This technique simulates the heart cell environment, providing heart tissue with primitive capillaries engineered from native and cardiac myocyte enriched heart cell populations.[43] Fusion of single-unit engineered heart tissue allows the production of larger constructs that may eventually serve as optimized tissue grafts for transplantation in the hearts of patients with end-stage heart failure, to optimize cardiac regeneration. Besides vascularization in situ, another obstacle in cardiac regeneration after MI is the fibrotic scar tissue in the infarcted area. One way to solve this is surgical resection of the scar, but this is a drastic approach. It would be more applicable to reduce fibrosis in advance by influencing, for example, matrix metalloproteinase levels and fibroblast behavior.

Conclusions

A new focus of cardiovascular research is stem cell therapy for myocardial regeneration in the search for causal treatment in ischemic heart failure. Cardiovascular disease is responsible for approximately 40% of the total mortality in the established market economies; half of these patients die from ischemic heart disease. Despite improved pharmacological therapies and the introduction of intracardiac defibrillators preventing sudden death, the mortality rate is substantial and morbidity is rising. Patients with advanced ischemic heart failure due to excessive loss of cardiomyocytes seem the best candidates for myocardial tissue replacement therapy, but

vascularization of the infarcted area is of paramount importance to enable migration and long-term survival of stem cells.

To date, the isolation of undifferentiated cells from the heart that express stem cell markers and early cardiac transcription factors has been established. In vitro these cells can be forced to differentiate into cardiomyocytes, but functionally the cells are still immature. However, undifferentiated cells expanded in vitro and transplanted into rodent hearts were able to reduce remodeling. The emphasis of future research will mainly concentrate on the many regulatory pathways which are involved in activation, migration, maintenance, proliferation, and differentiation of somatic cardiac stem cells. The newly formed tissue needs adequate vasculature in situ, and electrical and mechanical coupling with host cells is essential.

References

1. Orlic D, Kajstura J, Chimenti S et al. Bone marrow stem cells regenerate infarcted myocardium. Pediatr Transplant 2003; 7 (Suppl 3): 86–8.
2. van Vliet P, Sluijter JP, Doevendans PA, Goumans MJ. Isolation and expansion of resident cardiac progenitor cells. Expert Rev Cardiovasc Ther 2007; 5: 33–43.
3. Doevendans PA, Kubalak SW, An RH et al. Differentiation of cardiomyocytes in floating embryoid bodies is comparable to fetal cardiomyocytes. J Mol Cell Cardiol 2000; 32: 839–51.
4. Mummery C, Ward-van Oostwaard D, Doevendans P et al. Differentiation of human embryonic stem cells to cardiomyocytes: role of coculture with visceral endoderm-like cells. Circulation 2003; 107: 2733–40.
5. Chien KR. Stem cells: lost in translation. Nature 2004; 428: 607–8.
6. Menasche P, Hagege AA, Vilquin JT et al. Autologous skeletal myoblast transplantation for severe postinfarction left ventricular dysfunction. J Am Coll Cardiol 2003; 41: 1078–83.
7. van Laake LW, Hassink R, Doevendans PA, Mummery C. Heart repair and stem cells. J Physiol 2006; 577: 467–78.
8. Rosenthal N. Prometheus's vulture and the stem-cell promise. N Engl J Med 2003; 349: 267–74.
9. Anversa P, Kajstura J, Leri A, Bolli R. Life and death of cardiac stem cells: a paradigm shift in cardiac biology. Circulation 2006; 113: 1451–63.

10. Kajstura J, Leri A, Finato N et al. Myocyte proliferation in end-stage cardiac failure in humans. Proc Natl Acad Sci USA 1998; 95: 8801–5.

11. Beltrami AP, Urbanek K, Kajstura J et al. Evidence that human cardiac myocytes divide after myocardial infarction. N Engl J Med 2001; 344: 1750–7.

12. Urbanek K, Quaini F, Tasca G et al. Intense myocyte formation from cardiac stem cells in human cardiac hypertrophy. Proc Natl Acad Sci USA 2003; 100: 10440–5.

13. Quaini F, Urbanek K, Beltrami AP et al. Chimerism of the transplanted heart. N Engl J Med 2002; 346: 5–15.

14. Hierlihy AM, Seale P, Lobe CG, Rudnicki MA, Megeney LA. The post-natal heart contains a myocardial stem cell population. FEBS Lett 2002; 530: 239–43.

15. Martin CM, Meeson AP, Robertson SM et al. Persistent expression of the ATP-binding cassette transporter, Abcg2, identifies cardiac SP cells in the developing and adult heart. Dev Biol 2004; 265: 262–75.

16. Zhou S, Schuetz JD, Bunting KD et al. The ABC transporter Bcrp1/ABCG2 is expressed in a wide variety of stem cells and is a molecular determinant of the side-population phenotype. Nat Med 2001; 7: 1028–34.

17. Goodell MA, Brose K, Paradis G, Conner AS, Mulligan RC. Isolation and functional properties of murine hematopoietic stem cells that are replicating in vivo. J Exp Med 1996; 183: 1797–806.

18. Pfister O, Mouquet F, Jain M et al. CD31– but not CD31+ cardiac side population cells exhibit functional cardiomyogenic differentiation. Circ Res 2005; 97: 52–61.

19. van de Rijn M, Heimfeld S, Spangrude GJ, Weissman IL. Mouse hematopoietic stem-cell antigen Sca-1 is a member of the Ly-6 antigen family. Proc Natl Acad Sci USA 1989; 86: 4634–8.

20. Ronnstrand L. Signal transduction via the stem cell factor receptor/c-Kit. Cell Mol Life Sci 2004; 61: 2535–48.

21. Matsuura K, Nagai T, Nishigaki N et al. Adult cardiac Sca-1-positive cells differentiate into beating cardiomyocytes. J Biol Chem 2004; 279: 11384–91.

22. Oh H, Bradfute SB, Gallardo TD et al. Cardiac progenitor cells from adult myocardium: homing, differentiation, and fusion after infarction. Proc Natl Acad Sci USA 2003; 100: 12313–18.

23. Wang X, Hu Q, Nakamura Y et al. The role of the sca-1+/CD31– cardiac progenitor cell population in postinfarction left ventricular remodeling. Stem Cells 2006; 24: 1779–88.

24. Beltrami AP, Barlucchi L, Torella D et al. Adult cardiac stem cells are multipotent and support myocardial regeneration. Cell 2003; 114: 763–76.

25. Linke A, Muller P, Nurzynska D et al. Stem cells in the dog heart are self-renewing, clonogenic, and multipotent and regenerate infarcted myocardium, improving cardiac function. Proc Natl Acad Sci USA 2005; 102: 8966–71.

26. Laugwitz KL, Moretti A, Lam J et al. Postnatal isl1+ cardioblasts enter fully differentiated cardiomyocyte lineages. Nature 2005; 433: 647–53.

27. Messina E, De Angelis L, Frati G et al. Isolation and expansion of adult cardiac stem cells from human and murine heart. Circ Res 2004; 95: 911–21.

28. Smith RR, Barile L, Cho HC et al. Regenerative potential of cardiosphere-derived cells expanded from percutaneous endomyocardial biopsy specimens. Circulation 2007; 115: 896–908.

29. Dawn B, Stein AB, Urbanek K et al. Cardiac stem cells delivered intravascularly traverse the vessel barrier, regenerate infarcted myocardium, and improve cardiac function. Proc Natl Acad Sci USA 2005; 102: 3766–71.

30. Dimmeler S, Zeiher AM, Schneider MD. Unchain my heart: the scientific foundations of cardiac repair. J Clin Invest 2005; 115: 572–83.

31. Gnecchi M, He H, Liang OD et al. Paracrine action accounts for marked protection of ischemic heart by Akt-modified mesenchymal stem cells. Nat Med 2005; 11: 367–8.

32. Bogaert J, Maes A, Van de Werf F et al. Functional recovery of subepicardial myocardial tissue in transmural myocardial infarction after successful reperfusion: an important contribution to the improvement of regional and global left ventricular function. Circulation 1999; 99: 36–43.

33. Kattman SJ, Huber TL, Keller GM. Multipotent flk-1+ cardiovascular progenitor cells give rise to the cardiomyocyte, endothelial, and vascular smooth muscle lineages. Dev Cell 2006; 11: 723–32.

34. Moretti A, Caron L, Nakano A et al. Multipotent embryonic isl1+ progenitor cells lead to cardiac, smooth muscle, and endothelial cell diversification. Cell 2006; 127: 1151–65.

35. Zwaginga JJ, Doevendans P. Stem cell-derived angiogenic/vasculogenic cells: possible therapies for tissue repair and tissue engineering. Clin Exp Pharmacol Physiol 2003; 30: 900–8.

36. Urbich C, Dimmeler S. Endothelial progenitor cells functional characterization. Trends Cardiovasc Med 2004; 14: 318–22.

37. Hassink RJ, Brutel de la Riviere, Mummery CL, Doevendans PA. Transplantation of cells for cardiac repair. J Am Coll Cardiol 2003; 41: 711–17.

38. Smits AM, van Vliet P, Hassink RJ, Goumans MJ, Doevendans PA. The role of stem cells in cardiac regeneration. J Cell Mol Med 2005; 9: 25–36.

39. Boyle AJ, Whitbourn R, Schlicht S et al. Intracoronary high-dose CD34+ stem cells in patients

with chronic ischemic heart disease: a 12-month follow-up. Int J Cardiol 2006; 109: 21–7.

40. Abraham MR, Henrikson CA, Tung L et al. Antiarrhythmic engineering of skeletal myoblasts for cardiac transplantation. Circ Res 2005; 97: 159–67.

41. Alonso L, Fuchs E. Stem cells in the skin: waste not, Wnt not. Genes Dev 2003; 17: 1189–200.

42. Reya T, Clevers H. Wnt signalling in stem cells and cancer. Nature 2005; 434: 843–50.

43. Naito H, Melnychenko I, Didie M et al. Optimizing engineered heart tissue for therapeutic applications as surrogate heart muscle. Circulation 2006; 114 (1 Suppl): I72–8.

chapter 7

Myocardial Regeneration via Embryonic Stem Cell-Derived Cardiomyocytes

Manhal Habib and Lior Gepstein

Introduction

Adult cardiac muscle lacks significant capacity to regenerate, and therefore any significant heart cell loss such as occurs during myocardial infarction is mostly irreversible and may result in permanent impairment of myocardial performance and the development of progressive heart failure. The recent advances in molecular and stem cell biology and in tissue engineering have paved the way to the development of a new biomedicine discipline: regenerative medicine. This approach seeks to circumvent the low regenerative capacity of certain organs by using cell replacement strategies to restore the function of diseased or absent tissues. The hope is that these emerging strategies will enable the development of future cures for a variety of devastating disease states such as Parkinson's disease, stroke, heart failure, and diabetes. The heart represents an attractive candidate for these emerging technologies, and much attention has been directed in recent years to utilize cell therapy and tissue engineering to ameliorate cardiac injury.[1–3]

The overall objective of cell replacement therapy is to repopulate postinfarction scar tissue with a new pool of functional cells that can restore the mechanical properties of this compromised region. Although several cell types have been suggested as possible candidates for myocardial repair (as outlined in the different chapters and in a number of excellent reviews[1–3]), the inherent structural, electrophysiological, and contractile properties of cardiomyocytes strongly suggest that they may be the ideal donor cell type. In early studies, fetal cardiomyocytes transplanted into healthy mice hearts were demonstrated to survive, align, and form cell-to-cell contacts with host myocardium.[4] Cardiomyocyte transplantation in rodent models of myocardial infarction was associated with smaller infarcts, prevented cardiac dilatation and remodeling,[5] and also resulted in function improvements in some of these studies.[6] Despite these encouraging results, the clinical utility of this approach is significantly hampered by the paucity of cell sources for human cardiomyocytes.

Human Embryonic Stem Cells

One of the most exciting areas in basic research today involves the use of stem cells. All stem cells, irrespective of their specific source, share a number of properties.[7] First, they are capable of self-renewal, meaning that they can generate stem cells with similar properties. Second, stem cells are clonogenic, i.e. they can form a colony of cells that are derived from a single stem cell and have identical genetic constitution. Third, they can differentiate into one or more mature cell types.

The different stem cells can be categorized anatomically, functionally, or by cell surface markers, transcription factors, or other expressed proteins. One clear division of the stem cell family is between those in adult somatic tissue, known as adult stem cells, and those isolated from the preimplantation embryo, known as embryonic stem cells. Adult stem cells can be derived from non-embryonic sources such as peripheral blood, bone marrow, liver, gastrointestinal tract, and muscle. Although they were found to be more versatile than originally believed,[8] their differentiation potential is generally limited to defined cell lineages.

In contrast, cells in the early mammalian embryo have the potential to differentiate into derivatives of all three primary germ layers arising during development (ectoderm, endoderm, and mesoderm), a property that is termed pluripotency. A few days following fertilization, at the blastocyst stage, a hollow sphere of cells is formed that contains an outer cell layer (trophectoderm) and an inner cluster of cells termed the inner cell mass (ICM) (Figure 7.1). The latter cells will eventually give rise, through specialized progenitor cells, to all the tissues in the body, and are therefore truly pluripotent.[9]

In 1981, ICM cells isolated from mouse blastocysts were used to generate pluripotent stem cell lines that were termed embryonic stem cells (ESCs).[10,11] The mouse ESCs were demonstrated to be capable of prolonged in vitro proliferation and self-renewal, but also retained the ability to differentiate into all cell types in the body both in vitro and in vivo. Given the outstanding potential demonstrated by the mouse ESCs, it was not surprising that much effort was spent on the development of similar human lines. In 1998, the first human ESC (hESC) lines were established by Thomson et al[12] and shortly thereafter by Reubinoff et al.[13] The hESC lines were derived from the ICM cells of human blastocysts, produced by in vitro fertilization for clinical purposes and donated after informed consent. In the process of hESC isolation, the outer trophectoderm layer was selectively removed using specific antibodies (immunosurgery) or mechanical dissection, and the ICM cells were isolated, and plated on a mitotically inactivated mouse embryonic fibroblast (MEF) feeder layer (Figure 7.1). The resulting colonies were selected, passaged, and expanded for the creation of hESC lines.

The hESC lines were demonstrated to fulfill all the criteria defining embryonic stem cells, namely: derivation from the pre- or peri-implantation embryo, prolonged undifferentiated proliferation under special conditions, and the capacity to form derivatives of all three germ layers. Thus, when cultured on the MEF feeder layer, the hESCs could be propagated in the undifferentiated state. When removed from the feeder layer, and allowed to spontaneously differentiate, they form three-dimensional differentiating cell aggregates termed embryoid bodies (EBs), containing cell derivatives of all three germ layers (Figure 7.1).[14] The pluripotency of hESCs was also confirmed by subcutaneous injection of undifferentiated hESCs into immunodeficient mice.[12] This resulted in the formation of benign teratomas harboring advanced tissue derivatives of all three germ layers. The undifferentiated hESC lines and their clonal derivatives were shown to express high levels of telomerase and retain normal karyotype for prolonged culture periods.

Cardiomyocyte Differentiation of Human Embryonic Stem Cells

The most common method used for inducing in vitro differentiation of ESCs requires an initial aggregation step to form EBs[15] (Figure 7.1). Different protocols have been used in the murine ESC model for such in vitro differentiation, including the "mass-culture" technique, cultivation in methylcellulose, and the most common "hanging drop" technique.[16] During subsequent culture in adherent conditions a proportion of the EBs display easily identifiable, rhythmically contracting outgrowths.

The generation of a cardiomyocyte differentiating system from the hESC lines was first described by Kehat et al[17] from our laboratory. Following cultivation of EBs for 7–10 days in suspension, they are cultured in adherent conditions and observed microscopically for the

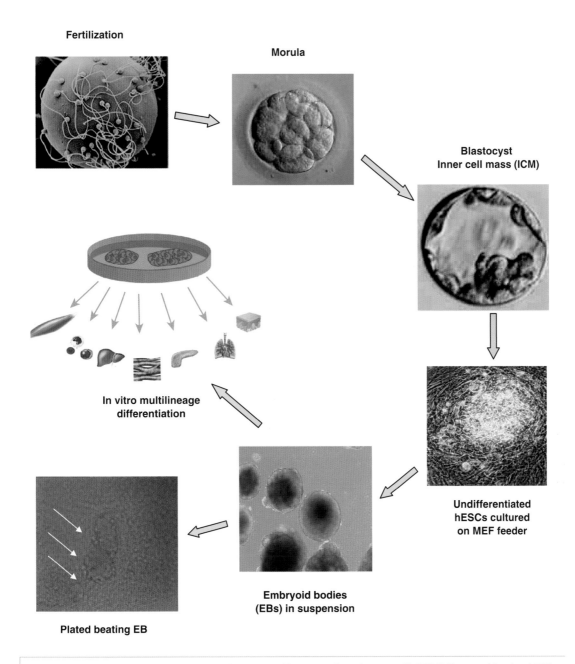

Fertilization

Morula

Blastocyst Inner cell mass (ICM)

In vitro multilineage differentiation

Undifferentiated hESCs cultured on MEF feeder

Embryoid bodies (EBs) in suspension

Plated beating EB

Figure 7.1 *Early embryonic development, derivation of human embryonic stem cell (hESC) lines, and in vitro hESC cardiomyocyte differentiation. The hESC lines were derived from human blastocysts. At this stage, the blastocyst comprises the trophectoderm and the inner cell mass (ICM). ICM cells are isolated, plated on the mouse embryonic fibroblast (MEF) feeder layer, and propagated for the generation of hESC lines. The hESC lines can be propagated in the undifferentiated state when grown on top of the MEF feeder layer. To induce differentiation, hESCs are removed from the feeder layer and cultivated in suspension where they form three-dimensional cell aggregates (embryoid bodies, EBs). This in vitro differentiating system can be used to generate a plurality of tissue types, including cardiomyocytes that appear as spontaneously contracting areas within the EBs.*

appearance of spontaneous contraction (Figure 7.1). Rhythmically contracting areas appear at 4–22 days after plating in ~10% of the EBs. Recently, other groups have reinforced our findings and generated hESC-derived cardiomyocytes (hESC-CMs) using different hESC lines.[18–20]

Phenotypic Characterization of hESC-Derived Cardiomyocytes

Several lines of evidence confirmed the cardiomyocyte nature of the cells within beating human EBs[17] (Figure 7.2). Reverse transcriptase-polymerase chain reaction (RT-PCR) studies demonstrated the expression of cardiac-specific transcription factors (GATA4 and *Nkx2-5*) and cardiac-specific structural genes (cTnI, cTnT, ANP, MLC2v, MLC2a). Initial analysis of gene expression pattern during in vitro hESC cardiomyocyte differentiation revealed a reproducible developmental temporal pattern.[21] This was manifested initially by a gradual decrease in the expression of undifferentiated stem cell markers, such as OCT4. This was followed, during the suspension phase, by the expression of known cardiogenic-inducing growth factors such as Wnt11 and bone morphogenetic protein 2 (BMP2). Next, the expression of cardiac-specific transcription factors (*Nkx2-5*, *Mef2c*, and GATA4) was detected followed by the expression of cardiac-specific structural genes (ANP (atrial natriuretic peptide) and MHC).

Immunostaining studies revealed the presence of typical sarcomeric proteins: atrial and ventricular myosin light chains (MLC2a and MLC2v), myosin heavy chain (MHC), tropomyosin, α-actinin, cardiac troponin T (cTnT), cTnI, and desmin. The existence of both MLC2a and MLC2v may suggest the presence of different cardiomyocyte cell types within the contracting EBs.

Morphological analysis revealed that while early-stage hESC-CMs were relatively small, round, or rod-shaped, their appearance changed to strands of more elongated cardiomyocytes during in vitro maturation.[22] These morphological changes were coupled with a similar ultrastructural maturation process characterized by a progressive increase in the amount and organization of the contractile material and the generation of

well-defined sarcomeres with recognizable A, I, and Z bands in late-stage myocytes. Interestingly, simultaneous with this ultrastructural maturation, the hESC-CMs gradually withdrew from the cell cycle. Hence, high levels of [³H]thymidine uptake were found in early-stage hESC-CMs, which was gradually reduced in intermediate-stage EBs and was almost absent in late-stage EBs.[22]

The hESC-CMs also portrayed a functional phenotype of early-stage human heart cells, including typical extracellular and intracellular electrical activity, intracellular calcium transients, and appropriate chronotropic response to adrenergic and cholinergic agents.[17–20,23] Thus, all the components of normal cardiac excitation–contraction coupling were demonstrated to be present within these cells, including the typical electrical activation, increase in $[Ca^{2+}]_i$, and the resulting contraction, albeit in an embryonic and somewhat "immature" phenotype.

Whole-cell patch clamp studies demonstrated that the hESC-CMs display cardiac-specific action-potential morphologies and ionic currents.[23] This study also revealed the basis for the spontaneous automaticity in these cells, namely the absence of significant inward rectifier K⁺ current and a prominent Na⁺ current with the presence of the HCN (hyperpolarization-activated cyclic nucleotide-gated cation channels) pacemaker current (I_f).

Our next step was to determine whether the hESC differentiating system is limited to the creation of isolated cardiomyocytes or whether a functional cardiac tissue is generated. High-resolution electrical activation maps of the beating EBs, generated with a microelectrode array (MEA) mapping technique (Figure 7.2), demonstrated the development of a functional cardiac syncytium with spontaneous pacemaker activity and action-potential propagation.[24]

Myocardial Regeneration Strategies Using hESC-Derived Cardiomyocytes

Although a number of cell types have been proposed for myocardial repair, the ideal donor cell

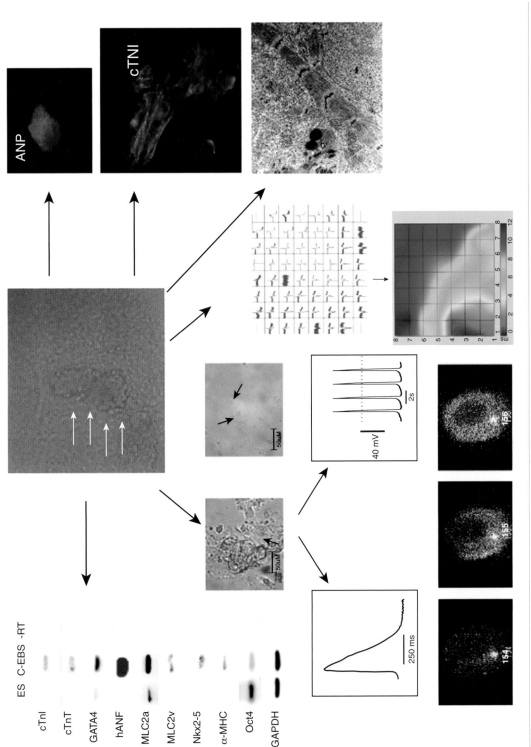

Figure 7.2   *Phenotypic characterization of the hESC-derived cardiomyocyte. The contracting areas within the EBs display molecular, structural, and functional properties of early-stage human cardiomyocytes. These properties include expression of cardiac-specific genes and transcription factors and positive immunocytochemical staining for cardiac-specific proteins (such as atrial natriuretic peptide (ANP) and cardiac troponin I (cTnI)). Transmission electron microscopy demonstrates the presence of an early sarcomeric ultrastructural pattern and intercalated discs typical of cardiomyocytes. The cells are also demonstrated to display cardiac-specific action-potentials and ionic transients (during patch clamp recordings), intracellular calcium transients (using laser confocal calcium imaging), and spontaneous pacemaker activity and electrical conduction at the tissue level using multielectrode recordings (see color-coded activation map).*

should probably exhibit the electrophysiological, structural, and contractile properties of cardiomyocytes, and should be able to integrate structurally and functionally with host tissue. In addition, it has to retain an initial proliferative potential that may enable improved colonization of the scar. Finally, the optimal candidate cell should have an autologous origin or retain minimal immunogenicity, and should be readily available in large quantities for transplantation.

Unfortunately, none of the currently available cell sources exhibit all of the aforementioned properties. The derivation of hESCs and their cardiomyocyte derivatives offers a number of theoretical advantages for myocardial cell-replacement strategies. hESCs are currently the only cell source that can provide, ex vivo, potentially an unlimited number of human cardiomyocytes for transplantation. Because of their inherent cardiac phenotype, hESC-CMs are more likely to achieve a functional connection with host myocardium. Another possible advantage is their ability to differentiate into a plurality of cell lineages, including vascular precursors[25,26] (for angiogenesis) and even specialized cardiomyocyte subtypes (pace-making, atrial, and ventricular cells) tailored for specific applications.[20] In addition, due to their clonal origin, the hESC-CMs could lend themselves to extensive characterization and genetic manipulation to promote desirable characteristics such as resistance to ischemia and apoptosis, improved contractile function, and specific electrophysiological properties.

In Vivo Transplantation and Functional Integration

The ultimate goal of cardiovascular regenerative medicine is to generate functional myocardial tissue that can engraft, survive, mature, and become well integrated with host myocardium, leading to restoration of the myocardial electromechanical properties. Hence, optimal functional improvement would require appropriate structural, electrophysiological, and mechanical coupling of donor cells to the existing network of host cardiomyocytes. For example, although

transplantation of skeletal myoblasts was shown to improve myocardial performance in animal studies, gap junctions were not observed between graft and host tissues. Moreover, as shown in an elegant study by Rubart et al[27] (using two-photon imaging of intracellular calcium transients in the intact heart), the vast majority of these donor-derived skeletal myocytes were functionally isolated from host myocardium. The inability of the skeletal myoblasts to integrate with host cardiomyocytes may unfavorably affect the myocardial electrophysiological substrate, by increasing tissue inhomogeneities, slowing conduction, and increasing the likelihood of re-entrant arrhythmias.[28] This issue may have clinical implications, as a disturbingly high incidence of ventricular arrhythmias were reported in some of the skeletal myoblast clinical trials.[29,30]

Yet, even the presence of gap junctions between host and donor tissues does not guarantee functional integration. For such integration to occur, currents generated in one cell passing through gap junctions must be sufficient to depolarize neighboring cells. In a recent study we tested the ability of hESC-CMs to integrate structurally and functionally with host cardiac tissue.[31] Initially, the in vitro ability of the hESC-CMs to form electromechanical connections with primary neonatal rat cardiomyocyte cultures was determined. Within 24 h we could start to detect microscopically, in all cocultures studied, synchronous mechanical activity. High-resolution activation mapping documented long-term, tight electrophysiological coupling between the two tissue types. The electrophysiological data were reinforced by the positive connexin 43 immunostaining (indicating the formation of gap junctions) between human and rat cells.

The potential role of ESCs for myocardial regeneration was initially demonstrated in the mouse model. Using genetically selected mESC-derived cardiomyocytes, Klug et al[32] demonstrated the successful formation of stable intracardiac grafts in the mouse heart. Later, studies in the infarcted rat heart suggested that transplantation of mESCs may lead to improvement in global left ventricular function, attenuation of the remodeling process, and augmentation of the neovascularization process.[33–35] More recently, Menard et al[36] reported that cardiac committed mESCs (pre-treated with BMP2) transplanted to the infarcted sheep heart differentiated to mature cardiomyocytes and improved cardiac function.

In vivo transplantation studies with hESCs are just emerging. Laflamme et al showed that hESC-CMs could form stable grafts in the uninjured left ventricular (LV) wall of nude rat hearts.[37] The grafted cells expressed multiple cardiac markers and were demonstrated to retain some proliferative capacity.

In contrast to several studies assessing the effect of cell transplantation on the global cardiac function, the in vivo functional integration of the grafted cells was only assessed in a handful of studies. Rubart et al[38] using two-photon imaging of intracellular calcium transients showed that transplanted fetal mice cardiomyocytes were able to functionally couple with neighboring host cardiomyocytes in the intact healthy adult mouse ventricle. Similarly, in a recent study we tested the in vivo ability of hESC-CMs to survive, function, and integrate within the host myocardium.[31] Spontaneously beating human EBs were transplanted into pig LV myocardium after the induction of complete atrioventricular block. The transplanted cardiomyocytes were demonstrated to function as a "biological pacemaker" as manifested by the appearance of a new ectopic ventricular rhythm arising from the site of cell transplantation. Recently, our findings were reinforced in a study by Xue et al, showing the ability of hESC-CMs to pace the guinea-pig heart.[39]

Despite these encouraging studies, several obstacles remain in the path to the clinical utilization of these cells: (1) strategies need to be developed to augment and direct hESC cardiac differentiation; (2) purification of the differentiating cardiomyocyte population should be achieved; (3) strategies need to be developed for optimizing hESC culturing techniques and for scaling up the entire process to derive clinically relevant numbers of cardiomyocytes; (4) transplantation techniques should be developed to

enable proper alignment of the graft tissue, high seeding and survival rates, and minimal damage to the host tissue; and (5) strategies aimed at preventing immune rejection of the cells should be established.

Directing cardiomyocyte differentiation

The current hESC cardiomyocyte differentiation system is essentially spontaneous and characterized by a relatively low cardiomyocyte yield. Since both undifferentiated hESCs and their cell derivatives express receptors for various growth factors, supplementation of the culturing system with the appropriate factors may have a favorable effect on directing differentiation of the hESCs towards a specific lineage. Nevertheless, the development of a directed cardiomyocyte differentiation system is limited by the relative paucity of data regarding the inductive clues that lead to commitment and differentiation of early cardiac-precursor cells in humans. Such differentiation strategies should therefore follow lessons learned from a number of developmental model organisms in the chick, amphibians, zebrafish, and the mouse.[40]

The heart arises from cells in the anterior–lateral plate mesoderm. The anterior endoderm that is in direct contact with the cardiac crescent is believed to provide the factors required for cardiac induction. For example, the avian endoderm (or its conditioned medium) was found to enhance mESC cardiogenesis. Recently, the visceral endoderm was also shown to play a role in hESC cardiogenesis. Coculturing of an hESC line that does not regularly differentiate to cardiomyocytes with END2 cells (a visceral endoderm-like line) provided the missing trigger for cardiac differentiation.[19]

In terms of defined endogenous factors, various genetic and biochemical perturbations in several organisms have shown a key role for bone morphogenetic proteins (BMPs), members of the transforming growth factor β (TGFβ) superfamily, in specifying and/or maintaining the myocardial lineage.[33] Along with BMPs and their antagonists, additional factors such as fibroblast growth factors (FGFs), TGFβ2, members of the Wnt/wingless signaling pathway, and a number of small molecules were implicated in cardiac induction of mESCs.[21] Possible strategies for increasing hESC cardiomyogenesis may thus include the use of different growth factors, over-expression of cardiac-specific transcription factors, coculturing with feeder layers, and potentially different mechanical factors.

Cardiomyocyte purification strategies

Although the aforementioned strategies may augment cardiomyocyte yield to a certain degree, it is still expected that most of the differentiating cells will not become cardiomyocytes. Given the heterogeneous cell mixture within the EBs, the derivation of a homogeneous cardiomyocyte population will ultimately depend on the establishment of a selection process. Although mechanical dissection of the contracting areas[31] and Percoll®-gradient centrifugation[18] have been used to enrich the cardiomyocyte population, the degree of purity that is achieved will probably be insufficient for clinical or research purposes. Such a strategy is required to prevent the presence of non-cardiomyocyte or remaining pluripotent stem cells within the cell-graft. The latter may be crucial to prevent the generation of teratomas.

An elegant and relatively simple selection scheme for the generation of a pure cardiomyocyte population was reported in the mouse model by Klug et al.[32] This approach is based on utilizing a tissue-specific promoter to drive the expression of a selectable marker. Undifferentiated mouse ESCs were transfected with a fusion gene encoding neomycin resistance under the regulation of the cardiac-specific α-MHC promoter. The mESCs were then allowed to differentiate in vitro and were subjected to antibiotic selection, resulting in >99% pure cardiomyocyte cultures.[32] Using a slightly different approach, Muller et al[41] derived transgenic mESC progeny expressing green fluorescent protein (GFP) driven by the cytomegalovirus (CMV) enhancer and a ventricle-specific promoter (MLC2v). The use of Percoll-gradient centrifugation and fluorescence activated cell sorting (FACS) yielded 97% pure cardiomyocyte fractions, of which 80% displayed ventricular action-potentials.

More recently, we were able to generate stable transgenic hESC clones expressing a marker gene (enhanced GFP, EGFP) under the transcriptional control of a cardiac-specific promoter (the hMLC2v promoter).[42] Our results demonstrated the appearance of EGFP-expressing cells during hESC differentiation that could be identified and FACS-sorted. The EGFP-expressing cells stained positively for cardiac-specific proteins, expressed cardiac-specific genes, displayed cardiac-specific action-potentials, and could form stable myocardial cell grafts following in vivo transplantation.

Line characterization, scaling up, and good manufacturing practice

Worldwide it is estimated that there are approximately 200 hESC lines. However, the ability of hESCs to differentiate into cardiomyocytes was shown in only a minority of these lines. Characterization of the wide range of hESC lines representing the diverse human genetic pool is required. Examination of hESCs for a minimal set of pluripotency markers, gene expression profile, and cytogenetic and epigenetic features may help in reducing the current heterogeneity between available hESC lines. Importantly, each cell line should also be evaluated for extended periods, assuring that no modifications occur during prolonged passaging.

The hESCs were derived in medium containing serum and were plated on top of a mouse feeder layer. From the perspective of therapeutic applications, a xeno-free and serum-independent culturing system is essential for minimizing the risk of xenozoonoses. Recently, support systems based on human cells such as human fetal fibroblasts, adult epithelial cells, or foreskin cells were described as an alternative to MEF feeders.[43] Also recently, some of the key regulators mediating ESC self-renewal were defined, and feeder-free cultivation systems were established.[44]

It is estimated that a large myocardial infarction that results in heart failure is associated with the loss of hundreds of millions of cardiomyocytes. Given the significant number of cardiomyocytes that are lost during the process of cell transplantation or die immediately thereafter, an even greater number of cells will be required. Strategies to increase the number of cardiomyocytes can theoretically be employed at several levels: (1) by increasing the initial number of undifferentiated hESCs, (2) by increasing the percentage of hESCs differentiating to the cardiac lineage, (3) by increasing the proliferative capacity of the hESC-CMs, (4) by upscaling the entire process using bioreactors and related technologies,[45] and (5) by improving colonization of the scar and long-term survival of the cells following engraftment.

Optimizing cell delivery and tissue engineering

Clinical translation of cell therapy approaches has been hampered by the large cell loss during the injection procedure and by the significant cell death following grafting into the hostile ischemic myocardium.[46] Hence, initially techniques should be developed to increase cell retention within the transplanted area. This may be achieved by improving the delivery techniques, by using improved injection media, and by developing different routes of administration. Similarly, strategies should be developed to increase the size of the in vivo cell-grafts. This may be accomplished by establishing strategies to reduce the degree of cell death following transplantation (for example by overexpression of antiapoptotic proteins or by inducing angiogenesis) or alternatively by augmenting the in vivo ability of the hESC-CMs to proliferate.

One potential strategy to overcome the aforementioned obstacles lies in the emerging field of tissue engineering. This multidisciplinary field applies the principles of engineering and life sciences to the development of biological substitutes aiming to restore, maintain, or improve tissue function. The use of cell-seeded scaffolds to promote tissue development is the hallmark of tissue engineering. The scaffold serves many purposes, including the delivery of biological signals to control and enhance tissue formation, to provide adequate biomechanical support for the cell graft, to control graft shape and size, to promote angiogenesis, and to protect from physical damage. Several tissue-engineering approaches are currently being explored for cardiac repair.

The most common approach is to seed cardiomyocytes onto biodegradable porous scaffolds that can be engrafted to the injured heart. This approach is based on the concept that the biodegradable scaffolds act as a useful initial alternative for the extracellular matrix and that seeded cells will eventually reform their native structure following scaffold biodegradation.

In vivo transplantation of degradable biopolymers into the injured heart of the rat has yielded promising results. Several cell-seeded biopolymers have been transplanted in the infarcted heart of the rat, including alginate,[47] fibrin glue, and polyurethane scaffolds, all of which resulted in a decrease in infarct size, induction of neovascularization, and attenuation of the remodeling process.

Insufficient graft vascularization is considered one of the main factors responsible for the limited graft survival and thickness of the engineered transplanted tissue. Enrichment of the degree of graft vascularization may significantly improve the survival of transplanted myocytes. Recent work from our group described the generation of a three-dimensional engineered, human vascularized, cardiac tissue. In this work, PLLA/PLGA (poly(L-lactide)/poly(D,L-lactide-coglycolide)) biodegradable scaffolds were seeded with hESC-CMs, endothelial cells, and embryonic fibroblasts. Ultrastructural analysis, immunostaining, RT-PCR, pharmacology, and confocal laser calcium imaging studies confirmed the presence of functional cardiac tissue coupled with a developing microvasculature system.[48]

Achieving immune tolerance

Prevention of the expected immune response against the transplanted cells is a major concern in all tissue regeneration strategies utilizing embryonic stem cells. The first question to be addressed is to determine precisely how immunogenic are tissues derived from hESCs. Drukker et al[49] found that hESCs express relatively low levels of human leukocyte antigen (HLA) class-I molecules with no expression of HLA class-II molecules or the ligands for natural killer (NK) cell receptors. This expression was only moderately increased after in vitro and in vivo differentiation, but was significantly augmented following γ-interferon treatment. The same group utilized the elegant human–mouse trimera model, enabling assessment of the alloimmune response of the human immune system to transplanted human cells, to elucidate the immunocostimulatory characteristics of the hESC. Engrafted undifferentiated and differentiated hESCs elicited only a minute immune response over the course of 1 month.[50] These results imply that immunosuppressive regimes for future hESC-based therapeutics may be significantly reduced in comparison to the conventional organ transplantation situation.

Despite the abovementioned results, it is still expected that hESC-CMs will be rejected following transplantation into the immunocompetent heart and that strategies should therefore be developed to overcome this immune rejection process. While a detailed discussion of this issue is beyond the scope of the current chapter and is discussed in detail in a number of excellent reviews,[51,52] we will briefly discuss some of the suggested strategies.

One approach to overcome the immunological barriers to stem cell transplantation is to minimize the alloantigenic differences between donor and recipient. This may be achieved by establishing "banks" of major histocompatibility complex (MHC) antigen-typed hESCs and then matching donors and recipients, as is carried out routinely for tissue and organ transplantation. An alternative solution may be the generation of a universal donor hESC line. This could be achieved by silencing genes associated with the assembly or transcriptional regulation of MHCs or by inserting or deleting other genes that can modulate the immune response. Another attractive theoretical strategy for inducing tolerance is hematopoietic chimerism, which may be achieved by transplantation of hematopoietic stem cells derived from hESCs. Following cell engraftment, the host will obtain tolerance due to the negative selection of alloreactive T cells in the thymus. Next, various differentiated derivatives of the specific hESC line could be safely transplanted without the risk for immune rejection.

Somatic Cell Nuclear Transfer Technology

One of the most promising strategies for achieving immune tolerance to the transplanted hESC derivatives is based on the generation of isogenic ESC lines tailored specifically for each patient. This may be achieved through somatic cell nuclear transfer technology (SCNT). The use of SCNT (also known as genomic replacement or therapeutic cloning) seems to be the theoretically perfect immunological solution to the problem of matching an hESC-derived graft with the intended host.[51,52]

SCNT is the initial step in the process of cloning, and it has been routinely used to generate cloned animals. When SCNT is used for creating genetically and immunologically compatible pluripotent stem cells, it is referred to as therapeutic cloning. The process of nuclear transfer-derived ESC production involves transferring the nucleus of a mature somatic cell into the cytoplasm of an oocyte from which the original nucleus has been removed. Once a blastocyst is formed, cells from the ICM can be utilized to produce pluripotent ESCs that are genetically identical to the nucleus donor's cells, with the exception of the mitochondrial DNA.

The first successful utilization of therapeutic cloning for the production of embryonic stem cell-like lines from somatic cells was reported in a bovine model,[53,54] and was followed by production in mouse models. These embryonic stem cell-like cell lines are believed to retain the same properties of unlimited differentiation and self-renewal as those of conventional embryonic stem cell lines derived from normal embryos produced by fertilization.[54] Nevertheless, cloning efficiency remains low, there are significant difficulties in extending the nuclear transfer approach to human oocytes, and there are also potential safety issues. In addition to the scientific and ethical concerns involved in SCNT, there are many other important practical considerations such as the time and cost that would be involved in carrying out genomic replacement for individual patients. This would require the customized generation of embryos, derivation of stem cell lines, and their differentiation to clinically useful tissues.

Summary

The development of hESC lines and their ability to differentiate into cardiomyocyte tissue hold great promise for several cardiovascular research and clinical areas. Most important, the ability to generate, for the first time, human cardiac tissue provides an exciting and promising cell source for the emerging disciplines of regenerative medicine, tissue engineering, and myocardial repair. Nevertheless, as described above, several milestones have to be achieved in order to fully harness the enormous research and clinical potential of this unique technology.

References

1. Murry CE, Field LJ, Menasche P. Cell-based cardiac repair: reflections at the 10-year point. Circulation 2005; 112: 3174–83.
2. Laflamme MA, Murry CE. Regenerating the heart. Nat Biotechnol 2005; 23: 845–56.
3. Dimmeler S, Zeiher AM, Schneider MD. Unchain my heart: the scientific foundations of cardiac repair. J Clin Invest 2005; 115: 572–83.
4. Soonpaa MH, Koh GY, Klug MG, Field LJ. Formation of nascent intercalated disks between grafted fetal cardiomyocytes and host myocardium. Science 1994; 264: 98–101.
5. Etzion S, Battler A, Barbash IM et al. Influence of embryonic cardiomyocyte transplantation on the progression of heart failure in a rat model of extensive myocardial infarction. J Mol Cell Cardiol 2001; 33: 1321–30.
6. Scorsin M, Hagege AA, Marotte F et al. Does transplantation of cardiomyocytes improve function of infarcted myocardium? Circulation 1997; 96: II188–93.
7. Weissman IL, Anderson DJ, Gage F. Stem and progenitor cells: origins, phenotypes, lineage commitments, and transdifferentiations. Annu Rev Cell Dev Biol 2001; 17: 387–403.
8. Krause DS, Theise ND, Collector MI et al. Multiorgan, multi-lineage engraftment by a single bone marrow-derived stem cell. Cell 2001; 105: 369–77.
9. Winkel GK, Pedersen RA. Fate of the inner cell mass in mouse embryos as studied by microinjection of lineage tracers. Dev Biol 1988; 127: 143–56.
10. Evans M, Kaufman M. Establishment in culture of pluripotent cells from mouse embryos. Nature 1981; 292: 154–6.
11. Martin G. Isolation of a pluripotent cell line from early mouse embryos cultured in medium conditioned by teratocarcinoma stem cells. Proc Natl Acad Sci USA 1981; 78: 7635.
12. Thomson JA, Itskovitz-Eldor J, Shapiro SS et al. Embryonic stem cell lines derived from human blastocysts. Science 1998; 282: 1145–7.
13. Reubinoff BE, Pera MF, Fong CY, Trounson A, Bongso A. Embryonic stem cell lines from human blastocysts: somatic differentiation in vitro. Nat Biotechnol 2000; 18: 399–404.
14. Itskovitz-Eldor J, Schuldiner M, Karsenti D et al. Differentiation of human embryonic stem cells into embryoid bodies compromising the three embryonic germ layers. Mol Med 2000; 6: 88–95.
15. Doetschman TC, Eistetter H, Katz M, Schmidt W, Kemler R. The in vitro development of blastocyst-derived embryonic stem cell lines: formation of visceral yolk sac, blood islands and myocardium. J Embryol Exp Morphol 1985; 87: 27–45.
16. Wobus AM, Wallukat G, Hescheler J. Pluripotent mouse embryonic stem cells are able to differentiate into cardiomyocytes expressing chronotropic responses to adrenergic and cholinergic agents and Ca2+ channel blockers. Differentiation 1991; 48: 173–82.
17. Kehat I, Amit M, Gepstein A et al. Development of cardiomyocytes from human ES cells. Methods Enzymol 2003; 365: 461–73.
18. Xu C, Police S, Rao N, Carpenter MK. Characterization and enrichment of cardiomyocytes derived from human embryonic stem cells. Circ Res 2002; 91: 501–8.
19. Mummery C, Ward-van Oostwaard D, Doevendans P et al. Differentiation of human embryonic stem cells to cardiomyocytes: role of coculture with visceral endoderm-like cells. Circulation 2003; 107: 2733–40.
20. He JQ, Ma Y, Lee Y, Thomson JA, Kamp TJ. Human embryonic stem cells develop into multiple types of cardiac myocytes: action potential characterization. Circ Res 2003; 93: 32–9.
21. Lev S, Kehat I, Gepstein L. Differentiation pathways in human embryonic stem cell-derived cardiomyocytes. Ann NY Acad Sci 2005; 1047: 50–65.
22. Snir M, Kehat I, Gepstein A et al. Assessment of the ultrastructural and proliferative properties of human embryonic stem cell-derived cardiomyocytes. Am J Physiol Heart Circ Physiol 2003; 285: H2355–63.
23. Satin J, Kehat I, Caspi O et al. Mechanism of spontaneous excitability in human embryonic stem cell derived cardiomyocytes. J Physiol 2004; 559: 479–96.
24. Kehat I, Gepstein A, Spira A, Itskovitz-Eldor J, Gepstein L. High-resolution electrophysiological assessment of human embryonic stem cell-derived cardiomyocytes: a novel in vitro model for the study of conduction. Circ Res 2002; 91: 659–61.

25. Caspi O, Lesman A, Basevitch Y et al. Tissue engineering of vascularized cardiac muscle from human embryonic stem cells. Circ Res 2007; 100: 263–72.

26. Levenberg S, Golub JS, Amit M, Itskovitz-Eldor J, Langer R. Endothelial cells derived from human embryonic stem cells. Proc Natl Acad Sci USA 2002; 99: 4391–6.

27. Rubart M, Soonpaa MH, Nakajima H, Field LJ. Spontaneous and evoked intracellular calcium transients in donor-derived myocytes following intracardiac myoblast transplantation. J Clin Invest 2004; 114: 775–83.

28. Abraham MR, Henrikson CA, Tung L et al. Antiarrhythmic engineering of skeletal myoblasts for cardiac transplantation. Circ Res 2005; 97: 159–67.

29. Menasche P, Hagege AA, Vilquin JT et al. Autologous skeletal myoblast transplantation for severe postinfarction left ventricular dysfunction. J Am Coll Cardiol 2003; 41: 1078–83.

30. Smits PC, van Geuns RJ, Poldermans D et al. Catheter-based intramyocardial injection of autologous skeletal myoblasts as a primary treatment of ischemic heart failure: clinical experience with six-month follow-up. J Am Coll Cardiol 2003; 42: 2063–9.

31. Kehat I, Khimovich L, Caspi O et al. Electromechanical integration of cardiomyocytes derived from human embryonic stem cells. Nat Biotechnol 2004; 22: 1282–9.

32. Klug MG, Soonpaa MH, Koh GY, Field LJ. Genetically selected cardiomyocytes from differentiating embryonic stem cells form stable intracardiac grafts. J Clin Invest 1996; 98: 216–24.

33. Behfar A, Zingman LV, Hodgson DM et al. Stem cell differentiation requires a paracrine pathway in the heart. FASEB J 2002; 16: 1558–66.

34. Hodgson DM, Behfar A, Zingman LV et al. Stable benefit of embryonic stem cell therapy in myocardial infarction. Am J Physiol Heart Circ Physiol 2004; 287: H471–9.

35. Min JY, Yang Y, Converso KL et al. Transplantation of embryonic stem cells improves cardiac function in postinfarcted rats. J Appl Physiol 2002; 92: 288–96.

36. Menard C, Hagege AA, Agbulut O et al. Transplantation of cardiac-committed mouse embryonic stem cells to infarcted sheep myocardium: a preclinical study. Lancet 2005; 366: 1005–12.

37. Laflamme MA, Gold J, Xu C et al. Formation of human myocardium in the rat heart from human embryonic stem cells. Am J Pathol 2005; 167: 663–71.

38. Rubart M, Pasumarthi KB, Nakajima H et al. Physiological coupling of donor and host cardiomyocytes after cellular transplantation. Circ Res 2003; 92: 1217–24.

39. Xue T, Cho HC, Akar FG et al. Functional integration of electrically active cardiac derivatives from genetically engineered human embryonic stem cells with quiescent recipient ventricular cardiomyocytes: insights into the development of cell-based pacemakers. Circulation 2005; 111: 11–20.

40. Olson EN, Schneider MD. Sizing up the heart: development redux in disease. Genes Dev 2003; 17: 1937–56.

41. Muller M, Fleischmann BK, Selbert S et al. Selection of ventricular-like cardiomyocytes from ES cells in vitro. FASEB J 2000; 14: 2540–8.

42. Huber I, Itzhaki I, Caspi I, Arbel G, Tzukerman M, Gepstein A, Habib M, Yankelson L, Kehat I, Gepstein L. Identification and selection of cardiomyocytes during human embryonic stem cell differentiation. FASEB J 2007; 21(10): 2551–63.

43. Richards M, Fong CY, Chan WK, Wong PC, Bongso A. Human feeders support prolonged undifferentiated growth of human inner cell masses and embryonic stem cells. Nat Biotechnol 2002; 20: 933–6.

44. Xu C, Inokuma MS, Denham J et al. Feeder-free growth of undifferentiated human embryonic stem cells. Nat Biotechnol 2001; 19: 971–4.

45. Zandstra PW, Bauwens C, Yin T et al. Scalable production of embryonic stem cell-derived cardiomyocytes. Tissue Eng 2003; 9: 767–78.

46. Muller-Ehmsen J, Peterson KL, Kedes L et al. Rebuilding a damaged heart: long-term survival of transplanted neonatal rat cardiomyocytes after myocardial infarction and effect on cardiac function. Circulation 2002; 105: 1720–6.

47. Leor J, Aboulafia-Etzion S, Dar A et al. Bioengineered cardiac grafts: a new approach to repair the infarcted myocardium? Circulation 2000; 102: III56–61.

48. Caspi O, Lesman A, Basevitz Y, Gepstein A, Arbel G, Habib M, Gepstein L, Levenberg S. Tissue Engineering of Vascularized Cardiac Muscle From Human Embryonic Stem Cells. Circ Res 2007; 100: 263–72.

49. Drukker M, Katz G, Urbach A et al. Characterization of the expression of MHC proteins in human embryonic stem cells. Proc Natl Acad Sci USA 2002; 99: 9864–9.

50. Drukker M, Katchman H, Katz G et al. Human embryonic stem cells and their differentiated derivatives are less susceptible to immune rejection than adult cells. Stem Cells 2006; 24: 221–9.

51. Odorico JS, Kaufman DS, Thomson JA. Multilineage differentiation from human embryonic stem cell lines. Stem Cells 2001; 19: 193–204.

52. Bradley JA, Bolton EM, Pedersen RA. Stem cell medicine encounters the immune system. Nat Rev Immunol 2002; 2: 859–71.

53. Cibelli JB, Stice SL, Golueke PJ et al. Transgenic bovine chimeric offspring produced from somatic cell-derived stem-like cells. Nat Biotechnol 1998; 16: 642-6.

54. Lanza RP, Chung HY, Yoo JJ et al. Generation of histocompatible tissues using nuclear transplantation. Nat Biotechnol 2002; 20: 689–96.

chapter 8

The Role of Arteriogenesis and Angiogenesis for Cardiac Repair

Wolfgang Schaper

Introduction

Heart failure is caused by the loss of contractile myocytes and/or the loss of contractile material from individual cells. The causes for this are, in the majority, of vascular origin. It appears logical that repairing the infarcted heart requires also a vascular approach besides the challenging task of restarting the arrested mitotic cycle of cardiac myocytes. The task is a formidable one because, with a moderate to severe myocardial infarct, about 30 grams of tissue have disappeared and have to be replaced, and for a chunk of tissue of that size a new vascular system has to be built. However, factors other than acute myocardial infarction contribute to heart failure, in particular the subtle chronic and cumulating loss of individual myocytes in pressure overload, be it from high blood pressure or from aortic valve stenosis[1] and from chronic ischemia as in hibernating myocardium,[2] resulting in substitution fibrosis.

It would appear that the prevention of chronic myocyte loss would constitute a reasonable basis for preventing or at least delaying heart failure, especially when all possibilities of vascular repair have been exhausted. This would require complete knowledge about the mechanism of myocyte death, which is, however, in debate. While there is agreement about ischemic cell death, also called oncosis, in acute transmural infarction starting with leaky cell membranes, mitochondrial calcium overload, and adenosine triphosphate (ATP) loss followed by leukocyte influx presenting the full picture of necrosis, the role of apoptosis is less clear.[3] Apoptosis requires ATP, which is not available in ischemia, and apoptosis does not, in contrast to necrosis, elicit an inflammatory response. The incidence of apoptotic cells in human cardiac needle biopsies is extremely low (when the TUNEL procedure (terminal deoxynucleotide transferase-mediated dUTP nick-end labeling), prone to false positives and artifacts, is carefully conducted), and hence does not offer an explanation for heart failure. However, the extra load under which the remaining "normal" myocardium is put when a significant number of cells has died leads to an increased turnover of proteins, an increased number of misfolded proteins, and an extra load on the mechanisms of debris disposal, demonstrated by increased amounts of unprocessed ubiqitinated proteins and increased amounts of lipofuscin. The accumulation of cell debris is caused by the limiting capacity of the enzyme isopeptidase, which prevents exocytosis and leads finally to autophagic cell death,[1,4] the most frequent type of death in pressure-overloaded human hearts and in "hibernating" myocardium. It would appear useful to study ways and means to increase the activity of isopeptidase for the prevention of autophagic cell death. On the other hand, chronic ischemia and the staged dropout of cells suffocating from the debris overload and lowered oxygen tensions should (but do not) mobilize the intramyocardial stem cells that Anversa and his co-workers described.[5] And chronic ischemia should also stimulate angiogenesis, which it fails to do.

Chronic Ischemic Myocardium: a Stimulus for Angiogenesis?

Hypoxic tissues activate the transcription factor HIF (hypoxia inducible factor),[6] which is composed of two parts, 1α and 1β, where, under normoxic conditions, 1α is constantly formed and immediately inactivated leading to no significant transcriptional activity. Under hypoxic conditions 1α is not broken down, and activates, among many other hypoxia-sensitive genes, vascular endothelial growth factor (VEGF), the angiogenic growth factor par excellence. *Hypoxic myocardium should therefore have the capacity to self-heal.* This, however, is not the case, at least on the capillary level. Studies of human hibernating myocardium have shown that the capillary density actually decreases.[7] Hibernating myocardium, as a response to chronic hypoxia, lowers its metabolic rate in relation to the reduced amount of oxygen it receives (it ceases to contract), thereby lowering the degree of hypoxia, which may, in part, explain the lack of angiogenic response. The hibernating myocyte not only downregulates its function, but also breaks down its contractile machinery and disassembles many of its mitochondria. This puts another strain on debris disposal and explains why hibernating myocytes disappear via the route of autophagic cell death. Whereas brief or repetitive hypoxia may lead to the formation of new capillaries, chronic lasting hypoxia may circumvent the angiogenic response in favor of removing the potential source of VEGF. The abovementioned possibility of preventing autophagic cell death may restore the angiogenic potency and open the way again to self-healing.

Chronic Ischemic Myocardium: a Stimulus for Arteriogenesis?

Arteriogenesis,[8] the formation of collateral arteries that circumvent a coronary arterial occlusion, can be a very efficient process provided that the time necessary for its formation (about 1 week) is available, which is not often the case, because an arterial thrombus can develop within minutes.

However, a slowly growing thrombus or a contracting thrombus leaving significant stenosis is an ideal circumstance for the growth of collateral arteries. Many cases have been reported in the literature of silent chronic coronary occlusions without infarctions, even with multiple occlusions, due to the timely development of collateral arteries.[9] Arteriogenesis proceeds almost always in the presence of ischemia, and the notion prevailed for a long time that ischemia is causally linked to arteriogenesis. However, this is now a matter of debate. Almost half a century ago, Fulton[10,11] concluded, on the basis of postmortem angiographies of human hearts, that the process of collateralization either started or extended in(to) the region of the non-ischemic part of the heart, which cast first doubts on the causative role of ischemia. Moreover, pre-existent collateral arterioles that have the capacity for growth are constantly perfused with arterial blood, and cannot become hypoxic themselves. Oxygen diffuses also through the arteriolar wall, and contributes to oxygenation of the myocardium closely surrounding it and prevents cell death there, even when somewhat remote tissue is fully necrotic. It is therefore unlikely that ischemia is causally related to arteriogenesis. The studies by Fujita et al,[12] who found that repetitive ischemia in a canine model of coronary occlusions and reperfusion stimulated the formation of coronary collateral vessels, can be interpreted differently: each occlusion increased collateral flow and with it fluid shear stress. Each reperfusion, leading to maximal vasodilatation, increased again the fluid shear stress in all arterioles including pre-existing collaterals. Furthermore, animals showing a low degree of ischemia at the first occlusion required significantly fewer occlusions to reach full collateral status, which would prevent an infarct in the case of permanent coronary occlusion. Increased fluid shear stress rather than ischemia had been the dominant influence.

Studies with collateral development in the vascular periphery have shown that the oxygen tension in skeletal muscles of the upper leg, where collateral development occurs after femoral artery occlusion, is normal.[13,14] Low oxygen partial pressures are found only in the lower leg where collaterals do not form. This means that tissue ischemia and arteriogenesis often occur at the same time (and rarely in the same space) but are not causally related.

Angiogenesis or Arteriogenesis? Is That the Question?

Angiogenesis describes the sprouting or longitudinal split of capillaries from pre-existent ones. This is a crucial process in wound healing, but a debate arose regarding whether this is a useful mechanism for tissues that have become ischemic because of occlusion of a feeder artery and where the number of capillaries is normal. Treatment with angiogenic growth factors that increase capillary density may not achieve much unless they also stimulate collateral artery growth, which is not yet clear. Acute or chronic ischemia does not lead to increased expression of angiogenic growth factors on the transcriptional level,[15] and pharmacologic administration of large doses of these factors leads only to moderate effects.[8] Complete restitution of function of the occluded artery by collateral vessels is possible with high flow and high fluid shear stresses, and no known growth factor or their combination was found to equal the effect of fluid shear stress.

An angiogenic response to slowly progressing coronary occlusion was described in the pig heart where no pre-existent arteriolar connections exist.[16] Collateral connections develop, but only by capillary sprouting, and by the creation of thin-walled giant capillary connections between adjacent territories that withstand the tangential wall tension only because the intravascular pressure remains low and because myocytes wrap around these vessels to help bear part of the wall stresses. The generalized angiogenic response in the chronic ischemic pig heart segment reduces the minimal resistance to flow, which constitutes about half of the total resistance determined by anatomy, and this may play a significant part in the survival scenario, but only in very slowly progressing coronary stenosis.[17,18] Depending on the presence or absence of pre-existing collateral arterioles the above question must be answered in the affirmative: both mechanisms are important. In the presence of pre-existent interconnecting arterioles, arteriogenesis is the dominant mechanism. In their absence, angiogenesis is of some limited help, because elevated left ventricular end-diastolic pressures encroach upon the low perfusion pressures in the capillary-originating collateral network, thereby lowering the threshold for ischemia.

Fluid Shear Stress is the Vascular Molding Force

The viscous drag that flowing blood exerts on the endothelium is the molding force for arterial size. Thoma[19] was the first to observe the relationship between blood flow velocity and arterial size in the developing chick vasculature. Later studies with arteriovenous shunts demonstrated a cause-and-effect relationship.[8,15,20]

Arteriogenesis relies on increased fluid shear stress, because arteriolar connections between side-branches upstream of the occluded artery and those downstream experience a steep gradient of pressure, which increases flow and fluid shear stress. However, enlargement of these collateral connections either functionally by vasomotion or structurally by growth reduces shear stress, which is inversely related to the third power of the vessel's radius. This is a self-limiting process, which stops growth when only 40% of the maximal physiological conductance of the arterial bed is replaced by collaterals. We removed this inhibition in the following experiment. By side-to-side anastomosis between the distal stump of the occluded artery, which functions as the collecting vessel of the collaterals bridging the occlusion, and the accompanying vein, very high collateral flows were generated, because the pressure gradient between artery and vein remained high. The high flows stimulated arteriogenesis to such a degree that maximal conductance of the collateral circulation was double that of the artery now replaced by collaterals. These studies were carried out in the pig, rabbit, and rat hindlimb. Similar studies appear difficult to perform in the heart because of intense ischemia resulting not only from the acute occlusion but also from the shunting of the collateral flow into the venous system. The lesson learned from these experiments is that blood flow should be kept high, which is best done by exercise. Indeed, Seiler[21] has shown that marathon training and running leads to the growth of collateral vessels in the normal human heart to such a degree that an acute coronary occlusion (e.g. by brief balloon inflation) would be tolerated without signs of ischemia. The downside of the idea of repairing the infarcted heart via stimulation of arteriogenesis is that it usually comes too late: the myocardial survival time after acute coronary occlusion is about 1 hour.[22] Pre-existent collateral vessels need about 3 days to grow and to deliver enough blood flow. This highlights the importance of rapid intervention to re-establish flow.

Translation of the Shear Stress Signal into Arterial Growth

A large literature covers the field of fluid shear stress and its translation into signals for remodeling of the arterial or arteriolar vessels. Fluid shear stress is a "weak" force in comparison to the pressure-derived forces of wall stress. Nevertheless, that weak force plays a major role in the vascular adaptation to flow load. Increased flow deforms the endothelial cell, and Ingber put forward the concept that deformation of the cytoskeleton (tensegrity) leads to the expression of genes responsible for arterial growth.[23,24] Other hypotheses describe the formation of a mechanosensory complex consisting of platelet endothelial cell adhesion molecule 1 (PECAM1), vascular endothelial (VE)-cadherin, and VEGF receptor 2 (VEGFR2), which activates phosphatidylinositol (PI) kinase and is said to be activated in the early stages of atherosclerosis.[25] Since atherosclerosis is a disease with predilections for foci with low shear stress, we assume that it is downregulated in regions of high shear stress, which is difficult to test because of the low expression of the complex in normal

arteries in vivo. Signals from the stressed endothelium also arise from integrins and from the focal adhesion kinase, and it is highly probable that these signals are conducted via the Rho pathway.[15,26] Ion channels such as the chloride and calcium channels change their open probability, which leads to changes in volume regulation.[27] Signals from the activated endothelium are also directed at the underlying layer of smooth muscle (Figure 8.1).

Monocytes Adhere to Shear-Activated Endothelium

Signals generated by stressed endothelial cells with smooth muscle cells as their target must be secreted molecules, because no cellular junctions exist between endothelial cells and smooth muscle cells. These secreted molecules must be small (such as NO), because there are barriers to diffusion including the extracellular matrix and the internal elastic lamina. We described some time ago that monocytes are attracted to stress-activated endothelial cells (Figure 8.2) by the secretion of monocyte chemoattractant protein 1 (MCP1),[28] and stick to the surface now covered by adhesion molecules such as intercellular adhesion molecule 1 (ICAM1) and vascular cell adhesion molecule (VCAM), also overexpressed by activated endothelium. These invading monocytes produce vascular growth factors and proteolytic enzymes that digest the internal elastic lamina and lead to more direct contact between the endothelial and smooth muscle cells, which start the cell cycle and proliferate. The importance of monocytes/ macrophages was tested in several experiments using phosphonate, fluorouracil, and genetic approaches. As a general conclusion of these experiments one can say that a reduction of monocyte number in the peripheral blood, caused either by bone marrow poisoning with 5-fluorouracil or by knockdown of circulating monocytes with phosphonate-loaded liposomes, leads to a significant retardation of collateral artery growth.[29] Animals with low monocyte numbers because of genetic defects (osteopetrosis) are inherently at a disadvantage with regard to

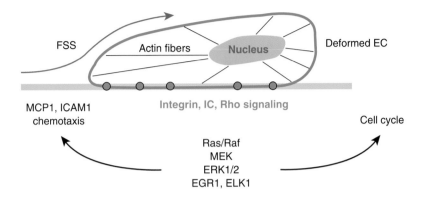

FSS   Actin fibers   Nucleus   Deformed EC

MCP1, ICAM1   Integrin, IC, Rho signaling
chemotaxis   Cell cycle

Ras/Raf
MEK
ERK1/2
EGR1, ELK1

Figure 8.1 *Summary of the molecular changes that occur when a steep pressure gradient develops along the length of a pre-existent arteriole connecting a branch proximal from an occlusion with one distal. This increases the blood flow velocity and with it the fluid shear stress. This leads to deformation of the cytoskeleton and applies physical forces upon the nucleus. Ion channels are activated and transmit signals leading to transcriptional changes that lead to attraction of monocytes, digestion of the internal elastic lamina, and proliferation of the smooth muscle of the media. EC, endothelial cell; IC, ion channel; Ras/Raf, MEK, ERK, EGR, ELK, members of mitogen activated kinase family; FSS, fluid shear stress; MCP1, monocyte chemoattractant protein; ICAM, intercellular adhesion molecule.*

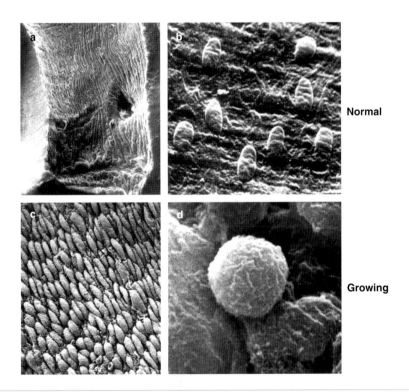

Normal

Growing

Figure 8.2 *Scanning electron microscopic images of the endothelial surface of a collateral arteriole before (a, b) and after (c, d) onset of growth. (a, b) Note the smooth endothelial surface with the oval shaped nuclei arranged along the axis of blood flow. (c) An increase of fluid shear stress and activation and swelling of the endothelium are demonstrated. (d) Attachment of a monocyte is visualized.*

arteriogenesis.[8] Increases in monocyte blood concentration, be it by transfusion or by the rebound following 5-fluorouracil withdrawal, lead to the acceleration of arteriogenesis.[29] The importance of monocyte attraction by the endothelial-secreted chemokine MCP1 was illustrated by the finding that genetic targeting of the MCP1 receptor (CCR2) leads to significant inhibition of arteriogenesis.[30]

Positive outward remodeling of small pre-existent collateral vessels into large arterial blood conductors is also achieved by monocytes/macrophages. In addition to proteolysis, cytotoxic activity is also needed, which is achieved by activation of iNOS (inducible NO synthase).

These latter mentioned experiments were carried out in the vascular periphery of rabbits, rats, or mice. Our previous experience with the collateral circulation of the heart has taught us that the fundamental processes of arteriogenesis apply to the vasculature of the heart, brain, and periphery as well.

The Role of Bone Marrow-Derived Stem Cells

With our 1976 publication we were the first to observe a role of monocytes in arteriogenesis.[31] In a canine model of slowly progressing coronary artery occlusion, we demonstrated the adhesion of monocytes to regions of shear stressed endothelium that had also changed its phenotype from a smooth lining with slightly protruding oval nuclei arranged in the axis of flow to a rough surface composed of swollen cells. Monocytes belong to the bone marrow-derived cells, and the question arose of what their function may be and whether they (or other bone marrow-derived cells) remain as monocytes or transform into cells of a different lineage, as suggested more recently by others. Our research has led us to the conclusion that although invading monocytes change their phenotype into that of macrophages, they do not transform into endothelial or into smooth muscle cells. We have described an experiment recently in which a wild-type mouse received, after "lethal" X-irradiation, bone marrow transplantation from

a mouse expressing green fluorescent protein.[32] After about 6 weeks, close to 90% of all bone marrow cells were green, which allowed tracing of these cells in vascular tissue. In growing collaterals these cells were found where we formerly also detected monocytes. In no case was there any transformation of a green cell into a smooth muscle cell or into an endothelial cell. Our study is the only one so far to use confocal immunofluorescence with three-dimensional reconstruction. This is important, because in cases of overlay of a green cell with an endothelial or smooth muscle cell misinterpretation is possible if microscopy is used only in fluorescent mode, as was the case in several earlier publications by others.[33,34] Bone marrow-derived cells not only attach to the endothelium but also reach the adventitia of growing collaterals via leaky venules, providing growth factors and proteolytic enzymes, necessary for positive remodeling of the artery. From these studies we concluded that bone marrow-derived cells play a very important role as producers of factors and enzymes, but they do not transform into cells of different lineages.

No Need to Implicate a Role of Endothelial Progenitor Cells

Circulating endothelial progenitor cells (EPCs) are widely discussed today as assisting in angiogenesis and arteriogenesis, by attaching to vascular regions in need of proliferation.[35] However, it is generally accepted that endothelial and smooth muscle cells are able to divide even in the absence of EPCs, i.e. in cell culture bathed in synthetic media. When we observe endothelial and smooth muscle cells under in vivo conditions where they divide in situ, connected firmly to their neighbors, and when we are able to see endothelial cells in situ gradually modifying their histological phenotype towards a proliferative one, we conclude that these dividing cells have not been recruited from the bloodstream but that local cells have responded to local cues. And the same is also true for smooth muscle cells that gradually change their phenotype from a contractile into a synthetic and finally into a proliferative phenotype and back when the major remodeling processes have reached a mature phase. Furthermore, smooth muscle cells are far more difficult targets for EPCs to reach from the bloodstream compared to endothelial cells. "Ockham's razor" applies here: the simplest explanation has the greater possibility of being true.

The Role of Angiogenic Growth Factors

Angiogenic growth factors have been tested clinically in patients with coronary and peripheral artery disease. Improvement using gene therapy approaches was reported,[33] especially in peripheral arterial disease. However, controlled clinical trials failed to reach statistical significance.[36,37] This was unexpected, because sensational successes were reported from animal experiments where the entire femoral artery had been excised, thereby mimicking late stages of peripheral artery disease in patients.[38,39] However, a close reading of the experimental papers, the basis for the clinical studies, showed some weaknesses on a methodological level. Especially the use of two methods for measuring blood flow, the non-invasive cuff method for lower leg blood pressure in rabbits and the laser Doppler imaging (LDI) method for measuring skin blood flow, were too non-specific to justify them as a basis for clinical studies. It is often overlooked that cuff pressure (sensitive to position), a derivative endpoint for post-occlusive flow, expected to be high after treatment, is low with peripheral vasodilatation. Laser Doppler imaging is only a reliable method to measure skin blood flow when applied to the dorsal skin of mouse paws, but not when applied to the entire lower body as performed by Aicher et al.[40]

On the other hand, the design of the clinical trials also left much to be desired. For the ischemic heart studies, single injections of growth factor protein into the coronary artery at routine cardiac catheterization was probably expecting too much. The present day state of the art for the treatment of coronary, peripheral, renal, and carotid artery occlusions is balloon dilatation and stent implantation, and the results obtained with these techniques, not to forget bypass surgery, have to be met and surpassed by molecular therapies. This would appear to be difficult to achieve in the foreseeable future. To restrict molecular approaches to cases where no stents can be placed, and no surgery performed with any expectations of success, is probably also doomed to fail, because the development of collateral arteries depends on the presence of at least one source of normal arterial pressure.

How to Vascularize "New" Adult Myocardium?

To replace a tough infarct scar with new cardiac myocytes is probably asking too much, and attempts at restarting the cardiac myocyte cell cycle will probably lead to generalized hyperplasia of the non-scarred myocardium. These new cells will probably be able to generate their own capillaries via HIF and VEGF. Increased tissue mass and a more capacious capillary network will generate more flow in the feeder arteries that experience a higher fluid shear stress, and mechanisms as described above will lead to the widening of these vessels.

Conclusions

Myocardium weakened by the loss of contractile units but hopefully soon assisted by new cardiac myocytes is in need of an enlarged vasculature to meet the demands of the added cells. This demand must be met with new capillaries and by increasing the capacity of the arterial system. To achieve this, angiogenesis and arteriogenesis have to be activated. The mechanisms for these two processes of adaptation differ. Angiogenesis requires activation of the hypoxia inducible factor, which leads to VEGF transcription and translation, which in turn leads to sprouting of new capillaries from existing ones. Arteriogenesis is a more complex mechanism, which requires activation of shear stressed endothelium, which results in upregulation of transcription factors, notably carp (cardiac ankyrin repeat protein), egr1 (early growth response 1), and STARS/ABRA (striated muscle activator of Rho signaling/actin-binding Rho activating protein), leading to upregulation of chemokine, adhesion molecule, and integrin transcription and translation. Monocytes adhere and penetrate the wall of pre-existent small arteriolar collateral vessels, where they assist in the remodeling and proliferation of smooth muscle and endothelial cells by partially destroying the existing structure to generate space for the new and much larger artery. The final result of the transformation is an up to 25 times larger arterial vessel, depending on the species studied. Apart from monocytes and T-lymphocytes we have not found evidence for the participation of other bone marrow-derived cells. Division and proliferation of endothelial and smooth muscle cells occurred in situ and responded only to local cues. The processes described here characterize a self-healing process that may occur spontaneously in the "new" myocardium generated by reversing the terminal differentiation of myocytes.

References

1. Kostin S, Pool L, Elsasser A et al. Myocytes die by multiple mechanisms in failing human hearts. Circ Res 2003; 92: 715–24.
2. Elsasser A, Schlepper M, Klovekorn WP et al. Hibernating myocardium: an incomplete adaptation to ischemia. Circulation 1997; 96: 2920–31.
3. Elsasser A, Suzuki K, Schaper J. Unresolved issues regarding the role of apoptosis in the pathogenesis of ischemic injury and heart failure. J Mol Cell Cardiol 2000; 32: 711–24.
4. Schaper J, Elsasser A, Kostin S. The role of cell death in heart failure. Circ Res 1999; 85: 867–9.
5. Anversa P, Leri A, Kajstura J. Cardiac regeneration. J Am Coll Cardiol 2006; 47: 1769–76.
6. Semenza GL, Agani F, Iyer N et al. Hypoxia-inducible factor 1: from molecular biology to cardiopulmonary physiology. Chest 1998; 114: 40S–5S.
7. Elsasser A, Schaper J. Hibernating myocardium: adaptation or degeneration? Basic Res Cardiol 1995; 90: 47–8.
8. Schaper W, Schaper J. Arteriogenesis. Boston: Kluwer Academic Publishers, 2004.
9. Schaper W, De Brabander M, Lewi P. DNA synthesis and mitoses in coronary collateral vessels of the dog. Circ Res 1971; 28: 671–9.
10. Fulton WF. Arterial anastomoses in the coronary circulation. II. Distribution, enumeration and measurement of coronary arterial anastomoses in health and disease. Scott Med J 1963; 8: 466–74.
11. Fulton WF. Anastomotic enlargement and ischaemic myocardial damage. Br Heart J 1964; 26: 1–15.
12. Fujita M, Yamanishi K, Araie E et al. Determinants of collateral development in a canine model with repeated coronary occlusion. Heart Vessels 1994; 9: 292–9.
13. Helisch A, Wagner S, Khan N et al. Impact of mouse strain differences in innate hindlimb collateral vasculature. Arterioscler Thromb Vasc Biol 2006; 26: 520–6.
14. Ito WD, Arras M, Winkler B et al. Angiogenesis but not collateral growth is associated with ischemia after femoral artery occlusion. Am J Physiol 1997; 273: H1255–65.
15. Eitenmuller I, Volger O, Kluge A et al. The range of adaptation by collateral vessels after femoral artery occlusion. Circ Res 2006; 99: 656–62.
16. De Brabander M, Schaper W, Verheyen F. Regenerative changes in the porcine heart after gradual and chronic coronary artery occlusion. Beitr Pathol 1973; 149: 170–85.
17. Gorge G, Schmidt T, Ito BR, Pantely GA, Schaper W. Microvascular and collateral adaptation in swine hearts following progressive coronary artery stenosis. Basic Res Cardiol 1989; 84: 524–35.
18. Roth DM, White FC, Bloor CM. Altered minimal coronary resistance to antegrade reflow after chronic coronary artery occlusion in swine. Circ Res 1988; 63: 330–9.
19. Thoma R. Untersuchungen über die Histogenese und Histomechanik des Gefäßsystems Stuttgart: F Enke, 1893.
20. Pipp F, Boehm S, Cai WJ et al. Elevated fluid shear stress enhances postocclusive collateral artery growth and gene expression in the pig hind limb. Arterioscler Thromb Vasc Biol 2004; 24: 1664–8.
21. Seiler C. The human coronary collateral circulation. Heart 2003; 89: 1352–7.
22. Htun P, Ito WD, Kirsch KP, Schaper J, Schaper W. Cardioprotection by aFGF and bFGF can be antagonized by Genistein and Suramin. J Mol Cell Cardiol 1997; 29: Fr64 (abstr).
23. Ingber DE. Tensegrity I. Cell structure and hierarchical systems biology. J Cell Sci 2003; 116: 1157–73.
24. Ingber DE. Tensegrity II. How structural networks influence cellular information processing networks. J Cell Sci 2003; 116: 1397–408.
25. Tzima E, Irani-Tehrani M, Kiosses WB et al. A mechanosensory complex that mediates the endothelial cell response to fluid shear stress. Nature 2005; 437: 426–31.

26. Tzima E. Role of small GTPases in endothelial cytoskeletal dynamics and the shear stress response. Circ Res 2006; 98: 176–85.

27. Ziegelhoeffer T, Scholz D, Friedrich C et al. Inhibition of collateral artery growth by mibefradil: possible role of volume-regulated chloride channels. Endothelium 2003; 10: 237–46.

28. Ito WD, Arras M, Winkler B et al. Monocyte chemotactic protein-1 increases collateral and peripheral conductance after femoral artery occlusion. Circ Res 1997; 80: 829–37.

29. Heil M, Ziegelhoeffer T, Pipp F et al. Blood monocyte concentration is critical for enhancement of collateral artery growth. Am J Physiol Heart Circ Physiol 2002; 283: H2411–19.

30. Heil M, Ziegelhoeffer T, Wagner S et al. Collateral artery growth (arteriogenesis) after experimental arterial occlusion is impaired in mice lacking CC-chemokine receptor-2. Circ Res 2004; 94: 671–7.

31. Schaper J, Koenig R, Franz D, Schaper W. The endothelial surface of growing coronary collateral arteries. Intimal margination and diapedesis of monocytes. A combined SEM and TEM study. Virchows Arch A (Pathol Anat) 1976; 370: 193–205.

32. Ziegelhoeffer T, Fernandez B, Kostin S et al. Bone marrow-derived cells do not incorporate into the adult growing vasculature. Circ Res 2004; 94: 230–8.

33. Isner JM, Kalka C, Kawamoto A, Asahara T. Bone marrow as a source of endothelial cells for natural and iatrogenic vascular repair. Ann NY Acad Sci 2001; 953: 75–84.

34. Iwaguro H, Yamaguchi J, Kalka C et al. Endothelial progenitor cell vascular endothelial growth factor gene transfer for vascular regeneration. Circulation 2002; 105: 732–8.

35. Asahara T, Murohara T, Sullivan A et al. Isolation of putative progenitor endothelial cells for angiogenesis. Science. 1997; 275: 964–7.

36. Henry TD, Abraham JA. Review of preclinical and clinical results with vascular endothelial growth factors for therapeutic angiogenesis. Curr Interv Cardiol Rep 2000; 2: 228–41.

37. Hendel RC, Henry TD, Rocha-Singh K et al. Effect of intracoronary recombinant human vascular endothelial growth factor on myocardial perfusion: evidence for a dose-dependent effect. Circulation 2000; 101: 118–21.

38. Bauters C, Asahara T, Zheng LP et al. Site-specific therapeutic angiogenesis after systemic administration of vascular endothelial growth factor. J Vasc Surg 1995; 21: 314–24; discussion 324–5.

39. Takeshita S, Rossow ST, Kearney M et al. Time course of increased cellular proliferation in collateral arteries after administration of vascular endothelial growth factor in a rabbit model of lower limb vascular insufficiency. Am J Pathol 1995; 147: 1649–60.

40. Aicher A, Heeschen C, Mildner-Rihm C et al. Essential role of endothelial nitric oxide synthase for mobilization of stem and progenitor cells. Nat Med 2003; 9: 1370–6.

chapter 9

Cytokine Treatment for Cardioprotection and Cardiac Regeneration

Nirat Beohar and Douglas W Losordo

Introduction

Myocardial infarction (MI) induces left ventricular (LV) dysfunction and remodeling as a consequence of a healing process during which necrotic cardiomyocytes are removed by an inflammatory reaction and replaced with connective tissue scar.[1,2] Although early revascularization reduces myocardial damage and improves survival after MI, approximately 30–35% of patients with successful restoration of epicardial flow demonstrate adverse cardiac remodeling, which is associated with worse long-term clinical outcomes.[3,4]

Novel strategies to replace lost myocardium, protect at-risk cardiomyocytes, or augment vascularity may preserve LV function and limit remodeling. Cytokine therapy has emerged as a non-invasive modality due to its potential ability to regenerate cardiomyoctyes, prevent cardiomyoctye loss through inhibition of apoptosis, induce neovascularization, and possibly improve interstitial matrix characteristics. These salutary effects of cytokine therapy can have a favorable impact on LV remodeling. Cytokine therapy may be applicable in conjunction with mechanical or cellular therapies or particularly for "no-option" patients – those with disabling ischemia despite optimal medical treatment, after all possibilities for conventional mechanical revascularization have been exhausted.

Growth Factors, Chemokines, Cardioprotectives, Transcription Factors, and Agents that Act on Intercellular Matrix (Table 9.1)

Therapeutic neovascularization

Agents for therapeutic neovascularization have traditionally included growth factors that act predominantly by stimulating endothelial cell proliferation and migration and enhancing endothelial cell survival under the toxic conditions (e.g. hypoxia) which necessitate angiogenesis. The vascular endothelial growth factor (VEGF) and fibroblast growth factor (FGF) families were the first factors shown to exert a therapeutic effect by promoting a favorable outcome in the setting of ischemia.[5,6] Subsequently, multiple isoforms of VEGF were identified that have varying success for stimulating neovascularization or lymphangiogenesis, depending upon heparin binding activity (determining local tissue retention) and affinity for the multiple VEGF receptors. The VEGF receptors 1 and 2 are both expressed on endothelial cells and hematopoietic stem cells. Particularly the expression of VEGF receptors on hematopoietic stem cells appears of major importance for VEGF-dependent regulation of endothelial progenitor cells. More recently, another member of the VEGF family, the placenta-derived growth factor (PlGF), is gaining increased attention as a potent direct

Table 9.1   Rebuilding the infarcted heart: growth factors, chemokines, cardioprotectives, transcription factors, and agents that act on intercellular matrix

	Molecular targets	*Effect on progenitor cells*
Growth factors	VEGF receptors expressed on endothelial	Mobilization of EPC
VEGF	cells, monocytes, hematopoietic stem	Improves survival and differentiation
	cells; stimulates proliferation,	of EPC
	migration, and tube formation	
PlGF	VEGF receptor 1 (cross-talk with	Mobilization of hematopoietic stem
	VEGF receptor 2)	cells and EPC
FGF	FGF receptors expressed on	Included in EPC culturing media
	endothelial cells, smooth muscle	
	cells, and myoblasts; stimulates	
	proliferation	
G-CSF	Activates G-CSF receptors on	Mobilization of hematopoietic stem
	hematopoietic and non-hematopoietic	cells (? Effects on resident cardiac
	cells, synergistic action with SDF1,	stem cells) and granulocytes
	Activation of Jak–Stat pathway	
	thereby inhibition of apoptosis	
GM-CSF	Activates monocytic cells,	Mobilization of hematopoietic stem
	stimulates arteriogenesis	cells and EPC
SCF	Acts through c-Kit	Acts synergistically with colony
		stimulating factors in mobilizing
		precursor cells
Angiopoietin 1	Tie2 receptor expressed on endothelial	Mobilizes EPC and hematopoietic
	cells; enhances vessel	progenitor cells
	maturation and stability	
HGF	c-Met receptor expressed on various	Attraction of tissue-resident cardiac
	cells including endothelial cells,	stem cells
	cardiac myocytes, progenitor cells	
IGF	IGF receptor expressed on vascular cells	Included in EPC culturing media
	and satellite cells; enhances	
	skeletal muscle regeneration	
Erythropoietin	Activates the Epo receptor, which	Mobilization of EPC
	is expressed on hematopoietic stem cells,	
	EPC, endothelial cells, and cardiac	
	myocytes; improves survival	
FL	Acts through Flt3 receptor	Proliferation, survival and
		differentiation of hematopoietic
		precursor cells
Chemokines		
MCP1	Promotes arteriogenesis by stimulating	Chemoattractant for EPC (?)
	CCR2 receptor on monocytic cells	
Cardioprotective agents		
Akt	Upregulates VEGF, FGF, IGFI, HGF and	
	inhibits apoptotic factors	
	(Bcl2 and caspases)	

Table 9.1 (Continued)

	Molecular targets	Effect on progenitor cells
Thymosin β4	Mediated through *Akt*1	
Transcription factors		
HIF1	Activation of gene expression (e.g. VEGF, VEGF receptor 2, erythropoietin, IGFII, and NO synthase)	
Extracellular matrix proteins		
CCN family (e.g. Cyr61)	Interaction with integrins	
Del1	Integrin binding ($\alpha_v\beta_5$) Upregulation of HOXD3	

VEGF, vascular endothelial growth factor; PlGF, placenta-derived growth factor; FGF, fibroblast growth factor; EPC, endothelial progenitor cells; HGF, hepatocyte growth factor; IGF, insulin-like growth factor; GM-CSF, granulocyte–macrophage colony stimulating factor; G-CSF, granulocyte colony stimulating factor; SCF, stem cell factor; SDF1, stem cell derived factor 1; FL, Flt3 ligand; MCP1, monocyte chemoattractant protein 1; CCR2, C-C chemokine receptor; HIF1, hypoxia inducible factor 1.

activator of VEGF receptor 1 and an amplifier of VEGF receptor 2 signaling. PlGF increases angiogenesis but also promotes a proinflammatory response that accelerates atherosclerosis, probably by activating VEGF receptor 1 positive monocytic cells.[7,8]

The FGF family consists of more than 20 multifunctional proteins that bind to and activate a diverse group of FGF receptors. Activation of the FGF receptors expressed on endothelial cells, smooth muscle cells, and muscle progenitors stimulates their proliferation. FGF1, FGF2, and FGF4 are also known to be potent angiogenic agents that can act synergistically with VEGF.

Hepatocyte growth factor (HGF) was first identified as a factor that promotes liver regeneration. More recently it has been shown to have potent angiogenic effects via promotion of endothelial cell activation. Its cognate receptor c-Met is expressed on multiple cell types including endothelial cells and hematopoietic stem cells.

Additional candidates for therapeutic neovascularization include sonic hedgehog,[9] secretoneurin,[10] angiopoietin 1,[11] erythropoietin,[12,13] and insulin-like growth factor (IGF),[14,15] and

others in earlier phases of development such as regulators of the wnt/frizzled pathway, as shown for the secreted frizzled-related protein FrzA, promote adult angiogenesis.[16,17]

Several potent proangiogenic factors appear to act indirectly via upregulation of other factors. The classic example of this mechanism is hypoxia inducible factor 1α (HIF1α), which upregulates VEGF, erythropoietin, and FGF2.[18–20] This has also been observed in members of the hedgehog (Hh) protein family, which are prototypical embryonic morphogens that can also be activated during postnatal life for tissue repair. For example, sonic hedgehog (Shh) is a potent inducer of neovascularization after ischemia,[9,21] acting both by local upregulation of cytokines and by mobilization and recruitment of local and bone marrow-derived progenitor cells.[22,23] Another more recently described means of augmenting neovessel formation involves modulation of the interstitial matrix environment. Prototypical examples include the extracellular matrix protein Del1, which coordinates integrin expression,[24] and Cyr61, which binds to $\alpha_v\beta_5$ to induce angiogenesis.[25]

Mobilization of bone marrow-derived stem (progenitor) cells

The therapeutic mobilization of stem cells from the bone marrow (BM) was initially postulated by hematologists as a means to accelerate recovery after cancer chemotherapy.[26] The discovery that BM includes various stem cells spawned the strategy of directly mobilizing and homing BM cells into the heart to regenerate injured tissue.[27] Resident side population cells[28] and lineage negative, c-*kit* positive cells[27] were shown to differentiate into endothelial cells, smooth muscle cells, and cardiomyocytes in a murine MI model. Recently, there has been a growing body of evidence that the endogenous mobilization of BM cells could be induced by local or systemic use of vascular endothelial growth factor (VEGF),[29–31] placental growth factor (PlGF),[8] G-CSF (granulocyte colony stimulating factor),[27] stromal cell derived factor 1 (SDF1),[32] and GM-CSF (granulocyte–monocyte colony stimulating factor).[33,34]

G-CSF is a potent hematopoietic cytokine that influences the proliferation, survival, maturation, and functional activation of granulocytes. It is involved in the mobilization of granulocytes, stem (progenitor) cells from the BM, into the circulation.[35] G-CSF is reported to have a direct action on non-hematopoietic cells expressing G-CSF receptors such as cardiomyocytes, endothelial cells, and neuronal cells.[36] The process of mobilization is not fully understood, but appears to be mediated through the binding of G-CSF to a specific cell-surface receptor, the G-CSF receptor, leading to the subsequent digestion of adhesion molecules by enzyme release, and through trophic chemokines. Stromal cell derived factor 1 (SDF1) and its receptor CXCR4 seem to play a central role.[37] Animal studies suggest that a combination of treatment with VEGF-A gene transfer followed by G-CSF mobilization of stem cells might be superior to either of the therapies alone.[38]

Stem cell factor (SCF) was cloned as a ligand for c-*kit*.[39] SCF exerts its activity at the early stages of hematopoiesis in the bone marrow and acts synergistically with colony stimulating factors. Flt3 is a receptor expressed predominantly on hematopoietic stem cells (HSCs) and progenitors and has many overlapping activities with c-*kit*. FL (Flt3 ligand) belongs to a family of hematopoietic cytokines, including SCF and macrophage colony stimulating factor (M-CSF), that are specific for class III tyrosine kinase receptors.[40] FL plays a central role in the proliferation, survival, and differentiation of early hematopoietic precursor cells. FL is usually not efficient as a single cytokine, but with G-CSF it exerts synergistic effects on the mobilization and engraftment of HSCs.[41]

GM-CSF is a cytokine that stimulates the growth and differentiation of granulocyte and macrophage precursor cells in vitro.[34] It induces peripheral monocytosis and prolongs the lifespan of monocytes via a reduction of apoptosis.

Cardioprotection

The survival factor Akt has also been shown to be capable of augmenting tissue perfusion[42,43] and restoring or preserving tissue integrity in ischemic myocardium, illustrating the potential benefit of exploiting signaling pathways. At 4 weeks after coronary artery ligation in mice, treatment with thymosin β4 resulted in a near doubling in LV ejection fraction (LVEF) (58% vs 28%).[44] This effect may be mediated through activation of Akt1, which has the dual function of upregulating expression of VEGF, FGF, IGFI, and HGF and inhibiting apoptotic factors (Bcl2 and caspases). In a rat infarct model, Akt1 overexpression restored 80–90% of lost myocardial volume and completely normalized systolic and diastolic cardiac function in a dose-dependent manner.[45] Interestingly, even the culture medium taken from Akt-overexpressing stem cells significantly limited infarct size and improved ventricular function.[46]

When given early after MI in a rat model, G-CSF decreases apoptotic death in cardiomyoctyes, which correlates with decreased infarct size. G-CSF has been shown to activate the Jak–Stat signal transduction pathway, which consequently stimulates the production of several antiapoptotic proteins.[47]

Additional considerations

The underlying mechanisms of cytokine action are complex. While the various stem (progenitor) cell populations within BM may exert a therapeutic effect by direct cellular differentiation of stem cells, paracrine action is also a major mechanism to mediate therapeutic effects of BM-derived cells.[48,49] Accumulating evidence suggests that various biologically active molecules such as antiapoptotic and angiogenic factors derived from recruited BM cells in the myocardium could help endangered myocardium survive, accelerate the recovery of ischemic and stunned myocardium, and amplify function in non-ischemic zones. Angiogenic factors released include VEGF-A, VEGF-C,[50] angiopoietins,[51] and matrix metalloproteinases.[52]

Cytokines also modulate adhesion molecules on the mobilized HSCs (lin–/Sca1+/c-Kit+ cells). It appears that the added benefit of cytokine combination is not restricted to the quantitative increase in mobilization but also induces qualitative changes that favor the homing of HSCs into myocardium. In addition, in a murine model of infarction with G-CSF-induced improvement in left ventricular function, enhanced arteriogenesis and an increase in intercellular adhesion molecule 1 (ICAM1) expression on endothelial cells were observed.[53]

Experimental Experience

Animal experience

Animal studies have shown a beneficial effect of G-CSF mobilization of stem cells on LV function after MI, regeneration of myocardium via the induction of myogenesis and vasculogenesis, and diminished postinfarction remodeling.[27,54] Orlic et al[27] injected splenectomized mice with recombinant rat SCF and recombinant human G-CSF to mobilize stem cells for 5 days, then ligated the coronary artery, and continued the treatment with SCF and G-CSF for 3 days. The LVEF improved significantly, possibly due to the formation of new myocytes, arterioles, and capillaries. Although this study demonstrated

regenerating cardiomyocytes and vessels by bromodeoxyuridine (BrdU) and Ki67 immunostaining, it did not prove direct transdifferentiation of mobilized BM cells into myocardial cells. These effects on improving LVEF and reducing remodeling were confirmed by Minatoguchi et al in their experiments with G-CSF after reperfused MI in rabbits.[55] In contrast, G-CSF failed to improve myocardial function in a rat arterial ligation MI model.[56] The mechanism of action of G-CSF in inducing cardiac homing of BM cells to regenerate hearts was challenged by the study of Harada et al.[47] Harada et al showed that G-CSF directly binds G-CSF receptors present on multiple myocardial cells and activates its downstream signals such as the Jak–Stat pathway, thereby reducing myocardial apoptosis, increasing angiogenesis, and favorably remodeling infarcted myocardium.

Beohar et al[57] used an ischemia reperfusion porcine model of myocardial infarction (90 minutes occlusion followed by reperfusion). An early treatment group (G-CSF 10 µg/kg/day every other day for 20 days beginning after reperfusion) and a delayed treatment group (given G-CSF 10 µg/kg/day daily for 10 days beginning 5 days post-MI) were compared to controls (MI only). At 56 days, cardiac magnetic resonance imaging (CMR) showed that the change in end-diastolic volume was 53% less in the early ($p = 0.005$) and 24% greater in the delayed ($p = NS$) group compared to controls. The delayed group also showed a 60% relative increase in normalized infarct mass (infarct mass/LV mass) ($p = 0.055$) and an 88% relative increase in the expansion index as compared to controls ($p = 0.003$). The delayed but not the early group had decreased arteriolar density in the mid-scar. Dawn et al[58] used an ischemia–reperfusion murine model. They found that a combination of G-CSF plus FL regenerated injured heart to a greater extent histopathologically and functionally than G-CSF plus SCF or G-CSF alone. G-CSF alone showed no benefit compared to controls.

Tomita et al[59] and Hou et al[60] reported that G-CSF administration prompted the migration of BM cells to the damaged heart and improved the ultrastructure of cardiomyocytes in adriamycin-induced dilated cardiomyopathy in rats.

Maekawa et al[61] reported a study using a model of MI that was produced in Wistar rats by ligation of the left coronary artery. The MI group was randomized to receive GM-CSF inducer (romurtide 200 μg/kg/day for 7 consecutive days) (MI/Ro) or saline (MI/C). The GM-CSF induction by romurtide facilitated infarct expansion in association with the promotion of monocyte recruitment and inappropriate collagen synthesis in the infarcted region during the early phase of MI.

Taken together, these data suggest that important differences in therapeutic effect may exist based on species, cytokine used, timing of cytokine administration, combination of cytokine therapy, and myocardial reperfusion.

The human experience

Trials of G-CSF treatment after ST-elevation myocardial infarction
The promising, although by no means consistent, results of animal studies of cytokine therapy, especially with G-CSF, along with the ease of its administration led to human clinical trials. All published clinical studies of G-CSF treatment after ST-elevation myocardial infarction (STEMI) are summarized in Tables 9.2 and 9.3. The initial small clinical phase I trials with G-CSF treatment after acute MI treated with percutaneous coronary intervention (PCI) supported the animal experience which showed that G-CSF treatment improved LV function (Tables 9.2 and 9.3).[36,63,65,66,70] In the FIRSTLINE-AMI trial, 6-months follow-up of 50 patients[66] and 1-year follow-up of 30 patients[70] have been published. The trial was a phase I randomized but open-label trial of G-CSF treatment initiated within 90 minutes after primary PCI for STEMI. The control group did not receive placebo injections, but had identical follow-up. The G-CSF-treated patients had a significant improvement in LV function with enhanced systolic wall thickening in the infarct zone and an increase in LVEF (Table 9.3). In contrast, the control group had less systolic wall thickening and a decrease in LVEF.[66]

Three double-blind randomized placebo-controlled G-CSF trials did not confirm the uncontrolled phase I trial results (Tables 9.2 and 9.3).[67–69] In the stem cells in myocardial infarction (STEMMI) trial, a total of 78 patients were treated with primary PCI for STEMI.[67] This study showed that G-CSF BM stem cell mobilization did not improve LV function or reduce infarct size. The placebo-treated patients had the same improvement in cardiac parameters, including LVEF, as seen in the G-CSF-treated groups. The results were comparable to CMR measurements obtained in studies of cardiac function after primary PCI.[71,72]

The double-blind, placebo-controlled REVIVAL-2 G-CSF trial[68] was designed to be almost identical to the STEMMI trial, except that baseline imaging studies were performed later and G-CSF treatment was initiated later (5 days after the primary PCI vs immediately after PCI). In the REVIVAL-2 study, there was no improvement in the primary endpoint of the change in infarct size by scintigraphy from baseline to follow-up. The size of infarct reduction was identical in the G-CSF group and the placebo group. The LVEF in the G-CSF group when compared with the placebo group also did not show any improvement (Tables 9.2 and 9.3). This is consistent with the STEMMI trial results, which did not demonstrate any effect of G-CSF treatment on change in infarct size.

The effect of mobilization of stem cells in patients with subacute STEMI and late revascularization between 6 hours and 7 days after onset of angina was investigated in the double-blind, placebo-controlled G-CSF-STEMI trial.[69] At 3-months follow-up, improvement in LVEF was identical in G-CSF and placebo groups (Table 9.3).

The discrepancy in results between the initial open-label and the double-blind placebo-controlled STEMMI and REVIVAL-2 trials emphasizes the need for blinding and placebo controls in the evaluation of new stem cell therapies. Treatment with primary PCI after STEMI in most studies results in a significant recovery of LV function. Additional treatment with mobilization of bone marrow stem cells by subcutaneous injections of G-CSF starting within 5 days after primary PCI had no influence on infarct size and LV function. Further studies addressing the

Table 9.2   Non-blinded studies of G-CSF therapy in patients with acute myocardial infarction

Study	Design	G-CSF dose and duration	Endpoint evaluation and duration of follow-up	Groups	Δ EF	Myocardial perfusion	Δ End-diastolic volume (ml)	Δ End-systolic volume (ml)	Δ Systolic wall thickening in infarct area
Kuethe et al[36]	Non-randomized, open-label	10 μg/kg/day, mean 7 days, starting 48 hours after reperfusion	SPECT, 3 months	G-CSF = 14	Δ = 7.8	↑	Δ = 3.7	NA	NA
				Control = 9	Δ = 3.2 p = NS	→ p = 0.037	Δ = 6.5 p = NS	NA	NA
Kang et al,[62] MAGIC	Randomized, open-label	10 μg/kg/day, 4 days	SPECT, 6 months	Cell infusion = 7	Δ = 6.4 p = 0.005 vs control	↑	NA	NA	NA
				G-CSF = 3	Δ = −1.0 p = NS vs control	→	NA	NA	NA
				Control = 1	Δ = NA	NA	NA	NA	NA
Suarez de Lezo et al[63]	Observational	10 μg/kg/day, 10 days	Left ventricular angiography, 3 months	G-CSF = 13	Δ = 6.2	↑	NA	NA	NA
Steinwender et al[64]	Non-randomized, open-label	10 μg/kg/day, 4 days, starting 2nd day after PCI	SPECT, echocardiography, 6 months	G-CSF = 20	Δ = 7.9	↑	Δ = 6.5	Δ = −7.9	NA

EF, ejection fraction; SPECT, single photon emission computed tomography; PCI, percutaneous coronary intervention; NS, not significant; NA, not applicable; ↑, increased; →, no change.

optimal time of G-CSF treatment and the need for combining G-CSF with factors that increase stem cell homing should be considered.

G-CSF treatment in patients with chronic ischemic heart disease   The use of G-CSF has also been tested as a therapeutic modality in chronic ischemic heart disease (Table 9.4). Hill et al[74] treated 16 patients with coronary artery disease (CAD) and angina with G-CSF (10 μg/kg

body weight) for 5 days, resulting in a large increase in CD34+ and CD34+/133+ stem cells. At 1-month follow-up, there was no change in LVEF, in LV wall motion at rest or after stress, in myocarial perfusion, or treadmill exercise times. Wang et al[73] prospectively treated 13 patients with severe occlusive coronary artery disease with G-CSF 5 μg/kg body weight for 6 days and compared them to a control group. There was no difference in the number of segments with perfusion defects

Table 9.3 Blinded studies of G-CSF therapy in patients with acute myocardial infarction (AMI)

Study	Design	GCSF dose and duration	Endpoint evaluation and duration of follow-up	Groups	Δ EF	Myocardial perfusion	Δ End-diastolic volume (ml)	Δ End-systolic volume (ml)	Δ Systolic wall thickening in infarct area
Valgimigli et al[65]	Randomized, single-blinded, placebo-controlled	G-CSF 5 µg/kg/day, 4 days, starting 37 ± 66 hours after symptoms	SPECT, 6 months	G-CSF = 10	Δ = 22 ± 10	↑	Δ = 6% ± 5	NA	NA
				Control = 10	Δ = 14 ± 9 p = 0.074	↑ p = NS	Δ = 11% ± 5 p = 0.058	NA	NA
Ince et al,[66] FIRSTLINE-AMI	Randomized, open-label, blinded evaluation	G-CSF 10 µg/kg/day, 6 days, starting within 89 ± 35 minutes	Echocardiography, 4-months	G-CSF = 25	4-month EF = 54% ± 8	NA	55 ± 5 Δ = 0	NA	Δ = 0.82 mm
				Control = 25	4-month EF = 43% ± 5 p < 0.001	NA	58 ± 4 Δ = 3 p = 0.002	NA	Δ = 0.26 mm p = < 0.001
Ripa et al[67] STEMMI	Randomized, double-blinded, placebo-controlled	G-CSF 10 µg/kg/day, 6 days, starting 1–2 days after AMI	Magnetic resonance imaging 6 months	G-CSF = 39	Δ = 8.5 (CMR)	NA	12.6	-6.9	Δ = 17%
				Control = 39	Δ = 8.2 (CMR) p = 0.9	NA	9.7 p = 0.7	-6.5 p = 1.0	Δ = 17% p = 1.0
Zohlnhöfer et al,[68] REVIVAL-2	Randomized, double-blinded, placebo-	G-CSF 10 µg/kg/day, 5 days, starting	Primary: infarct size by sestamibi scintigraphy at 4–6 months	G-CSF = 56	Δ = + 0.5% ± 3.8	Decrease in infarct size = 6.2% ± 9.1	Δ = -0.9 (ml/m²)	-0.6 (ml/m²)	NA

Table 9.3 (Continued)

Study	Design	GCSF dose and duration	Endpoint evaluation and duration of follow-up	Groups	Δ EF	Myocardial perfusion	Δ End-diastolic volume (ml)	Δ End-systolic volume (ml)	Δ Systolic wall thickening in infarct area
	controlled	5 days after AMI	Secondary: LVEF by magnetic resonance imaging at 4–6 months	Control = 58	Δ = +2.0% ± 4.9 $p = 0.14$	Decrease in infarct size = 4.9% ± 8.9 $p = 0.56$	Δ = −1.8 (ml/m²)	−2.4 (ml/m²)	NA
Engelmann et al,[69] G-CSF-STEMI trial	Randomized, double-blinded, placebo-controlled	G-CSF 10 μg/kg/day, 5 days, starting 6 hours–7 days from symptoms	Magnetic resonance imaging at 3 months	G-CSF = 23	Δ = +6.2% ± 9.0	→	2 ± 42	−5 ± 26	0.5 mm ± 2.0
				Control = 21	Δ = +5.3% ± 9.8 $p = 0.77$	→ $p = $ NS	13 ± 46 $p = $ NS	−2 ± 35 $p = $ NS	0.9 mm ± 2.1 $p = $ NS

LVEF, left ventricular ejection fraction; CMR, cardiac magnetic resonance imaging; ↑, increased; →, no change; all p values are G-CSF therapy vs control.

at rest and stress from baseline to 2-months follow-up in both groups. Surprisingly, LVEF decreased in the G-CSF group from baseline to follow-up as evaluated by CMR and single photon emission computed tomography (SPECT) (p = NS). This finding could indicate an adverse effect of G-CSF on the myocardium, perhaps as the conseqeunce of an inflammatory response in the microcirculation by the mobilized leukocytes and subsequent development of myocardial fibrosis. A marked improvement in angina score and reduction in the need for nitroglycerine at the 2-months follow-up visit was seen after G-CSF treatment.[73] These effects were limited to the nine patients with a pronounced mobilization into the peripheral circulation of CD34+ stem cells from the bone marrow by G-CSF treatment. This finding supports the notion that stem cell mobilization is needed to acheive a clinical benefit.

Trials of VEGF protein for the treatment of coronary artery disease
Therapy with VEGF protein has been shown in preclinical studies to enhance collateral blood flow in an animal model of chronic myocardial ischemia.[77–80] Several phase I studies have been performed to assess the safety and feasibility of recombinant VEGF protein for therapeutic angiogenesis in patients with intractable myocardial ischemia who were not candidates for mechanical revascularization. Patients in these studies showed improvements in myocardial perfusion, increased collateral vessel formation on follow-up angiography, and a reduction in Canadian Cardiovascular Society (CCS) angina classification.[81,82]

The potential of recombinant VEGF for therapeutic angiogenesis was subsequently tested in a double-blind placebo-controlled trial (n = 178) of patients with inoperable CAD and stable angina.[83] Subjects were randomized to receive placebo or one of two doses of recombinant VEGF: 17 ng/kg/min (low-dose) and 50 ng/kg/min (high-dose). The primary endpoint of the trial was change in exercise treadmill times from baseline to day 60 between groups. Intracoronary and intravenous infusion of recombinant VEGF was well tolerated. The study failed to show a significant benefit in

exercise time in patients treated with recombinant VEGF at 60 days after treatment. There was a trend towards improved outcomes in the high-dose group at 120 days after treatment. Possible explanations for the findings of this study include an inadequate dose of recombinant VEGF, mixed routes of administration, and early time points to assess efficacy. This study also demonstrated the potential importance of the placebo effect in uncontrolled trials of therapeutic angiogenesis, especially when angina is used as a clinical endpoint.

Ripa et al[84] performed a clinical study to evaluate the safety and clinical effect of VEGF-A$_{165}$ gene transfer followed by bone marrow stimulation with G-CSF in patients with severe occlusive CAD. The combined treatment with VEGF-A$_{165}$ gene and G-CSF failed to induce vasculogenesis and did not improve the symptoms in patients with chronic myocardial ischemia.[84] However, the treatment was safe, and in opposition to the trial by Wang et al,[73] there was no deterioration in LVEF after G-CSF treatment as assessed by CMR and SPECT.

Trials of GM-CSF therapy
Seiler et al[34] recently reported the effects of intracoronary and systemic administration of GM-CSF in patients with CAD who were either not candidates for or refused coronary artery bypass graft surgery. In this randomized, double-blind, placebo-controlled study, an invasive measure of collateral artery blood flow (estimated by coronary artery pressure distal to balloon occlusion) before and after administration of GM-CSF or placebo indicated improved collateral flow in the GM-CSF group at 2 weeks, but not in the placebo group, with reduced electrocardiogram (ECG) signs of myocardial ischemia during coronary balloon occlusion. The low quantity of BM stem cells mobilized with GM-CSF in this study could indicate that the coronary vascular benefit determined may have resulted from direct cytokine effects on angiogenesis or on collateral vascular dilator tone with improved regional blood flow. No clinically relevant endpoints (e.g. exercise-induced myocardial ischemia or LV contractile response to stress) were assessed in this study.

Timing-dependent effects of cytokine therapy

The results of Beohar et al[57] in a porcine MI model suggest that G-CSF administration immediately post-MI may favorably impact on remodeling while late treatment may be harmful. The differential effects observed in this study based on dose timing of post-MI G-CSF administration suggest that a therapeutic window exists. Differing patterns of efficacy are also evident in four recent human trials depending on the dose timing and duration of G-CSF therapy following acute MI.[62,67,68,70]

The time-dependent effects of G-CSF post-MI may be direct, cytokine-mediated, or related to BM-derived stem cell recruitment. Early after MI induction in rats, the numbers of G-CSF receptors on cardiomyocytes are markedly increased.[47] When given early after MI, G-CSF decreased apoptotic death through the Jak–Stat signal transduction pathway in cardiomyoctyes, which correlated with decreased infarct size. Such a protective effect of G-CSF may be lost 5 days post-MI when myocardial necrosis has already progressed. Of note, the beneficial effect of G-CSF on LV function was attenuated when the initiation of therapy was delayed by several days.

An important issue might be a mismatch between the activation of homing factors in the necrotic myocardium and circulating stem cells, and thereby due to inadequately timed G-CSF treatment. The homing factor SDF1 is thought to play a crucial role in the induction of stem cell engraftment to ischemic tissue.[85] In a murine model of MI, these cytokines were upregulated immediately after MI and downregulated over a 7-day period. The delayed administration of G-CSF (56 days post-MI) only positively affected remodeling when SDF1 expression was enhanced in the infarcted tissue. This implies that the success of post-MI G-CSF therapy may rely upon the early, cytokine-mediated localization of mobilized stem cells to the injured myocardium.[85,86] Although pretreatment with growth factors prior to the induction of MI can augment stem cell recruitment, this treatment strategy is not clinically applicable for acute MI.[87]

In humans it has recently been demonstrated that plasma SDF1 and the vascular growth factors VEGF-A and FGF increase slowly during the first week after MI and reach a maximum concentration after 3 weeks.[88] Therefore, the G-CSF mobilization of stem cells within the first days after MI might not be optimal due to a low concentration of the homing factor SDF1 within the myocardium. Wang et al[89] demonstrated that in human myocardium after short-term acute ischemia there was no induction of SDF1 or vascular growth factor genes. Therefore, a more optimal time point for G-CSF stem cell therapy to induce vasculogenesis in ischemic or necrotic myocardium might be 1–3 weeks after a STEMI.

The ultimate lineage and properties of cells mobilized from the BM in the early stages following MI may differ from those mobilized several days later. Alternatively, the local milieu in the infarct zone early or late after infarction might differentially influence stem cell lineage and their effects. Moreover, G-CSF is known to stimulate the development of committed progenitor cells into neutrophils and macrophages,[90] and consequently unregulated inflammatory cell production could theoretically worsen cardiac remodeling following MI.[91]

Because in most of the trials a 10–20-fold mobilization of stem cells from the BM into the peripheral circulation has been seen, inadequate stem cell mobilization is unlikely to be reponsible for failure to demonstrate a benefit.

The impact of coronary reperfusion

Post-MI administration of G-CSF has been shown to improve LV function and limit remodeling in small and large animal models[55,92–94] and more recently in human trials.[70] However, most of the animal models employed chronic arterial ligation. The models used by Beohar et al[57] and Dawn et al[58] more closely resemble the typical clinical scenario of acute MI followed by early reperfusion. The time course of homing signal release and the ability of stem cells to be delivered into the area of infarction may be different after early reperfusion. Adverse post-MI LV remodeling has been shown to improve as a result of early and sustained reperfusion.[72,74] It is also possible that the benefits of myocardial reperfusion may overshadow the effects of post-MI G-CSF.

Table 9.4 Mobilization of stem cells by G-CSF in patients with chronic ischemic heart disease

Study	Design	Cytokine dose and duration	Endpoint evaluation and follow-up	Groups	ΔEF	Myocardial perfusion	End-diastolic volume (ml)	End-systolic volume (ml)	Myocardial ischemia
Wang et al[73]	Non-randomized	G-CSF 5 µg/kg/day, 6 days	SPECT/MRI, echocardiography, 2 months	G-CSF = 13	Δ = -4	↑	Δ = -7	Δ = 2	↓
				Control = 16					
Hill et al[74]	Non-randomized	G-CSF 10 µg/kg/day, 5 days	MRI, 1 month	G-CSF = 16	Δ = -3	↑	Δ = 15	Δ = 14	↑
					Δ = -0.3	↑	NA	NA	↑
Boyle et al[75]	Non-randomized	G-CSF 10 µg/kg/day, 4 days	Angiography, 12 months	Cell infusion = 5	Δ = 4.2	↑a	NA	NA	↓
Ripa et al[76]	Non-randomized	G-CSF 10 µg/kg/day, 6 days	SPECT/MRI, echocardiography, 3 months	G-CSF = 16	↑	↑	↑	↑	↑
				Control = 16	↑	↑	↑	↑	↑

MRI, magnetic resonance imaging; ↑, increased; →, no change; ↓, decreased; ªincrease in coronary blood flow.

Safety of Cytokine Therapy

Prior hematological studies raised concerns on the safety of using G-CSF/GM-CSF in unstable patients. In fact, recent clinical trials[62,74] using G-CSF/GM-CSF in patients with acute MI or angina revealed an apparent increase in acute coronary syndromes and in-stent restenosis. In all trials, subcutaneous injections of G-CSF were well tolerated. A few patients did report mild musculoskeletal pain.

Safety data from a total of 167 patients treated with G-CSF early after STEMI have been published. Two patients died in the follow-up period,[36,68] one after a splenic rupture[63] and the other after subacute stent thrombosis.[67,76] One trial[62] has indicated that G-CSF treatment might increase the progression of atherosclerosis and in-stent restenosis in patients treated with primary PCI. In this study, the peripheral circulating stem cells were collected after 3 days of G-CSF treatment and then injected into the coronary artery during PCI. In a recent unblinded uncontrolled study, G-CSF treatment was initiated 2 days after primary PCI and the collected stem cells injected 4 days later into the infarct-related coronary artery.[64] In this trial a 40% restenosis rate was seen at follow-up. In addition, two of the 20 patients studied suffered a myocardial infarction related to in-stent restenosis between 2 and 6 months after therapy. To the contrary, the STEMMI trial,[67] the FIRSTLINE-AMI trial,[66,70] and the REVIVAL-2 trial[68] demonstrated identical restenosis rates in G-CSF-treated and control groups. This discrepancy in restenosis rates could be because Kang et al[62] performed PCI at a time when the G-CSF-induced increase in leukocytes may have been at a peak level, which could heighten the inflammatory response in the culprit lesion.

It is conceivable that cytokines mobilize unwanted inflammatory cells and promote the secretion of inflammatory mediators such as monocyte chemoattractant protein 1 (MCP1) and C-reactive protein (CRP), contributing to the rupture of atherosclerotic plaques and aggravation of vascular inflammation. The clinical trials of patients with acute MI showed no worsening of myocardial inflammation in those treated with G-CSF.[36,65–70,76] Another potential concern is

that patients with more severe CAD may be more susceptible to inflammation and plaque destabilization after G-CSF therapy. Indeed, serious vascular adverse events were reported in two patients (13%) by Hill et al[74] and one patient (20%) by Boyle et al.[75] In a different study, a total of 29 patients[73,84] received G-CSF without any serious vascular adverse events. The limited experience to date does not allow for meaningful conclusions regarding the safety of G-CSF treatment in chronic ischemic heart disease.[95]

None of the clinical trials with G-CSF treatment in ischemic heart disease has shown a proarrhythmic effect. A recent experiment in mice actually showed a reduced inducibility of ventricular arrhythmias after G-CSF treatment when compared with controls.[96] VEGF protein therapy also has safety concerns. Its use in a porcine model resulted in significant hypotension, probably due to the upregulation of nitric oxide synthase.[97,98]

There are three important theoretical long-term concerns regarding therapeutic angiogenesis. First, it is possible that the induction of angiogenesis may increase the risk of neoplastic disease and malignancy. However, no clinical trial has revealed evidence that angiogenic cytokines increase the risk of tumor development. Second, the induction or worsening of retinopathy has been another concern in clinical trials of therapeutic angiogenesis. However, the trials of therapeutic angiogenesis have not demonstrated an untoward effect of angiogenic cytokines on the development of retinopathy.[99] The third major concern regarding therapeutic angiogenesis for vascular disease is that the induction of angiogenesis may stimulate the development and progression of atherosclerotic plaques leading to an increase in unstable vascular syndromes. While inhibitors of angiogenesis may lead to regression of atherosclerotic plaque in small animal models of fatty streak formation, the converse has not been shown in clinical trials of angiogenesis. Angiogenic therapy may, in fact, preserve endothelial integrity and thereby suppress intimal thickening.[100] Clinical trials of angiogenesis have not shown an increase in adverse cardiovascular events in patients treated with angiogenic cytokines compared to controls.

It is important to remember that patients with end-stage vascular disease are generally elderly, and are at risk for malignancy and retinopathy because of their underlying risk factors and comorbidities (age, smoking, diabetes). Therefore, candidates for trials of vascular gene therapy are likely to develop such complications as part of the natural history of their disease states and not necessarily because of therapy with angiogenic agents. Nevertheless, painstaking efforts must continually be taken to ensure that candidates for clinical trials of angiogenesis and cytokine combinations are thoroughly screened for malignant and premalignant conditions as well as retinopathy, and monitored until these risks are completely understood.

Future Directions

Cytokine therapy for cardiac repair offers hope as an attractive approach for patients and physicians. Although the outcomes of human clinical trials with G-CSF alone after acute MI have been disappointing, these results do not exclude the possibility that G-CSF may be effective as a component of a treatment strategy combining several cytokines with or without stem cells. Also, in patients with chronic CAD the combination SDF1 gene and G-CSF therapy holds promise.

A better appreciation of the myocardial cellular environment after MI may be critical for successful myocardial regeneration. Growth factors such as IGFI and HGF have angiogenic and antiapoptotic properties as well as an ability to induce the expression of collagen-degrading metalloproteinases that create an extracellular matrix receptive to cell migration. When selecting cytokines for future combination therapy the complexity of the targets and the injury milieu will need to be more fully understood.

Many questions remain concerning mechanisms involved in cytokine therapy such as the relationship between the magnitude of stem cell mobilization and the extent of myocardial regeneration, the ideal type of BM cells mobilized, signaling pathways, the effects on resident cardiac stem cells,[101] and the effect on matrix reorganization. It

also needs to be determined whether cytokine therapy can serve as a complement or as an alternative to cell therapy.

Summary

The burden of ischemic cardiovascular disease continues to grow. Despite all the advancements in the acute and long-term managment of CAD, there is still a need for novel strategies to further improve clinical outcomes. Although short-term cell mobilization with G-CSF appears safe in patients with acute MI, more experience is needed in patients with chronic CAD. In patients with acute MI, there is significant recovery of the LV function after primary PCI. However, convincing additional benefit from G-CSF treatment on LV function or myocardial perfusion has yet to be shown.

A large body of data suggests the safety and feasibility of therapeutic angiogenesis. However, proving the efficacy of therapeutic angiogenesis will require large phase III randomized placebo-controlled trials. Several challenges remain prior to their inception. The ideal agent for the induction of therapeutic angiogenesis needs to be identified. VEGF, FGF, and stem (progenitor) cells have been the most actively studied, but future studies are being planned on other potential angiogenic factors such as hepatocyte growth factor and sonic hedgehog. Additionally, recent preclinical data suggest that a combination of stem (progenitor) cells with angiogenic cytokines may be more effective at inducing angiogenesis.[38] The ideal form of the angiogenic cytokine needs to be elucidated. The optimal dose and timing of therapy of each of the potential angiogenic agents remain to be determined. Finally, a consensus needs to be established regarding the best clinical endpoint to assess and ideal time point to assess the efficacy of these therapies.

References

1. Pfeffer MA, Braunwald E. Ventricular remodeling after myocardial infarction. Experimental observations and clinical implications. Circulation 1990; 81: 1161–72.

2. Frangogiannis NG, Smith CW, Entman ML. The inflammatory response in myocardial infarction. Cardiovasc Res 2002; 53: 31–47.

3. Bolognese L, Neskovic AN, Parodi G et al. Left ventricular remodeling after primary coronary angioplasty: patterns of left ventricular dilation and long-term prognostic implications. Circulation 2002; 106: 2351–7.

4. Giannuzzi P, Temporelli PL, Bosimini E et al. Heterogeneity of left ventricular remodeling after acute myocardial infarction: results of the Gruppo Italiano per lo Studio della Sopravvivenza nell'Infarto Miocardico-3 Echo Substudy. Am Heart J 2001; 141: 131–8.

5. Yanagisawa-Miwa A, Uchida Y, Nakamura F et al. Salvage of infarcted myocardium by angiogenic action of basic fibroblast growth factor. Science 1992; 257: 1401–3.

6. Takeshita S, Zheng LP, Brogi E et al. Therapeutic angiogenesis. A single intraarterial bolus of vascular endothelial growth factor augments revascularization in a rabbit ischemic hind limb model. J Clin Invest 1994; 93: 662–70.

7. Carmeliet P, Moons L, Luttun A et al. Synergism between vascular endothelial growth factor and placental growth factor contributes to angiogenesis and plasma extravasation in pathological conditions. Nat Med 2001; 7: 575–83.

8. Luttun A, Tjwa M, Moons L et al. Revascularization of ischemic tissues by PlGF treatment, and inhibition of tumor angiogenesis, arthritis and atherosclerosis by anti-Flt1. Nat Med 2002; 8: 831–40.

9. Pola R, Ling LE, Aprahamian TR et al. Postnatal recapitulation of embryonic hedgehog pathway in response to skeletal muscle ischemia. Circulation 2003; 108: 479–85.

10. Kirchmair R, Gander R, Egger M et al. The neuropeptide secretoneurin acts as a direct angiogenic cytokine in vitro and in vivo. Circulation 2004; 109: 777–83.

11. Asahara T, Chen D, Takahashi T et al. Tie2 receptor ligands, angiopoietin-1 and angiopoietin-2, modulate VEGF-induced postnatal neovascularization. Circ Res 1998; 83: 233–40.

12. Anagnostou A, Lee ES, Kessimian N, Levinson R, Steiner M. Erythropoietin has a mitogenic and positive chemotactic effect on endothelial cells. Proc Natl Acad Sci USA 1990; 87: 5978–82.

13. Heeschen C, Aicher A, Lehmann R et al. Erythropoietin is a potent physiologic stimulus for endothelial progenitor cell mobilization. Blood 2003; 102: 1340–6.

14. Miele C, Rochford JJ, Filippa N, Giorgetti-Peraldi S, Van Obberghen E. Insulin and insulin-like growth factor-I induce vascular endothelial growth factor mRNA expression via different signaling pathways. J Biol Chem 2000; 275: 21695–702.

15. Kajstura J, Fiordaliso F, Andreoli AM et al. IGF-1 overexpression inhibits the development of diabetic cardiomyopathy and angiotensin II-mediated oxidative stress. Diabetes 2001; 50: 1414–24.

16. Losordo DW, Dimmeler S. Therapeutic angiogenesis and vasculogenesis for ischemic disease. Part I: angiogenic cytokines. Circulation 2004; 109: 2487–91.

17. Losordo DW, Dimmeler S. Therapeutic angiogenesis and vasculogenesis for ischemic disease: part II: cell-based therapies. Circulation 2004; 109: 2692–7.

18. Wang GL, Jiang BH, Rue EA, Semenza GL. Hypoxia-inducible factor 1 is a basic-helix-loop-helix-PAS heterodimer regulated by cellular O_2 tension. Proc Natl Acad Sci USA 1995; 92: 5510–14.

19. Melillo G, Musso T, Sica A et al. A hypoxia-responsive element mediates a novel pathway of activation of the inducible nitric oxide synthase promoter. J Exp Med 1995; 182: 1683–93.

20. Shyu KG, Vincent KA Luo Y et al. Naked DNA encoding an hypoxia-inducible factor 1a (HIF-1a)/VP16 hybrid transcription factor enhances angiogenesis in rabbit hindlimb ischemia: an alternate method for therapeutic angiogenesis utilizing a transcriptional regulatory system. Circulation 1998; 98: I–68.

21. Pola R, Ling LE, Silver M et al. The morphogen Sonic hedgehog is an indirect angiogenic agent upregulating two families of angiogenic growth factors. Nat Med 2001; 7: 706–11.

22. Kusano KF, Allendoerfer KL, Munger W et al. Sonic hedgehog induces arteriogenesis in diabetic vasa nervorum and restores function in diabetic neuropathy. Arterioscler Thromb Vasc Biol 2004; 24: 2102–7.

23. Kusano KF, Pola R, Murayama T et al. Sonic hedgehog myocardial gene therapy: tissue repair through transient reconstitution of embryonic signaling. Nat Med 2005; 11: 1197–204.

24. Zhong J, Eliceiri B, Stupack D et al. Neovascularization of ischemic tissues by gene delivery of the extracellular matrix protein Del-1. J Clin Invest 2003; 112: 30–41.

25. Babic AM, Kireeva ML, Kolesnikova TV, Lau LF. CYR61, a product of a growth factor-inducible immediate early gene, promotes angiogenesis and tumor growth. Proc Natl Acad Sci USA 1998; 95: 6355–60.

26. Morstyn G, Campbell L, Souza LM et al. Effect of granulocyte colony stimulating factor on neutropenia induced by cytotoxic chemotherapy. Lancet 1988; 1: 667–72.

27. Orlic D, Kajstura J, Chimenti S et al. Mobilized bone marrow cells repair the infarcted heart, improving function and survival. Proc Natl Acad Sci USA 2001; 98: 10344–9.

28. Jackson KA, Majka SM, Wang H et al. Regeneration of ischemic cardiac muscle and vascular endothelium by adult stem cells. J Clin Invest 2001; 107: 1395–402.

29. Asahara T, Masuda H, Takahashi T et al. Bone marrow origin of endothelial progenitor cells responsible for postnatal vasculogenesis in physiological and pathological neovascularization. Circ Res 1999; 85: 221–8.

30. Kalka C, Masuda H, Takahashi T et al. Vascular endothelial growth factor(165) gene transfer augments circulating endothelial progenitor cells in human subjects. Circ Res 2000; 86: 1198–202.

31. Hattori K, Heissig B, Wu Y et al. Placental growth factor reconstitutes hematopoiesis by recruiting VEGFR1(+) stem cells from bone-marrow microenvironment. Nat Med 2002; 8: 841–9.

32. Yamaguchi J, Kusano KF, Masuo O et al. Stromal cell-derived factor-1 effects on ex vivo expanded endothelial progenitor cell recruitment for ischemic neovascularization. Circulation 2003; 107: 1322–8.

33. Takahashi T, Kalka C, Masuda H et al. Ischemia- and cytokine-induced mobilization of bone marrow-derived endothelial progenitor cells for neovascularization. Nat Med 1999; 5: 434–8.

34. Seiler C, Pohl T, Wustmann K et al. Promotion of collateral growth by granulocyte-macrophage colony-stimulating factor in patients with coronary artery disease: a randomized, double-blind, placebo-controlled study. Circulation 2001; 104: 2012–17.

35. Anderlini P, Donato M, Chan KW et al. Allogeneic blood progenitor cell collection in normal donors after mobilization with filgrastim: the M.D. Anderson Cancer Center experience. Transfusion 1999; 39: 555–60.

36. Kuethe F, Figulla HR, Herzau M et al. Treatment with granulocyte colony-stimulating factor for mobilization of bone marrow cells in patients with acute myocardial infarction. Am Heart J 2005; 150: 115.

37. Flomenberg N, DiPersio J, Calandra G. Role of CXCR4 chemokine receptor blockade using AMD3100 for mobilization of autologous hematopoietic progenitor cells. Acta Haematol 2005; 114: 198–205.

38. Kawamoto A, Murayama T, Kusano K et al. Synergistic effect of bone marrow mobilization and vascular endothelial growth factor-2 gene therapy in myocardial ischemia. Circulation 2004; 110: 1398–405.

39. Zsebo K, Williams D, Geissler EN et al. Stem cell factor is encoded at the Sl locus of the mouse and is the ligand for the c-kit tyrosine kinase receptor. Cell 1990; 63: 213–24.

40. Lyman SD, James L, Vanden Bos T et al. Molecular cloning of a ligand for the flt3/flk-2 tyrosine kinase receptor: a proliferative factor for primitive hematopoietic cells. Cell 1993; 75: 1157–67.

41. Neipp MTZ, Zorina T, Domenick MA et al. Effect of FLT3 ligand and granulocyte colony-stimulating factor on expansion and mobilization of facilitating cells and hematopoietic stem cells in mice: kinetics and repopulating potential. Blood 1998; 92: 3177–88.

42. Dimmeler S, Zeiher AM. Akt takes center stage in angiogenesis signaling. Circ Res 2000; 86: 4–5.

43. Shiojima I, Walsh K. Role of Akt signaling in vascular homeostasis and angiogenesis. Circ Res 2002; 90: 1243–50.

44. Bock-Marquette I, Saxena A, White MD, Dimaio JM, Srivastava D. Thymosin beta4 activates integrin-linked kinase and promotes cardiac cell migration, survival and cardiac repair. Nature 2004; 432: 466–72.

45. Mangi AA, Noiseux N, Kong D et al. Mesenchymal stem cells modified with Akt prevent remodeling and restore performance of infarcted hearts. Nat Med 2003; 9: 1195–201.

46. Gnecchi M, He H, Noiseux N et al. Evidence supporting paracrine hypothesis for Akt-modified mesenchymal stem cell-mediated cardiac protection and functional improvement. FASEB J 2006; 20: 661–9.

47. Harada M, Qin Y, Takano H et al. G-CSF prevents cardiac remodeling after myocardial infarction by activating the Jak-Stat pathway in cardiomyocytes. Nat Med 2005; 11: 305–11.

48. Kamihata H, Matsubara H, Nishiue T et al. Implantation of bone marrow mononuclear cells into ischemic myocardium enhances collateral perfusion and regional function via side supply of angioblasts, angiogenic ligands, and cytokines. Circulation 2001; 104: 1046–52.

49. Gnecchi M, He H, Liang OD et al. Paracrine action accounts for marked protection of ischemic heart by Akt-modified mesenchymal stem cells. Nat Med 2005; 11: 367–8.

50. Wartiovaara U, Salven P, Mikkola H et al. Peripheral blood platelets express VEGF-C and VEGF which are released during platelet activation. Thromb Haemost 1998; 80: 171–5.

51. Huang YQ, Li JJ, Karpatkin S. Identification of a family of alternatively spliced mRNA species of angiopoietin-1. Blood 2000; 95: 1993–9.

52. Coussens LM, Tinkle CL, Hanahan D, Werb Z. MMP-9 supplied by bone marrow-derived cells contributes to skin carcinogenesis. Cell 2000; 103: 481–90.

53. Deindl E, Zaruba MM, Brunner S et al. G-CSF administration after myocardial infarction in mice attenuates late ischemic cardiomyopathy by enhanced arteriogenesis. FASEB J 2006; 20: 956–8.

54. Kawamoto A, Gwon HC, Iwaguro H et al. Therapeutic potential of ex vivo expanded endothelial progenitor cells for myocardial ischemia. Circulation 2001; 103: 634–7.

55. Minatoguchi S, Takemura G, Chen XH et al. Acceleration of the healing process and myocardial regeneration may be important as a mechanism of improvement of cardiac function and remodeling by postinfarction granulocyte colony-stimulating factor treatment. Circulation 2004; 109: 2572–80.

56. Werneck-de-Castro JP, Costa ESRH, de Oliveira PF et al. G-CSF does not improve systolic function in a rat model of acute myocardial infarction. Basic Res Cardiol 2006; 101: 494–501.

57. Beohar N, Flaherty JD, Davidson CJ et al. Granulocyte-colony stimulating factor administration after myocardial infarction in a porcine ischemia-reperfusion model: functional and pathological effects of dose timing. Catheter Cardiovasc Interv 2007; 69: 257–65.

58. Dawn B, Guo Y, Rezazadeh A et al. Postinfarct cytokine therapy regenerates cardiac tissue and improves left ventricular function. Circ Res 2006; 98: 1098–105.

59. Tomita S, Ishida M, Nakatani T et al. Bone marrow is a source of regenerated cardiomyocytes in doxorubicin-induced cardiomyopathy and granulocyte colony-stimulating factor enhances migration of bone marrow cells and attenuates cardiotoxicity of doxorubicin under electron microscopy. J Heart Lung Transplant 2004; 23: 577–84.

60. Hou XW, Son J, Wang Y et al. Granulocyte colony-stimulating factor reduces cardiomyocyte apoptosis and improves cardiac function in adriamycin-induced cardiomyopathy in rats. Cardiovasc Drugs Ther 2006; 20: 85–91.

61. Maekawa Y, Anzai T, Yoshikawa T et al. Prognostic significance of peripheral monocytosis after reperfused acute myocardial infarction: a possible role for left ventricular remodeling. J Am Coll Cardiol 2002; 39: 241–6.

62. Kang HJ, Kim HS, Zhang SY et al. Effects of intracoronary infusion of peripheral blood stem-cells mobilised with granulocyte-colony stimulating factor on left ventricular systolic function and restenosis after coronary stenting in myocardial infarction: the MAGIC cell randomised clinical trial. Lancet 2004; 363: 751–6.

63. Suarez de Lezo J, Torres A, Herrera I et al. [Effects of stem-cell mobilization with recombinant human granulocyte colony stimulating factor in patients with percutaneously revascularized acute anterior myocardial infarction]. Rev Esp Cardiol 2005; 58: 253–61.

64. Steinwender C, Hofmann R, Kammler J et al. Effects of peripheral blood stem cell mobilization with granulocyte-colony stimulating factor and their transcoronary transplantation after primary stent implantation for acute myocardial infarction. Am Heart J 2006; 151: 1296.e7–13.

65. Valgimigli M, Rigolin GM, Cittanti C et al. Use of granulocyte-colony stimulating factor during acute myocardial infarction to enhance bone marrow stem cell mobilization in humans: clinical and angiographic safety profile. Eur Heart J 2005; 26: 1838–45.

66. Ince H, Petzsch M, Kleine HD et al. Preservation from left ventricular remodeling by front-integrated revascularization and stem cell liberation in evolving acute myocardial infarction by use of granulocyte-colony-stimulating factor (FIRST-LINE-AMI). Circulation 2005; 112: 3097–106.

67. Ripa RS, Jorgensen E, Wang Y et al. Stem cell mobilization induced by subcutaneous granulocyte-colony stimulating factor to improve cardiac regeneration after acute ST-elevation myocardial infarction: result of the double-blind, randomized, placebo-controlled stem cells in myocardial infarction (STEMMI) trial. Circulation 2006; 113: 1983–92.

68. Zohlnhofer D, Ott I, Mehilli J et al. Stem cell mobilization by granulocyte colony-stimulating factor in patients with acute myocardial infarction: a randomized controlled trial. JAMA 2006; 295: 1003–10.

69. Engelmann MG, Theiss HD, Hennig-Theiss C et al. Autologous bone marrow stem cell mobilization induced by granulocyte colony-stimulating factor after subacute ST-segment elevation myocardial infarction undergoing late revascularization: final results from the G-CSF-STEMI (Granulocyte Colony-Stimulating Factor ST-Segment Elevation Myocardial Infarction) trial. J Am Coll Cardiol 2006; 48: 1712–21.

70. Ince H, Petzsch M, Kleine HD et al. Prevention of left ventricular remodeling with granulocyte colony-stimulating factor after acute myocardial infarction: final 1-year results of the Front-Integrated Revascularization and Stem Cell Liberation in Evolving Acute Myocardial Infarction by Granulocyte Colony-Stimulating Factor (FIRSTLINE-AMI) Trial. Circulation 2005; 112 (9 suppl): I73–80.

71. Baks T, van Geuns RJ, Biagini E et al. Recovery of left ventricular function after primary angioplasty for acute myocardial infarction. Eur Heart J 2005; 26: 1070–7.

72. Stone GW, Grines CL, Cox DA et al. Comparison of angioplasty with stenting, with or without abciximab, in acute myocardial infarction. N Engl J Med 2002; 346: 957–66.

73. Wang Y, Tagil K, Ripa RS et al. Effect of mobilization of bone marrow stem cells by granulocyte colony stimulating factor on clinical symptoms, left ventricular perfusion and function in patients with severe chronic ischemic heart disease. Int J Cardiol 2005; 100: 477–83.

74. Hill JM, Syed MA, Arai AE et al. Outcomes and risks of granulocyte colony-stimulating factor in patients with coronary artery disease. J Am Coll Cardiol 2005; 46: 1643–8.

75. Boyle AJ, Whitbourn R, Schlicht S et al. Intracoronary high-dose CD34+ stem cells in patients with chronic ischemic heart disease: a 12-month follow-up. Int J Cardiol 2006; 109: 21–7.

76. Ripa RS, Wang Y, Jargensen E et al. Safety of bone-marrow stem cell mobilization induced by granulocyte-colony stimulating factor: clinical 30 days blinded results from the stem cells in myocardial infarction (STEMMI) trial. Heart Drug 2005; 5: 177–82.

77. Banai S, Jaklitsch MT, Shou M et al. Angiogenic-induced enhancement of collateral blood flow to ischemic myocardium by vascular endothelial growth factor in dogs. Circulation 1994; 89: 2183–9.

78. Pearlman JD, Hibberd MG, Chuang ML et al. Magnetic resonance mapping demonstrates benefits of VEGF-induced myocardial angiogenesis. Nat Med 1995; 1: 1085–9.

79. Harada K, Friedman M, Lopez JJ et al. Vascular endothelial growth factor administration in chronic myocardial ischemia. Am J Physiol 1996; 270: H1791–802.

80. Lopez JJ, Laham RJ, Stamler A et al. VEGF administration in chronic myocardial ischemia in pigs. Cardiovasc Res 1998; 40: 272–81.

81. Henry TD, Rocha-Singh K, Isner JM et al. Intracoronary administration of recombinant human vascular endothelial growth factor to patients with coronary artery disease. Am Heart J 2001; 142: 872–80.

82. Henry TD, Abraham JA. Review of preclinical and clinical results with vascular endothelial growth factors for therapeutic angiogenesis. Curr Interv Cardiol Rep 2000; 2: 228–41.

83. Henry TD, Annex BH, McKendall GR et al. The VIVA trial: Vascular endothelial growth factor in Ischemia for Vascular Angiogenesis. Circulation 2003; 107: 1359–65.

84. Ripa RS, Wang Y, Jorgensen E et al. Intramyocardial injection of vascular endothelial growth factor-A165 plasmid followed by granulocyte-colony stimulating factor to induce angiogenesis in patients with severe chronic ischaemic heart disease. Eur Heart J 2006; 27: 1785–92.

85. Askari AT, Unzek S, Popovic ZB et al. Effect of stromal-cell-derived factor 1 on stem-cell homing and tissue regeneration in ischaemic cardiomyopathy. Lancet 2003; 362: 697–703.

86. Lee MS, Lill M, Makkar RR. Stem cell transplantation in myocardial infarction. Rev Cardiovasc Med 2004; 5: 82–98.

87. Norol F, Merlet P, Isnard R et al. Influence of mobilized stem cells on myocardial infarct repair in a nonhuman primate model. Blood 2003; 102: 4361–8.

88. Wang Y, Johnsen HE, Mortensen S et al. Changes in circulating mesenchymal stem cells, stem cell homing factor, and vascular growth factors in patients with acute ST elevation myocardial infarction treated with primary percutaneous coronary intervention. Heart 2006; 92: 768–74.

89. Wang Y, Gabrielsen A, Lawler PR et al. Myocardial gene expression of angiogenic factors in human chronic ischemic myocardium: influence of acute ischemia/cardioplegia and reperfusion. Microcirculation 2006; 13: 187–97.

90. Suda T, Suda J, Kajigaya S et al. Effects of recombinant murine granulocyte colony-stimulating factor on granulocyte-macrophage and blast colony formation. Exp Hematol 1987; 15: 958–65.

91. Vandervelde S, van Luyn MJ, Tio RA, Harmsen MC. Signaling factors in stem cell-mediated repair of infarcted myocardium. J Mol Cell Cardiol 2005; 39: 363–76.

92. Orlic D, Hill JM, Arai AE. Stem cells for myocardial regeneration. Circ Res 2002; 91: 1092–102.

93. Iwanaga K, Takano H, Ohtsuka M et al. Effects of G-CSF on cardiac remodeling after acute myocardial infarction in swine. Biochem Biophys Res Commun 2004; 325: 1353–9.

94. Ohtsuka M, Takano H, Zou Y et al. Cytokine therapy prevents left ventricular remodeling and dysfunction after myocardial infarction through neovascularization. FASEB J 2004; 18: 851–3.

95. Wilson RF, Henry TD. Granulocyte colony-stimulating factor and granulocyte-macrophage colony-stimulating factor: double-edged swords. J Am Coll Cardiol 2005; 46: 1649–50.

96. Kuhlmann MT, Kirchhof P, Klocke R et al. G-CSF/SCF reduces inducible arrhythmias in the infarcted heart potentially via increased connexin 43 expression and arteriogenesis. J Exp Med 2006; 203: 87–97.

97. Hariawala MD, Horowitz JR, Esakof D et al. VEGF improves myocardial blood flow but produces EDRF-mediated hypotension in porcine hearts. J Surg Res 1996; 63: 77–82.

98. Horowitz JR, Rivard A, van der Zee R et al. Vascular endothelial growth factor/vascular permeability factor produces nitric oxide-dependent hypotension. Evidence for a maintenance role in quiescent adult endothelium. Arterioscler Thromb Vasc Biol 1997; 17: 2793–800.

99. Vale PR, Rauh G, Wuensch DI, Pieczek A, Schainfeld RM. Influence of vascular endothelial growth factor on diabetic retinopathy. Circulation 1998; 17: I–353.

100. Van Belle E, Tio FO, Chen D et al. Passivation of metallic stents after arterial gene transfer of phVEGF165 inhibits thrombus formation and intimal thickening. J Am Coll Cardiol 1997; 29: 1371–9.

101. Urbanek K, Rota M, Cascapera S et al. Cardiac stem cells possess growth factor-receptor systems that after activation regenerate the infarcted myocardium, improving ventricular function and long-term survival. Circ Res 2005; 97: 663–73.

chapter 10

Surgical and Catheter-Based Intramyocardial Delivery of Stem Cells to the Human Heart

Emerson Perin and Guilherme Silva

Introduction

Stem cell therapy has emerged as a promising new therapy in cardiology. The efficacy of such therapies depends largely on successful delivery. As with any cell delivery method, the main objective is to achieve the concentration of stem cells necessary to repair the damaged region being targeted. To this end, the ideal modality should be safe; cost-effective; useful in a wide range of clinical disease settings and scenarios; easily, adequately, and effectively targeted; and conducive to long-lasting therapeutic effects.

Our current understanding of stem cell biology and kinetics gives us important clues as to how they should be delivered. Intramyocardial injection is the preferred route of delivery in patients with chronic total occlusion of coronary arteries and in disease settings that involve weaker homing signals, such as chronic congestive heart failure. Theoretically, it should also be the most suitable route for delivering larger cells such as skeletal myoblasts and mesenchymal stem cells (MSCs), which are prone to plugging microvessels. Another potential delivery strategy is the mobilization of stem cells from the bone marrow by means of cytokine therapy, with or without peripheral harvesting. However, intramyocardial injections, either directly during open heart surgery or percutaneously through

the transendocardial route, theoretically offer the advantage of higher cell retention. This chapter will address surgical (transepicardial) and catheter-based (transcoronary venous and transendocardial) intramyocardial strategies for stem cell delivery and the experimental and clinical evidence supporting each of them.

Transepicardial Injection

Transepicardial injection of stem cells has been used to deliver stem cells to infarct border zones or areas of infarcted or scarred myocardium during open surgical revascularization procedures. Because this approach requires a sternotomy, it is highly invasive and associated with surgical morbidity. However, it could be easily justified during a planned open-heart procedure, especially since not all areas of the myocardium (such as the septum) can be reached using a direct external approach.

The main advantage of transepicardial injection is its proven safety and ease of performance in patients with chronic myocardial ischemia (Table 10.1). However, direct injection in the setting of acute myocardial infarction (AMI) has not been widely tested in clinical trials. Another disadvantage to this method is its high cost and lack of optimal targeting. The surgeon

Table 10.1 Cell therapy trials using transepicardial delivery during coronary artery bypass grafting (CABU). Adapted from reference 1

Study	Disease type	Number of patients treated	LVEF	Cell type	Dose	Outcomes[a]
Hamano et al[2]	MI[b]	5	–	MNCs	$0.3–2.2 \times 10^9$	Perfusion ↑
Menasche et al[3]	ICM (3–228 months after MI)	10[c]	24 ± 4%	Myoblasts	$8.7 ± 1.9 \times 10^8$	Regional wall motion ↑; global LVEF ↑
Herreros et al[4]	ICM (3–168 months after MI)	11[d]	36 ± 8%	Myoblasts	$1.9 ± 1.2 \times 10^8$	Regional wall motion ↑; global LVEF ↑; viability in infarct area ↑
Siminiak et al[5]	ICM (4–108 months after MI)	10[d]	25–40%	Myoblasts	$0.04–5.0 \times 10^7$	Regional wall motion ↑; global LVEF ↑
Chachques et al[6]	ICM (time after MI not reported)	20[c]	28 ± 3%	Myoblasts	$3.0 ± 0.2 \times 10^8$	Regional wall motion ↑; global LVEF ↑; viability in infarct area ↑
Stamm et al[7,8]	ICM (3–12 weeks after MI)	12[c]	36 ± 11%	CD133+	$1.0–2.8 \times 10^6$	Global LVEF ↑; LVEDV ↓; perfusion ↑

[a]Effects reported only within cell therapy groups; [b]MI patients had no revascularization options; [c]CABG of uninjected areas only; [d]CABG of injected and uninjected areas; LVEF, left ventricular ejection fraction; MI, myocardial infarction; MNCs, bone marrow-derived mononuclear cells; ICM, ischemic cardiomyopathy; CD133+, bone marrow-derived CD133 + cells; LVEDV, left ventricular end-diastolic volume. Values are means ± SD.

chooses to inject stem cells either in the border of the infarcted tissue or within the scarred myocardium based solely on subjective visual assessment. Thus, transepicardial injection is easy to perform but is associated with high cost and risk. Despite its limitations, however, one can easily envision clinically indicated routine bypass surgery as an opportunity for the surgeon to inject stem cells into areas that cannot be grafted.

Transcoronary Venous Injection

Transcoronary venous injection uses a percutaneously placed catheter system to deliver cells into the coronary sinus. This technique uses intravascular ultrasound to guide the catheter and needle away from the pericardial space and coronary artery and into the adjacent myocardium. Initial studies have confirmed the feasibility and safety of this approach in swine models,[9] and to date, feasibility studies have had a good safety profile. This technique has also been used to deliver skeletal myoblasts to scarred myocardium in cardiomyopathy patients.[5]

This technique may be one of the more technically challenging delivery modes because of the tortuousness of the coronary veins. In addition, site-specific targeting is not possible with this approach.

Transendocardial Injection

Transendocardial injection is the most promising delivery modality in the setting of chronic myocardial ischemia. This technique is performed by means of a percutaneous femoral approach. Once an injection-needle catheter has been advanced in a retrograde fashion across the aortic valve and positioned against the endocardial surface, cells can be injected directly into any area of the left ventricular (LV) wall. Three catheter systems are currently available for transendocardial cell delivery: the Stiletto™ (Boston Scientific, Natick, MA), the BioCardia catheter delivery system (BioCardia, South San Francisco, CA), and the Myostar™ (Biosense Webster, Diamond Bar, CA).

The Stiletto is used with the aid of fluoroscopic guidance, usually in two planes. The main drawbacks of this technique are the two-dimensional orientation, the inherent lack of precision associated with fluoroscopy, and the inability to characterize the underlying myocardium. To address these deficiencies, preclinical experiments have coupled the Stiletto catheter with real-time cardiac magnetic resonance imaging (MRI), which allows online assessment of full-thickness myocardium and perfusion. Although not currently practical in terms of clinical application, this simultaneous use of MRI offers three-dimensional spatial orientation and a unique opportunity to track intramyocardial retention of cells labeled with iron-fluorescent particles, which can be detected in the beating heart after direct injection. The Stiletto is still investigational; few preclinical studies have been performed,[10] and no safety data have been assessed in humans. Nevertheless, it may be promising when associated with other imaging technologies or if targeting of myocardial therapy is not necessary.

The BioCardia delivery system uses a catheter with a deflectable, helical infusion needle at its tip. Initial preclinical and clinical experience with this system for stem cell delivery has provided preliminary evidence of its safety and feasibility. The BioCardia catheter with the helical ("screw-in") infusion needle might offer the advantage of more stable needle position during injection and, theoretically, less backflow of the injectate. However, the BioCardia catheter does not offer additional navigational or targeting tools.

The Myostar is an injection catheter that uses non-fluoroscopic magnetic guidance to target injections within a three-dimensional electromechanical map (EMM) of the endocardial surface of the left ventricle. This LV "shell" is constructed by acquiring a series of points at multiple locations on the endocardial surface, which are gated to a surface electrocardiogram. The Myostar catheter is then guided by ultralow magnetic fields (10^{-6}–10^{-5}T) that are generated by a triangular magnetic pad positioned beneath the patient.[11] The magnetic fields intersect with a location sensor just proximal to the deflectable tip of a 7F mapping catheter, which helps determine the real-time position and orientation of the catheter tip inside the left ventricle.

Using data obtained by the Myostar catheter, the NOGA™ EMM system analyzes both the contractility and the electrical viability of the endocardium. Data are obtained only when the catheter tip is in stable contact with the endocardium, which the system determines automatically. For contractility, the NOGA system uses an algorithm to calculate and analyze the movement of the catheter tip or the location of an endocardial point throughout systole and diastole. That movement is then compared with the movement of neighboring points in an area of interest. The resulting value, called linear local shortening (LLS), is expressed as a percentage that represents the degree of mechanical function of the LV region at that endocardial point.

The mapping catheter also incorporates electrodes that measure endocardial electrical signals in the form of unipolar (UniV) or bipolar voltage. Several clinical studies have validated the concept of electrical viability, which contends that measurement of endocardial voltage potentials provides a reliable and accurate assessment of myocardial viability.[12–17] In general, a UniV of 4.5 mV should indicate non-viable myocardium with nearly 100% certainty. A UniV of 4.5–8.4 mV indicates various degrees of viability, which is compatible with the relatively non-uniform nature of myocardial necrosis. A UniV of 6.9 mV can identify viable myocardial segments by means of delayed hyperenhancement MRI with 93% sensitivity and 88% specificity.[18] The NOGA system assigns voltage values to each point acquired during LV mapping, and an electrical map is constructed concurrently with the mechanical map. Thus, each data point has an LLS value and a voltage value. When the map is complete, the NOGA workstation integrates all of the data points and presents them in a three-dimensional, color-coded reconstruction of the endocardial surface. The system also provides 9- and 12-segment bull's-eye views that show average values for the LLS and voltage data in each myocardial segment. These maps can be spatially manipulated in real time on a Silicon Graphics workstation (Mountain View, CA). The three-dimensional representations acquired during the cardiac cycle can also be used to calculate LV volumes and ejection fraction (LVEF).

The EMM thus provides a three-dimensional platform that guides the catheter in navigating the left ventricle and provides orientation for transendocardial injections. It also serves as a diagnostic platform that can distinguish ischemic areas (which have low LLS but preserved UniV) from areas of infarct (which have low LLS and low UniV). Moreover, the Myostar catheter allows assessment of myocardial viability at any point at which the catheter touches the endocardial surface. The operator thus has the ability to target therapy to viable tissue (useful in situations of chronic ischemia, where neoangiogenesis may play an important role) or non-viable tissue (such as when the target is an area of scarring). Because myocardial involvement in human ischemic heart disease is often

patchy, the ability to distinguish underlying tissue characteristics is important in stem cell delivery. The NOGA/Myostar system has been widely tested in both animals and humans and has an excellent safety profile.

Clinical applications of transendocardial stem cell delivery

Transendocardial delivery of stem cells has been tested in a few clinical studies, mainly in patients with chronic myocardial ischemia (Table 10.2). Tse et al[20] transendocardially injected autologous bone marrow mononuclear cells (ABMMNCs) into eight patients with severe ischemic heart disease and preserved LV function, as indicated by the LVEF. After 3 months of follow-up study, the researchers observed an improvement in the patients' symptoms, and MRI showed improved perfusion and contractility in the ischemic region. Fuchs et al[21] conducted a clinical feasibility study in which filtered, unfractionated autologous bone marrow-derived (not mononuclear) cells were transendocardially injected into 10 patients with severe chronic, symptomatic myocardial ischemia not amenable to conventional revascularization. For each patient, 12 targeted 0.2-ml injections were administered into ischemic, non-infarcted myocardium that was preidentified with single photon emission computed tomography (SPECT) perfusion imaging. The patients experienced no serious adverse effects (arrhythmia, infection, myocardial inflammation, or increased scar formation). The treadmill exercise duration (available for nine patients) did not change significantly (391 ± 155 seconds vs 485 ± 198 seconds; $p < 0.11$), but there was improvement in their Canadian Cardiovascular Society angina scores (3.1 ± 0.3 vs 2.0 ± 0.94; $p < 0.001$) and stress scores involving segments within the injected regions (2.1 ± 0.8 vs 1.6 ± 0.8; $p < 0.001$).

Our group performed the first clinical trial in which transendocardially injected ABMMNCs were used to treat end-stage ischemic heart failure patients with severe systolic dysfunction.[22,23] The trial involved 21 patients, the first 14 of whom formed the treatment group and the last seven of whom formed the control group.

Table 10.2   Cell therapy trials using electromechanical mapping (EMM)-guided transendocardial delivery. Adapted from reference 1

Study	Disease type	Number of patients treated	LVEF	Cell type	Dose	Outcomes
Smits et al[19]	ICM (24–132 months after MI)	5	36 ± 11%	Myoblasts	$2.0 ± 1.1 × 10^8$	Regional wall motion ↑[a]; global LVEF ↑[a]
Tse et al[20]	MI[b]	8	58 ± 11%	MNCs	From 40 ml BM	Angina ↓[a]; perfusion ↑[a]; regional wall motion ↑[a]
Fuchs et al[21]	MI[b]	10	47 ± 10%	NCs	$7.8 ± 6.6 × 10^7$	Angina ↓[a]; perfusion ↑[a]
Perin et al[22,23]	MI[b]	14 (7 controls)[c]	30 ± 6%	MNCs	$3.0 ± 0.4 × 10^7$	Angina ↓; NYHA class ↓; perfusion ↑; regional wall motion ↑[a]; global LVEF ↑

[a]Effects reported only within cell therapy groups; [b]MI patients had no revascularization options; [c]non-randomized control group; BM, bone marrow; NCs, bone marrow-derived nucleated cells; NYHA, New York Heart Association. Values are means ± SD.

Baseline evaluations included complete clinical and laboratory tests, exercise stress studies, two-dimensional Doppler echocardiography, SPECT perfusion scanning, and 24-hour Holter monitoring. Bone marrow-derived mononuclear cells were harvested from each treated patient, isolated, washed, and resuspended in saline for injection by a NOGA/Myostar injection catheter (15 injections of 0.2 ml each, totaling $30 × 10^6$ cells per patient). EMM was performed to identify viable myocardium (UniV < 6.9 mV), and the results were integrated with the SPECT findings to define the treatment area. Only points with preserved viability were injected. All patients underwent non-invasive follow-up tests at 2 months and invasive studies at 4 months, using standard protocols and the same procedures as at baseline.[14] The demographic and exercise test variables did not differ significantly between the treatment and control groups. No procedural complications occurred, and no periprocedural arrhythmias were identified. At 2 months, quantitative SPECT analysis showed that patients in the treatment group had a significant reduction in the total reversible defect compared to patients in the control group ($p=0.02$). At 4 months, the LVEF had improved significantly from a baseline of 20% to 29% ($p=0.003$) in the treated patients, and the end-systolic volume was reduced ($p=0.03$). EMM revealed significant mechanical improvement of the injected segments ($p<0.0005$). In addition, the treated group's exercise capacity was also significantly improved. Importantly, the significant improvement seen at

2 and 4 months was maintained at 6 and 12 months.[23] Thus, transendocardial injection of ABMMNCs was safe overall and showed preliminary effectiveness. This trial provided the first objective evidence of perfusional and functional improvement in patients with severe ischemic heart failure treated solely with cell therapy and myocardial perfusion.

The transendocardial route has also been used for delivery of skeletal myoblasts. In studying the safety and feasibility of this method in five patients with ischemic heart failure, Smits et al[19] documented an improvement in global LVEF.

Future perspectives: transendocardial delivery of stem cells after AMI

In the setting of chronic ischemia, the transendocardial route has important advantages over intracoronary stem cell infusion. First, the transendocardial route provides a means by which tissues with various degrees of viability and ischemia can be mapped in detail, allowing the stem cell injections to be precisely targeted (for example, to the border zone of an infarct). Second, patients may require injection into areas not supplied by patent coronary arteries. Thus, based on current clinical experience, EMM-guided transendocardial injection is likely to be the first choice for cell delivery in treating patients with chronic myocardial ischemia, as this technique integrates anatomic precision with detailed tissue characterization.

Compared to the setting of chronic myocardial ischemia, in acute ischemic injury it would be logical to expect upregulation of homing signals and increased cell retention even after successful revascularization of AMI. The intracoronary route should therefore be the simplest way to administer cells after AMI. However, Vulliet et al[24] observed AMI and subacute myocardial microinfarctions after intracoronary arterial injection of bone marrow MSCs in dogs. These findings were particularly worrisome because they were obtained in healthy dogs with normal epicardial coronary arteries. Microcirculatory plugging is believed to have caused the microinfarctions. Transendocardial injection might therefore be more appropriate for delivering larger cells such as MSCs after AMI.

Transendocardial stem cell delivery guided by endomyocardial mapping after AMI has not yet been tested in the clinic. Nevertheless, our work at the Texas Heart Institute in a canine model of acute ischemia entails an excellent safety profile with no documented injection-related pericardial effusion or malignant arrhythmias (Perin E, Silva G, Assad JA et al, unpublished data). Transendocardial injections of MSCs into dogs 7 days after AMI were associated with significant functional improvement, as assessed by two-dimensional echocardiography. Further testing to assess the safety of transendocardial cell injections after AMI is warranted.

Conclusions

Despite many unresolved issues, the clinical potential of stem cell therapy for cardiovascular disease is enormous. The expectations of both patients and clinicians for this new therapeutic modality are high, however, and optimization of these techniques for routine use will require continued cooperation and close collaboration between basic and clinical researchers. Future studies should focus on unanswered questions related to optimal treatment dose, timing, and, most important, mode of delivery in various clinical scenarios.

References

1. Wollert KC, Drexler H. Clinical applications of stem cells for the heart. Circ Res 2005; 96: 151–63.
2. Hamano K, Nishida M, Hirata K et al. Local implantation of autologous bone marrow cells for therapeutic angiogenesis in patients with ischemic heart disease: clinical trial and preliminary results. Jpn Circ J 2001; 65: 845–7.
3. Menasche P, Hagege AA, Vilquin JT et al. Autologous skeletal myoblast transplantation for severe postinfarction left ventricular dysfunction. J Am Coll Cardiol 2003; 41: 1078–83.
4. Herreros J, Prosper F, Perez A et al. Autologous intramyocardial injection of cultured skeletal muscle-derived stem cells in patients with non-acute myocardial infarction. Eur Heart J 2003; 24: 2012–20.

5. Siminiak T, Kalawski R, Fiszer D et al. Autologous skeletal myoblast transplantation for the treatment of postinfarction myocardial injury: phase I clinical study with 12 months of follow-up. Am Heart J 2004; 148: 531–7.

6. Chachques JC, Herreros J, Trainini J et al. Autologous human serum for cell culture avoids the implantation of cardioverter-defibrillators in cellular cardiomyoplasty. Int J Cardiol 2004; 95 (Suppl 1): S29–33.

7. Stamm C, Kleine HD, Westphal B et al. CABG and bone marrow stem cell transplantation after myocardial infarction. Thorac Cardiovasc Surg 2004; 52: 152–8.

8. Stamm C, Westphal B, Kleine HD et al. Autologous bone-marrow stem-cell transplantation for myocardial regeneration. Lancet 2003; 361: 45–6.

9. Thompson CA, Nasseri BA, Makower J et al. Percutaneous transvenous cellular cardiomyoplasty. A novel nonsurgical approach for myocardial cell transplantation. J Am Coll Cardiol 2003; 41: 1964–71.

10. Dick AJ, Guttman MA, Raman VK et al. Magnetic resonance fluoroscopy allows targeted delivery of mesenchymal stem cells to infarct borders in swine. Circulation 2003; 108: 2899–904.

11. Sarmento-Leite R, Silva GV, Dohman HF et al. Comparison of left ventricular electromechanical mapping and left ventricular angiography: defining practical standards for analysis of NOGA maps. Tex Heart Inst J 2003; 30: 19–26.

12. Botker HE, Lassen JF, Hermansen F et al. Electromechanical mapping for detection of myocardial viability in patients with ischemic cardiomyopathy. Circulation 2001; 103: 1631–7.

13. Fuchs S, Hendel RC, Baim DS et al. Comparison of endocardial electromechanical mapping with radionuclide perfusion imaging to assess myocardial viability and severity of myocardial ischemia in angina pectoris. Am J Cardiol 2001; 87: 874–80.

14. Gyongyosi M, Sochor H, Khorsand A, Gepstein L, Glogar D. Online myocardial viability assessment in the catheterization laboratory via NOGA electroanatomic mapping: quantitative comparison with thallium-201 uptake. Circulation 2001; 104: 1005–11.

15. Keck A, Hertting K, Schwartz Y et al. Electromechanical mapping for determination of myocardial contractility and viability. A comparison with echocardiography, myocardial single-photon emission computed tomography, and positron emission tomography. J Am Coll Cardiol 2002; 40: 1067–74; discussion 1075–8.

16. Koch KC, vom Dahl J, Wenderdel M et al. Myocardial viability assessment by endocardial electroanatomic mapping: comparison with metabolic imaging and functional recovery after coronary revascularization. J Am Coll Cardiol 2001; 38: 91–8.

17. Wiggers H, Botker HE, Sogaard P et al. Electromechanical mapping versus positron emission tomography and single photon emission computed tomography for the detection of myocardial viability in patients with ischemic cardiomyopathy. J Am Coll Cardiol 2003; 41: 843–8.

18. Perin EC, Silva GV, Sarmento-Leite R et al. Assessing myocardial viability and infarct transmurality with left ventricular electromechanical mapping in patients with stable coronary artery disease: validation by delayed-enhancement magnetic resonance imaging. Circulation 2002; 106: 957–61.

19. Smits PC, van Geuns RJ, Poldermans D et al. Catheter-based intramyocardial injection of autologous skeletal myoblasts as a primary treatment of ischemic heart failure: clinical experience with six-month follow-up. J Am Coll Cardiol 2003; 42: 2063–9.

20. Tse HF, Kwong YL, Chan JK et al. Angiogenesis in ischaemic myocardium by intramyocardial autologous bone marrow mononuclear cell implantation. Lancet 2003; 361: 47–9.

21. Fuchs S, Satler LF, Kornowski R et al. Catheter-based autologous bone marrow myocardial injection in no-option patients with advanced coronary artery disease: a feasibility study. J Am Coll Cardiol 2003; 41: 1721–4.

22. Perin EC, Dohmann HF, Borojevic R et al. Transendocardial, autologous bone marrow cell transplantation for severe, chronic ischemic heart failure. Circulation 2003; 107: 2294–302.

23. Perin EC, Dohmann HF, Borojevic R et al. Improved exercise capacity and ischemia 6 and 12 months after transendocardial injection of autologous bone marrow mononuclear cells for ischemic cardiomyopathy. Circulation 2004; 110 (11 Suppl 1): II213–18.

24. Vulliet PR, Greeley M, Halloran SM, MacDonald KA, Kittleson MD. Intra-coronary arterial injection of mesenchymal stromal cells and microinfarction in dogs. Lancet 2004; 363: 783–4.

chapter 11

The Role of Non-invasive Imaging and Cell Labelling Techniques in the Clinical Assessment of Stem Cell Therapy

Dara L Kraitchman

Introduction

Non-invasive imaging can play several potential roles in cardiac regenerative therapy. In preclinical models, postmortem evaluation, both grossly and microscopically, can be performed to determine therapeutic efficacy. However, in cardiac clinical trials of stem cell therapy, obtaining cardiac tissue for sampling, such as from biopsy, is rarely performed due to the invasive nature. Thus, many preclinical studies have employed traditional imaging techniques to measure cardiac morphology, function, perfusion, and flow by echocardiography, radionuclide imaging, and/or cardiovascular magnetic resonance imaging (MRI) to optimize stem cell therapy protocols. These imaging studies provide surrogate measures of morbidity and mortality for measuring the success of cellular therapies in clinical trials. Recently, cellular labeling methods have been extended to the many types of stem cells in animal models of cardiovascular disease that open new avenues for cell targeting and tracking in combination with these non-invasive imaging techniques. It can be envisioned that cellular labeling techniques will be extended to cardiovascular stem cell clinical trials in the near future to enhance the interpretation of both negative and positive outcomes and ultimately for the tailoring of stem cell therapies to individual patients.

Non-invasive Imaging

Morphological and functional aspects of myocardial anatomy, contractile function, metabolism, and perfusion can all be evaluated by non-invasive imaging. While the success or failure of stem cell therapies in patients was initially determined largely based on the assessment of clinical improvement, non-invasive imaging offers a more rigorous and quantitative method to determine the efficacy of a particular stem cell therapy. To date, cardiovascular cellular therapy clinical trials have relied on a variety of non-invasive imaging techniques to assess response to treatment (Table 11.1). While a general overview of the advantages and disadvantages of each technique can be summarized (Table 11.2), the choice of imaging modality is often dictated by the institutional preference or financial considerations rather than the answers which one is seeking with non-invasive imaging.

X-ray imaging techniques

Cardiac catheterization is often used to assess or reestablish vessel patency after acute myocardial ischemia. In combination with ventriculography, a crude assessment of contractile function can be made. However, X-ray angiography is an invasive technique and cannot provide a full

Table 11.1 Currently used imaging modalities for cardiac cellular therapy trials

Clinical trial	Cell type	Angio	Echo	SPECT	PET	MRI
				Imaging modality		
BOOST[1-4]	BMC	x				x
Brehm et al[5]	BMC	x	x	x	x	
Fernandez-Aviles et al[6]	BMC	x	x			x
Fuchs et al[7]	BMC		x	x		
Galinanes et al[8]	BMC		x			
Hamano et al[9]	BMC	x	x			
IACT[10]	BMC	x		x	x	
Janssens et al[11]	BMC				x	x
Katritsis et al[12]	BMC		x			
Kuethe et al[13]	BMC	x	x			
Lunde et al[14]	BMC	x		x		x
Perin et al[15,16]	BMC		x	x		
Silva et al[17]	BMC		x	x		
Strauer et al[18]	BMC	x	x			
Tse et al[19]	BMC					x
Assmus et al[20]	BMC/CPC	x	x			x
TOPCARE-AMI[21-23]	BMC/CPC	x	x		x	x
Bartunek et al[24]	CD133+	x			x	x
Goussetis et al[25]	CD133+/CD34+	x	x	x		
Stamm et al[26,27]	CD133+	x	x			
Chen et al[28]	MSC		x		x	
Chachques et al[29]	Myoblasts		x			
Dib et al[30]	Myoblasts		x		x	
Herreros et al[31]	Myoblasts		x		x	
Ince et al[32]	Myoblasts		x			
Menasche et al[33]	Myoblasts		x		x	
POZNAN[34]	Myoblasts		x			
Siminiak et al[35]	Myoblasts		x			
Smits et al[36]	Myoblasts	x	x			x

BMC, bone marrow-derived mononuclear or nucleated cells; CPC, circulating blood-derived progenitor cells; MSC, bone marrow-derived mesenchymal stem cells; CD133+/CD34+, bone marrow-derived CD133+ or CD34+ cells; Angio, X-ray angiography; echo, echocardiography; PET, positron emission tomography; SPECT, single photon emission computed tomography; MRI, magnetic resonance imaging.

tomographic or three-dimensional (3D) assessment of cardiac remodeling postinfarction. Cardiac computed tomography (CCT) has gained inroads in the assessment of cardiac function over the last several years. However, concerns about radiation exposure, especially when considering the administration of potentially radiosensitive stem cells, have limited the widespread adoption of CCT for the serial assessment of myocardial function.

Table 11.2   Advantages and disadvantages of cardiovascular imaging techniques

Imaging technique	Advantages	Disadvantages
X-ray imaging	• High spatial and temporal resolution • Wide availability • High diagnostic accuracy for stenotic lesions	• Radiation exposure • Iodinated contrast agent exposure • Invasiveness
Echocardiography	• Low cost • Wide availability	• Limited imaging windows • Poor spatial resolution • Poor ability to determine blood flow
SPECT	• Low cost • Wide availability	• Radiation exposure • Poor specificity • Attenuation artifacts • Poor ability to determine wall motion • Poor spatial resolution
PET	• Quantitative evaluation • Metabolic information	• Radiation exposure • High cost • Limited accessibility to radiotracers • Poor ability to determine wall motion • Poor spatial resolution
MRI	• High spatial resolution • No ionizing radiation • High repeatability and diagnostic accuracy • Ability to determine wall motion, myocardial viability, and perfusion	• High cost • Limited availability

Echocardiography

Echocardiography is an inexpensive, readily accessible technique to assess wall motion abnormalities. Thus, the majority of cardiac stem cell clinical trials have used echocardiography to assess the response to cell therapy (Table 11.1). Due to limited acoustical windows, two-dimensional echocardiographic measurements of global contractile function, such as end-diastolic volume, end-systolic volume, and ejection fraction, are based on geometric assumptions about the heart. Because wall thinning and changes in cardiac geometry often accompany postinfarction remodeling, the variance of the global function measurements can be large.[37] Therefore, clinical trials that rely on echocardiographic assessment of cardiac contractile function will require larger patient populations than some other non-invasive imaging techniques to demonstrate a statistically significant improvement in cardiovascular function in patients treated with stem cells.

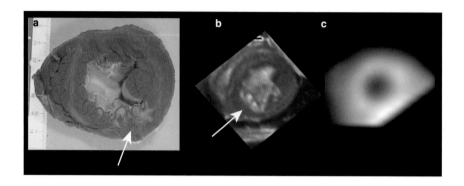

Figure 11.1 *A subendocardial infarction in a reperfused myocardial infarction in a dog is shown post-mortem by triphenyl tetrazolium staining as non-staining areas (arrow, a) and in vivo as hyperintensity regions (arrow, b) by delayed contrast-enhanced magnetic resonance imaging. However, [⁹⁹mTc]sestamibi single photon emission computed tomography (SPECT) imaging (c) fails to detect the subendocardial infarction. (Adapted from reference 42.)*

Radionuclide imaging

Radionuclide imaging is a well-accepted method for assessing myocardial metabolism and blood flow by the injection of specific radioisotopes. Single photon emission computed tomography (SPECT) scanners are widely available in the United States and Europe. Positron emission tomography (PET) scanners are less prevalent than SPECT scanners. Both PET and SPECT scanners now incorporate computed tomography (CT), which enables the determination of anatomical detail to assist with localizing radiotracer uptake. SPECT imaging can be used for determination of myocardial viability. Electrocardiogram (ECG)-gated SPECT scans have also been used to determine left ventricular function. Serial technetium-99m-labeled methoxyisobutyl isonitrile ([⁹⁹mTc]sestamibi) or [⁹⁹mTc]tetrafosmin SPECT imaging has been used to identify the "area at risk" and myocardial salvage after thrombolytic therapy.[38,39] [⁹⁹mTc]sestamibi/tetrafosmin is taken up in a dose dependent manner based on the number and activity of the mitochrondria.[40] Another frequently used SPECT radioisotope is Thallium-201 (²⁰¹Tl). ²⁰¹Tl is a potassium analog that is rapidly cleared from the circulation and taken up by the potassium–sodium adenosine triphosphatase (ATPase) pump and, thus, demonstrates intact cell membranes or viable myocytes.

Unlike ²⁰¹Tl, [⁹⁹mTc]sestamibi does not redistribute over time. When combined with pharmacological stress agents, such as adenosine, dipyridamole, or dobutamine, SPECT imaging is recommended for predicting ventricular functional recovery after revascularization therapy, prognosis, and risk assessment for future events after acute myocardial infarction.[41] Because the spatial resolution of SPECT imaging is limited, small subendocardial defects can often be missed, leading to false interpretation of the extent of myocardial ischemia or infarction (Figure 11.1).[43] In addition, attenuation artifacts due to the breast and the lack of quantitative methods limit the specificity of SPECT relative to PET.

PET imaging is approved for clinical use for a variety of cardiac applications. The short-half life of many of the PET radioisotopes necessitates production of the tracers in a cyclotron in close proximity to the scanners. 2-[¹⁸F]fluoro-2-deoxy-D-glucose ([¹⁸F]FDG), the most widely used radiopharmaceutical, is a glucose analog that in the brain was shown to be phosphorylated and thereby trapped within the cell to detect metabolic activity. While the action of [¹⁸F]FDG in the heart is more complex, due to reductions in blood flow and hence delivery, it is frequently used to determine myocardial viability.[44,45] Were it not for this limited accessibility and high cost of cardiac PET, [¹⁸F]FDG PET would probably be the preferred radionuclide method for assessing myocardial viability with a sensitivity and specificity of the order of 89% and 73%, respectively.[46,47] The ability to perform a quantitative evaluation with PET is a major strength over SPECT imaging. Other tracers, such as rubidium-82 chloride, carbon-11 acetate, and oxygen-15 water, have seen limited use in the determination of blood flow or oxygen consumption. All-in-all, the major drawbacks of radionuclide imaging techniques are the high radiation exposure for the patient and the limited spatial resolution, which is unable to resolve the transmural extent of viability in the ventricular wall.

Magnetic resonance imaging

MRI offers several advantages over echocardiographic, X-ray angiographic, and radionuclide imaging methods, including increased spatial resolution and enhanced soft-tissue visualization for exquisite anatomical detail. ECG-gated imaging is performed to obtain video loops for the analysis of wall motion abnormalities. As a tomographic technique, global measurements of left heart function, such as ventricular mass, ejection fraction, and ventricular volumes, are not affected by geometric assumptions. The use of gadolinium-based contrast agents enables the determination of myocardial perfusion and viability.[48–51] Specialized methods of non-invasively "tagging" the heart wall with markers[52,53] enables the determination of transmural wall motion. Because of the high reproducibility of MRI measurements, the diagnostic accuracy of measurements of infarct size are markedly improved over other imaging techniques.[54] The lack of ionizing radiation with MRI makes this the imaging technique of choice for serial assessment of infarct size. First-pass perfusion imaging can be performed during rest and pharmacologic stress and analyzed visually or quantitatively to obtain an index of myocardial perfusion reserve. The ability to obtain myocardial perfusion, viability, and function in a single examination (Figure 11.2) has been shown to enhance diagnostic accuracy compared with each individual test.[55]

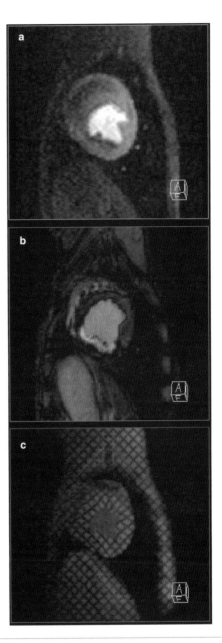

Figure 11.2   *First-pass perfusion magnetic resonance imaging (MRI) (a) demonstrates an area of microvascular obstruction in the short-axis plane in the left circumflex territory. Delayed contrast-enhanced MRI (b) in the short-axis plane demonstrates a non-transmural myocardial infarction (hyperintense area from 6 o'clock to 9 o'clock). The non-viable myocardium is larger than the "no-reflow" zone identified by first-pass perfusion MRI. Tagged MRI (c) at late systole in the short-axis planes demonstrates less tag bending or contraction in the left circumflex territory relative to the left anterior descending coronary artery territory.*

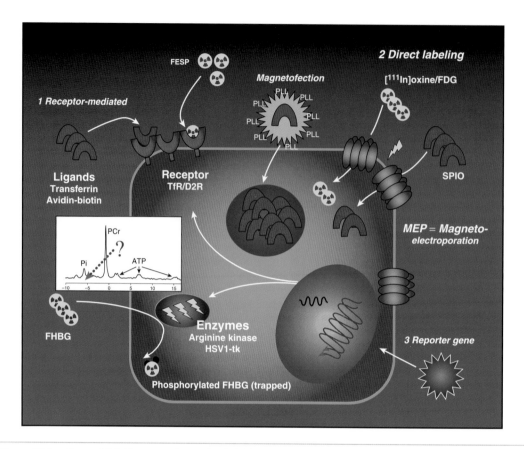

Figure 11.3 *Stem cell labeling strategies can be divided into three major areas: (1) receptor-mediated; (2) direct labeling; and (3) reporter gene probes. At present, preclinical labeling techniques are primarily focused on using radioisotopes (FHBG, FESP, [¹¹¹In]oxine) and superparamagnetic iron oxides (SPIOs) in concert with reporter gene methods and direct labeling techniques. FESP, [¹⁸F]fluoroethylspiperone; FHBG, 9-[3-fluoro-1-hydroxy-2-(propoxymethyl)]guanine; PLL, poly-L-lysine; FDG, 2-[¹⁸F]fluoro-2-deoxy-D-glucose. (Adapted from reference 57.)*

Recently, cardiovascular clinical stem cell trials have taken advantage of this enhanced accuracy and repeatability of MRI to study stem cell efficacy in a small number of patients. In particular, Janssens et al[11] were able to look at the improvement in cardiovascular function in acute myocardial infarction patients receiving intracoronary administration of bone marrow mononuclear cells, relative to the degree of transmural infarction.[11] Further speculation exists as to whether patients with "no-reflow zones", who have a worse overall prognosis,[56] should be administered intracoronary stem cell treatments. Nonetheless, one major limitation to cardiovascular MRI is safety concerns surrounding the imaging of patients in the high magnetic field with pacemakers, implantable cardiac defibrillators, and left ventricular assist devices. Presently, this restricts MRI to clinical trials in the acute myocardial infarction population due to the wide prevalence of these devices in patients with heart failure.

Labeling Strategies

Labeling of cells for imaging requires an imaging-visible macromolecule, that is either linked to the cell exogenously or in vivo to allow detection with the imaging instrument. Labeling of cells for imaging can be divided into three major classifications: (1) protein or receptor-bound labeling; (2) direct labeling; and (3) reporter gene transfection methods (Figure 11.3). Historically, cellular labeling was first developed based on labeling strategies that had been developed for radionuclide imaging and subsequently expanded to other imaging modalities.

When developing a cellular labeling agent, there are many considerations that come into play. Ideally, the labeling method is simple to implement and biocompatible. Thus, the label is non-species specific but specific for a particular lineage of cells. When considering biocompatibility, the label must be present in sufficient quantity for detection, but minimally alter the cell viability, metabolism and function. In addition, should the label be lost from the cell, the label must remain non-toxic and be excreted by a normal elimination pathway. In order to meet these minimum criteria, most cellular labeling schemes have been largely limited to detection by radionuclide and MR imaging and to a lesser extent by ultrasonography.

Candidate contrast agents for labeling

The most commonly used candidate for MRI cellular labeling in cardiovascular applications is superparamagnetic iron oxide particles (SPIOs). SPIOs cause a large magnetic field disturbance that leads to proton dephasing far away from the labeled cell, which is advantageous for enhancing detection of a limited number of cells. Typically, this susceptibility artifact is seen as a hypointense signal on images. Two additional advantages of SPIOs are the ability to target specific cells and the rapid clearance of SPIOs into the normal recirculating iron pool when released from dying stem cells and, thus, low toxicity.

Radiotracers for cellular labeling offer the benefit over other imaging labels in that the background signal is essentially non-existent. Thus, radionuclide imaging is exquisitively sensitive with the ability to detect picomolar quantities, i.e. small numbers of radiolabeled stem cells. Typically, DNA is most sensitive to the negative effects of radiation. Thus, strategies to enhance the distance between the radioisotope and the cell nucleus are paramount. In turn, this limits the amount of radiotracer that can be used to directly label a stem cell.

Intracellular uptake of radiopaque contrast agents is associated with a high level of toxicity. Therefore, to date, no direct labeling of stem cells with X-ray-visible agents has been performed. New strategies to contain contrast agents within nanolayers surrounding the stem cells offer a method to reduce label toxicity and explore imaging-visible agents that have not previously been considered.[58,59]

Protein/receptor-bound labeling

For protein- or receptor-bound labeling, peptide ligands or monoclonal antibodies are linked to radio tracers or contrast agents. The vast majority of receptor-based labeling has been for targeting specific vascular markers rather than cellular imaging. One commonly used method, the biotin–streptavidin system, shows promise for cellular imaging.[60] Classically, the contrast agent or tracer, such as indium-111, was biotinylated, and the streptavidin portion of the biotin–streptavidin complex demonstrated the high affinity of streptavidin for inflammation for the diagnosis of infection or angiogenesis in tumors.[61] Recently, streptavidin has been conjugated to iron oxide nanoparticles, and targeted to cells engineered to express biotinylated receptors.[60] Another method, which has been primarily employed for the atherosclerotic plaque imaging, is to create nanoparticles that incorporate contrast agents in the core, such as perfluorocarbons for ultrasonographic imaging, or on the surface, such as radiotracers, fluorescent dyes, or MRI contrast agents, in addition to antibody–receptor complexes on the surface for targeting.[62–64] To achieve sufficient sensitivity, a large number of particles must be bound to the cell, or each complex for labeling must contain a large number of contrast agent particles or tracer.

While targeting can be very specific to a particular receptor, species differences in cell surface receptors result in difficulty translating preclinical studies to the bedside without reengineering the particle. Furthermore, the lack of specific, unique cell receptors on the stem cell that do not dynamically change with stem cell differentiation has stymied these techniques. Another concern of protein/receptor-based labeling is whether the labeling agent remains bound to the cell. In addition, if the binding results in internalization of the label, often the sensitivity to the label is markedly diminished. Thus, preclinical cardiac stem cell studies using receptor-based labeling have not yet been performed.

Direct labeling

Direct labeling methods provide the additional advantage over receptor-based techniques in that the label is internalized by the cell and thereby concerns about binding and unbinding of the label are diminished. In clinical oncological applications, SPIOs are readily phagocytized by Kupffer cells, specialized macrophages, after intravenous injection.[65,66] Consequently, after SPIO administration, normal anatomy is obscured by hypointense regions, whereas neoplastic cells fail to take up the SPIOs and appear non-enhanced.

One drawback of SPIO cellular imaging is that methods to encourage non-phagocytic stem cells to take up SPIO had to be developed. Currently, the most widely used method is "magnetofection" – the incubation of SPIOs with transfection agents, e.g. poly-L-lysine or protamine sulfate.[67-69] The transfection agent (TA) coats the SPIO and results in endocytosis of the SPIO–TA complex, where it is stably maintained in lysosomes. Intracellular iron concentrations of 10–15 pg/cell are found after 24–48 hours of incubation. The technique works for a wide variety of stem cells and does not appear to be species specific (Figure 11.4).[71-76] While metabolism and cell viability are not altered by SPIO–TA labeling, there are reports of effects on cellular differentiation that may be cell or transfection agent specific.[77,78] To overcome this potential problem, magnetoelectroporation, based on electroporation techniques to incorporate proteins and DNA into cells, was developed as a method to directly label stem cells without transfection agents.[79] Unlike standard electroporation, small pulsed voltages are used to minimize cellular disruption. An added benefit of magnetoelectroporation (MEP) is that labeling of stem cells can be achieved very rapidly with minimal processing. In addition, since only a single Food and Drug

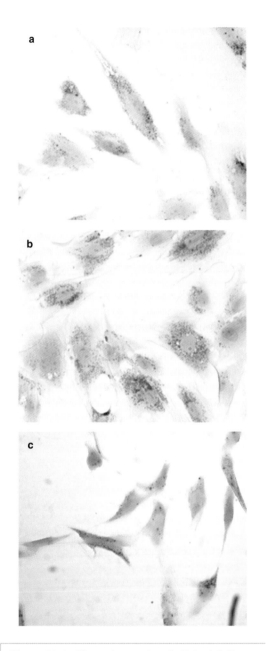

Figure 11.4 *Photomicrographs of cellular labeling of mesenchymal stem cells with superparamagnetic iron oxide (Feridex®; Berlex Laboratories, Inc) and poly-L-lysine magnetofection in human after 48 hours incubation (a), pig after 48 hours incubation (b), and dog after 24 hours incubation (c). The amount of iron oxide uptake is qualitatively dependent on the incubation time. Prussian blue staining for the iron oxide demonstrates its perinuclear location. (Adapted from reference 70.)*

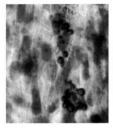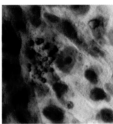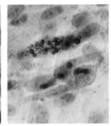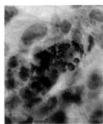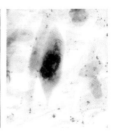

Figure 11.5   *Oil red O staining, in which fat stains red, of in vitro adipogenic differentiation of canine mesenchymal stem cells (MSCs) demonstrates similar differentiate capacity between unlabeled (left) and [^{111}In]oxine-labeled MSCs ranging from 5 to 30 μCi of [^{111}In]oxine/million cells (concentration increasing towards the right). (Reproduced with permission from reference 86.)*

Administration (FDA)-approved MR contrast agent is used, the likelihood of translation to the clinical realm is enhanced.

New studies are being performed investigating gadolinium- and fluorine-based agent direct labeling techniques sometimes combined with the magnetoelectroporation technique.[81] Using a higher relaxivity gadolinium agent, a hyperintense signal from magnetofected adipose-derived human mesenchymal stem cells (MSCs) in the brain was shown that has not been possible using conventional, clinically approved gadolinium chelates.[80,81]

Radionuclide isotopes used for direct labeling include [^{18}F]FDG, ^{99m}Tc, and indium-111 (^{111}In) oxine. The last, [^{111}In]oxine, has been approved for leukocyte labeling for diagnosis of inflammation and infection by SPECT imaging with a long record of patient safety.[82,83] The long half-life of [^{111}In]oxine of 2.8 days makes it ideal for serial imaging of stem cell retention, engraftment, and biodistribution. Direct labeling with most radiotracers is performed in vitro with passive diffusion of the tracer into the cell. Once intracellular, cleavage of products, i.e. the oxine portion of [^{111}In]oxine or phosphorylation as in [^{18}F]FDG, ensures that the radioisotope is trapped within the cell. [^{111}In]oxine has been used to label endothelial progenitor cells, hematopoietic stem cells, embryonic cardiomyoblasts, blood mononuclear cells, and mesenchymal stem cells in a variety of animals.[84–88] The clear advantage of radiolabeled stem cells is the enhanced ability to detect cells in the range of 1000–10 000 cells,

which is far below the detection limit of SPIO-labeled stem cells in the heart.[86,88] As with direct labeling with SPIOs, the dosimetry of direct radiolabeling must be carefully titrated to avoid loss in cell viability or function (Figure 11.5).[86,88,89] More extensive toxicity testing in each stem cell candidate type will be required prior to translation of the direct radiolabeling methods to clinical trials.

Recently, a new method of cellular labeling has been developed that enables the use of radiopaque stem cell labeling.[59] Rather than placing the contrast agent within the cell, nanolayers containing alginate, an algae-based product under development for cellular matrices and tissue engineering in the heart,[90,91] and the radiopaque agent are used to coat stem cells with a protective layer. Preliminary work demonstrates high conspicuity of the radiopaque capsules (Figure 11.6) for up to 2 weeks, which offers a new method to monitor mesenchymal stem cell delivery and engraftment with X-ray fluoroscopy and CT.[92]

Reporter gene methods

Reporter gene probes fall into three major classifications: (1) enzyme-based; (2) receptor-based; or (3) transporter-based. The advantage of reporter genes over direct cell labeling is that if the reporter gene can be stably integrated into the cell genome, then the cell (and subsequent daughter cells) can be traced by expression of the reporter probe. The greatest advances to date have been made with optical- and radiotracer-based reporter

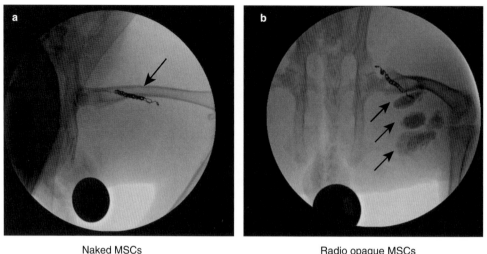

Naked MSCs   Radio opaque MSCs

Figure 11.6 *In a rabbit model of hind limb ischemia created by percutaneous placement of thrombogenic platinum coils (arrow), naked mesenchymal stem cells (MSCs) are not visible (a), whereas five injections of 5000 radiopaque encapsulated MSCs each (arrows demonstrate three injections) can be readily visualized on X-ray fluoroscopy (b).*

genes. In the simplest form, the gene product is expressed ubiquitously. By integrating a cardiospecific promoter,[93] one could theorectically detect cellular differentiation down a cardiac lineage. However, the long-term expression of reporter genes has remained problematic. One of the most widely used reporter gene constructs is the mutant form of the herpes simplex virus type 1 thymidine kinase (*HSV1-sr39tk*).[94] The production of thymidine kinase by the cells enables the phosphorylation of a wide range of substrates. In particular, 9-[3-fluoro-1-hydroxy-2-(propoxymethyl)]guanine (FHBG) can be used for PET or SPECT imaging to follow *HSV1-sr39tk* expression. The phosphorylation of FHBG by thymidine kinase traps the FHBG inside the cell. Unlike direct labeling, the cell does not need to be loaded with the radioisotope ex vivo. The radiotracer is administered intravenously and SPECT or PET imaging is used to detect the uptake of tracer by the exogenously transfected stem cell. Therefore, repeated scans can be performed by administering a new, small dose of this short-lived tracer as long as thymidine kinase is expressed. A triple reporter gene including thymidine kinase has been engineered to examine embryonic stem cell proliferation and teratoma formation in the heart.[95]

An enzyme reporter gene approach for MR spectroscopy (MRS) has been developed that involves transfection of skeletal muscle with a gene that produces a non-mammalian enzyme, arginine kinase. ^{31}P MRS can then be performed to detect the distinct phosphoarginine peak from transfected cells. While concerns about immune reactions are often raised with gene therapy, the use of a non-mammalian enzyme may enhance detection, but at the cost of increased immunogenicity.

MRI-based reporter gene systems are only starting to be developed. One such reporter is transfection to produce lysine-rich peptides. The amide residues of these proteins can be used for a specialized type of proton transfer imaging to alter signal intensity in the regions expressing the gene product. Preliminary studies using transfected xenografts placed in the brain provided proof-of-principle of this technique and offer the promise for a non-radioactive reporter gene method for imaging.[96]

Receptor-based reporter genes are also in early development, using MRI and radiolabels in the brain. Transfection of cells with a vector that causes overexpression of ferritin genes resulted in sequestration of iron within cells, leading to hypointensities on transfected cells on MRI.[97] Similarly, reporter genes to overexpress the transferrin receptor have been engineered without the normal regulatory iron inhibitory feedback.[98,99] Whether iron accumulation will result in toxicity in either of these reporter gene constructs is not clear.

A transporter-based reporter gene construct for the heart has been studied by Bengel and colleagues using the sodium–iodide symporter (NIS).[100,101] Transfection of cells with NIS in the heart results in expression of a new channel protein that can be used in conjunction with radiolabeled iodine for detection by either SPECT or PET. In general, radioactive iodine uptake is negligible in the normal heart due to the lack of endogenous NIS. As a result, this reporter gene offers the ability to yield a higher maximal signal uptake than with the thymidine kinase reporter.[101] The wider availability of radiolabeled iodine and SPECT scanners is another advantage of this potential reporter system. However, studies with ex vivo transfection of stem cells are only in the initial stages of implementation.

Preclinical and Clinical Applications

Many preclinical animal studies of direct labeling and, more recently, reporter gene labeling of stem cells have been reported. Of particular interest is a study by Hou et al using direct labeling of stem cells to study cell retention.[102] Using bone marrow mononuclear cells labeled with [¹¹¹In]oxine and intramyocardial, intracoronary, or retrograde coronary sinus administration in a swine myocardial infarction model, the highest cellular retention was achieved by direct intracardiac injection. A similar study using three routes of injection but without cellular labeling for non-invasive imaging by Freyman et al[103] reached a different conclusion. While one might

speculate on the different results, the ability to directly visualize the cell injections after delivery in the Hou study increases confidence in these results. Higher confidence in the initial delivery of the stem cell product could be envisioned with stem cell labeling in clinical cardiovascular trials. Moreover, studies like this have the potential to shift stem cell administration practices from largely an intracoronary route to a transmyocardial route.

In addition to examining cell retention by labeling, serial preclinical studies with labeled stem cells enable tracking of the cell biodistribution. In multiple animal studies using radiolabeled stem cells,[84–87,102,104] retention of stem cells in the lungs after intravenous delivery was noted to some extent and correlated to the physical size of the stem cell, with mesenchymal stem cells being the largest and most prone to pulmonary embolization.[86,102,104,105] Thus, these studies may offer suggestions for optimizing the route of cellular administration.

The first clinical trials with labeled stem cells in acute myocardial infarction were performed using bone marrow cells labeled with [¹⁸F]FDG.[106] Enriching the bone marrow for CD34+ cells resulted in enhanced retention of the cells in the heart after intracoronary administration. Therefore, the optimal cell type as well as route of administration for greater efficacy may best be sought based on patient studies with labeled stem cells. SPIO-labeled stem cells have not been used in cardiovascular clinical trials to date. However, dendritic cells exogenously labeled with [¹¹¹In]oxine and SPIOs have been tracked by SPECT and MRI in eight patients, providing the first application of SPIO-labeled cells in patients.[107] In this study, SPIO labeling demonstrated that ultrasound guidance of dendritic cell therapy was insufficient for targeting.[107] Thus, many of the outcome discrepancies of the early clinical cardiac stem cell trials may be based solely on the variability in delivery of the therapeutic, which cannot be ascertained.

In a similar vein, SPIO direct labeling of stem cells has enabled the tracking of intramyocardial injections of stem cells.[74,76,108–112] These studies are providing insight into the optimal location

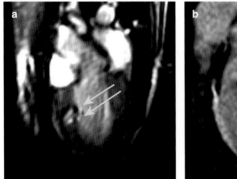
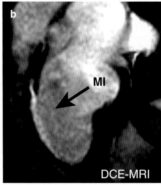
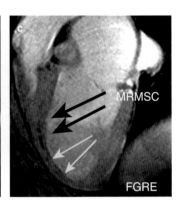

Figure 11.7 *Two injections of superparamagnetic iron oxide (SPIO)-labeled mesenchymal stem cells (MRMSCs) under MRI fluoroscopy at 72 hours after reperfused myocardial infarction (MI) appear as hypointense ovoid lesions (yellow arrows) in long-axis real-time cardiac MRI (a). At 8 weeks postinfarction, delayed-contrast enhanced (DCE)-MRI demonstrates a rim of subendocardial infarction in a canine model of reperfused MI with hypointensitites in fast, gradient echo (FGRE) MRI. (b) Stem cell injections are now centered on the epicardial rim of the infarcted tissue, suggesting active migration of the cells from the infarcted to the peri-infarcted tissue. At 8 weeks after MRMSC injection, the original two injections are still present (black arrows) as well as two injections of 100 000 MRMSCs in the ventricular apex (yellow arrows) (c). Therefore, approximately 100 000 MRMSCs can be visualized both in low resolution real-time imaging and after 8 weeks. (Adapted from reference 70.)*

and timing for stem cell injections. As in pre-clinical studies with histologically labeled stem cells, a large number of stem cells are destroyed shortly after injection. But most studies with direct SPIO labeling of stem cells have demonstrated persistence of the label for 2–6 months after administration.[111,112] Histological validation has shown that at least a portion of the remaining imaging-visible signal can still be attributed to the labeled stem cells.[74,86,111] Nonetheless, there is evidence to suggest that the stem cells may not need to permanently engraft to exert a long-term effect on cardiovascular functional improvement or remodeling.[113]

The impetus for MR fluoroscopic delivery systems was to enhance the success of transmyocardial delivery by direct confirmation of labeled stem cells.[109,111] In fact, approximately 25% of intramyocardial injections performed using X-ray angiography may be unsuccessful for the unskilled cardiac interventionalist.[74] In addition, these studies will potentially provide insight into the optimal location for stem cell delivery as cell migration and retention can be serially tracked (Figure 11.7). Meanwhile, conventional MRI

measurements of cardiac function, viability, and/or perfusion can be determined relative to stem cell injection sites.[110]

A recent development is the use of cross-modality platforms to guide injections and follow the response to therapy. Dual isotope imaging can be performed such that the stem cells can be labeled with a particular radiotracer and tracked alongside blood flow or metabolism measurements using traditional radiotracers (Figure 11.8).[87,114] Another alternative is to register the MRI delayed-contrast enhanced images of viability with radionuclide imaging to determine the location of cell specific homing (Figure 11.9).[86] Since many of the stem cell therapies are administered under X-ray angiographic guidance, the fusion of X-ray with MRI (XFM) may provide another convenient method for direct transmyocardial injection while avoiding areas that are non-viable, or enhance safety by avoiding puncturing areas with thinned myocardium.[115] Since these systems are already available, they provide an alternative to the purchase of dedicated electromechanical mapping systems for this purpose.[15,16]

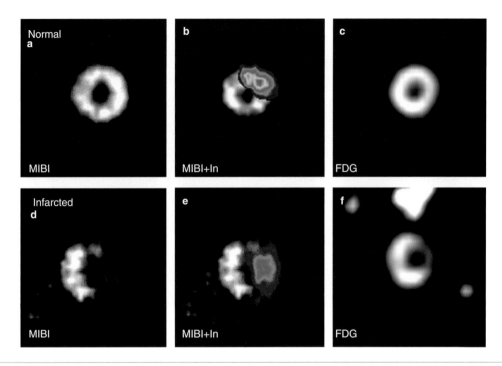

Figure 11.8   *Cardiac short-axis images in a normal rat (top, a–c) and an infarcted rat (bottom, d–f). Cardiac perfusion deficit using [^{99m}Tc]sestamibi (MIBI) SPECT is shown as a gray scale in the infarcted rat (d) but not the normal rat (a). [^{111}In]oxine-labeled rat embryonic myoblasts were injected by direct visualization into the peri-infarction area. The location of ^{111}In signal from SPECT images is shown as a color scale in fused images with MIBI SPECT (b, e). Decreased metabolism is shown in the infarcted heart by [^{18}F]FDG positron emission tomography (PET) (f) but not in the normal rat (c). Dual isotope imaging allows the registration of perfusion and metabolic abnormalities with the stem cell locations. (Adapted from reference 87.)*

Future Expectations

One of the largest challenges in the application of stem cell labeling to non-invasive imaging is the development of imaging agents that can be rapidly translated to clinical applications. For the most part, direct labeling techniques will find the fewest regulatory impediments and have been used in small scale studies. Initial results are encouraging, and point to treatment failures being correlated with the inability to target stem cells to the heart.

A remaining issue for stem cell labeling and imaging is the ability to detect small numbers of stem cells. Technological improvements to scanner hardware have enabled the detection of single cells after labeling in static tissue.[116,117] In clinical

practice, these techniques require at least several thousand[86,118] to several hundred thousand cells.[70,111] Presently, direct radiolabeling of stem cells provides a higher sensitivity to detect small numbers of cells compared to MRI (Figure 11.10). While tracking single cells may be a laudable goal, it is unlikely that the presence or absence of a cell will determine the clinical outcome. Therefore, the hope of stem cell labeling and imaging is to provide a means of improving cardiac regenerative therapy protocols for the community as a whole as well as the tailoring of individual therapies.

Reporter gene probes could open a whole new window onto the mechanism of stem cell action. With the use of cardiac specific promoters, the

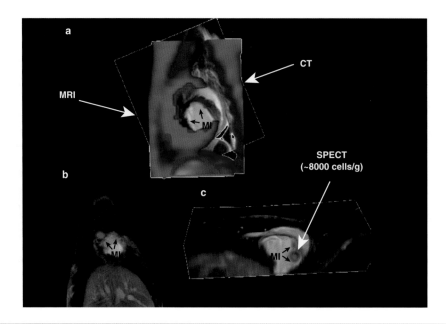

Figure 11.9   *Registration of SPECT/CT with MR images of the heart demonstrating focal uptake of MSCs in the peri-infarcted region. (a) Short-axis view of alignment of CT (gold) with MRI (gray scale) and SPECT (red) showing focal uptake in the septal region of the MI in a representative dog. (b, c) Focal uptake on SPECT (red) in another animal demonstrating localization of the MSCs to the infarcted myocardium (MI) in the short-axis (b) and long-axis (c) views. (Reproduced with permission from reference 86.)*

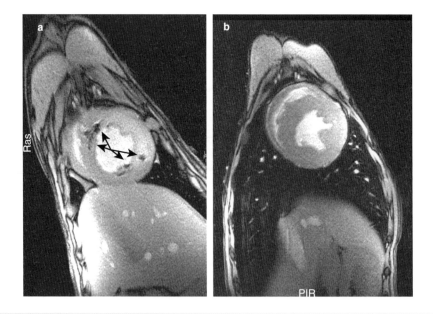

Figure 11.10   *Direct intramyocardial injections of 7 million SPIO-labeled mesenchymal stem cells (MSCs) per injection appear as hypointensities on high spatial resolution short-axis MRIs in a reperfused myocardial infarction in the dog (a). However, no hypointensities are seen after intravenous injection of ~150 million dual [^{111}In]oxine and SPIO-labeled MSCs in a reperfused myocardial infarction in the dog (b). The [^{111}In]oxine-labeled MSCs could be seen on SPECT imaging demonstrating the enhanced sensitivity to radioisotope direct labeling over MRI direct labeling techniques (Figure 11.9).*

fate of the stem cell as far as differentiation or action as a paracrine effect could be further probed. The caveat is that, similar to MRI, the detection limit will be diminished if the radioisotope is linked to a specific cellular event.

References

1. Wollert KC, Meyer GP, Lotz J et al. Intracoronary autologous bone-marrow cell transfer after myocardial infarction: the BOOST randomised controlled clinical trial. Lancet 2004; 364: 141–8.
2. Drexler H, Meyer GP, Wollert KC. Bone-marrow-derived cell transfer after ST-elevation myocardial infarction: lessons from the BOOST trial. Nat Clin Pract Cardiovasc Med 2006; 3 (Suppl 1): S65–8.
3. Meyer GP, Wollert KC, Lotz J et al. Intracoronary bone marrow cell transfer after myocardial infarction: eighteen months' follow-up data from the randomized, controlled BOOST (BOne marrOw transfer to enhance ST-elevation infarct regeneration) trial. Circulation 2006; 113: 1287–94.
4. Schaefer A, Meyer GP, Fuchs M et al. Impact of intracoronary bone marrow cell transfer on diastolic function in patients after acute myocardial infarction: results from the BOOST trial. Eur Heart J 2006; 27: 929–35.
5. Brehm M, Strauer BE. Stem cell therapy in postinfarction chronic coronary heart disease. Nat Clin Pract Cardiovasc Med 2006; 3 (Suppl 1): S101–4.
6. Fernandez-Aviles F, San Roman JA, Garcia-Frade J et al. Experimental and clinical regenerative capability of human bone marrow cells after myocardial infarction. Circ Res 2004; 95: 742–8.
7. Fuchs S, Satler LF, Kornowski R et al. Catheter-based autologous bone marrow myocardial injection in no-option patients with advanced coronary artery disease: a feasibility study. J Am Coll Cardiol 2003; 41: 1721–4.
8. Galinanes M, Loubani M, Davies J et al. Autotransplantation of unmanipulated bone marrow into scarred myocardium is safe and enhances cardiac function in humans. Cell Transplant 2004; 13: 7–13.
9. Hamano K, Nishida M, Hirata K et al. Local implantation of autologous bone marrow cells for therapeutic angiogenesis in patients with ischemic heart disease: clinical trial and preliminary results. Jpn Circ J 2001; 65: 845–7.
10. Strauer BE, Brehm M, Zeus T et al. Regeneration of human infarcted heart muscle by intracoronary autologous bone marrow cell transplantation in chronic coronary artery disease: the IACT Study. J Am Coll Cardiol 2005; 46: 1651–8.
11. Janssens S, Dubois C, Bogaert J et al. Autologous bone marrow-derived stem-cell transfer in patients with ST-segment elevation myocardial infarction: double-blind, randomised controlled trial. Lancet 2006; 367: 113–21.
12. Katritsis DG, Sotiropoulou PA, Karvouni E et al. Transcoronary transplantation of autologous mesenchymal stem cells and endothelial progenitors into infarcted human myocardium. Catheter Cardiovasc Interv 2005; 65: 321–9.
13. Kuethe F, Richartz BM, Sayer HG et al. Lack of regeneration of myocardium by autologous intracoronary mononuclear bone marrow cell transplantation in humans with large anterior myocardial infarctions. Int J Cardiol 2004; 97: 123–7.
14. Lunde K, Solheim S, Aakhus S et al. Intracoronary injection of mononuclear bone marrow cells in acute myocardial infarction. N Engl J Med 2006; 355: 1199–209.
15. Perin EC, Dohmann HF, Borojevic R et al. Transendocardial, autologous bone marrow cell transplantation for severe, chronic ischemic heart failure. Circulation 2003; 107: 2294–302.
16. Perin EC, Dohmann HF, Borojevic R et al. Improved exercise capacity and ischemia 6 and 12 months after transendocardial injection of autologous bone marrow mononuclear cells for ischemic cardiomyopathy. Circulation 2004; 110 (11 Suppl 1): II213–18.
17. Silva GV, Perin EC, Dohmann HF et al. Catheter-based transendocardial delivery of autologous bone-marrow-derived mononuclear cells in patients listed for heart transplantation. Tex Heart Inst J 2004; 31: 214–19.
18. Strauer BE, Brehm M, Zeus T et al. Repair of infarcted myocardium by autologous intracoronary mononuclear bone marrow cell transplantation in humans. Circulation 2002; 106: 1913–18.
19. Tse HF, Kwong YL, Chan JK et al. Angiogenesis in ischaemic myocardium by intramyocardial autologous bone marrow mononuclear cell implantation. Lancet 2003; 361: 47–9.
20. Assmus B, Honold J, Schachinger V et al. Transcoronary transplantation of progenitor cells after myocardial infarction. N Engl J Med 2006; 355: 1222–32.
21. Assmus B, Schachinger V, Teupe C et al. Transplantation of progenitor cells and regeneration enhancement in acute myocardial infarction (TOPCARE-AMI). Circulation 2002; 106: 3009–17.
22. Britten MB, Abolmaali ND, Assmus B et al. Infarct remodeling after intracoronary progenitor cell treatment in patients with acute myocardial infarction (TOPCARE-AMI): mechanistic insights from serial contrast-enhanced magnetic resonance imaging. Circulation 2003; 108: 2212–18.
23. Schachinger V, Assmus B, Britten MB et al. Transplantation of progenitor cells and regeneration enhancement in acute myocardial infarction: final one-year results of the TOPCARE-AMI Trial. J Am Coll Cardiol 2004; 44: 1690–9.

24. Bartunek J, Vanderheyden M, Vandekerckhove B et al. Intracoronary injection of CD133-positive enriched bone marrow progenitor cells promotes cardiac recovery after recent myocardial infarction: feasibility and safety. Circulation 2005; 112 (9 Suppl): I178–83.

25. Goussetis E, Manginas A, Koutelou M et al. Intracoronary infusion of CD133+ and CD133-CD34+ selected autologous bone marrow progenitor cells in patients with chronic ischemic cardiomyopathy: cell isolation, adherence to the infarcted area, and body distribution. Stem Cells 2006; 24: 2279–83.

26. Stamm C, Kleine HD, Westphal B et al. CABG and bone marrow stem cell transplantation after myocardial infarction. Thorac Cardiovasc Surg 2004; 52: 152–8.

27. Stamm C, Westphal B, Kleine HD et al. Autologous bone-marrow stem-cell transplantation for myocardial regeneration. Lancet 2003; 361: 45–6.

28. Chen SL, Fang WW, Ye F et al. Effect on left ventricular function of intracoronary transplantation of autologous bone marrow mesenchymal stem cell in patients with acute myocardial infarction. Am J Cardiol 2004; 94: 92–5.

29. Chachques JC, Herreros J, Trainini J et al. Autologous human serum for cell culture avoids the implantation of cardioverter-defibrillators in cellular cardiomyoplasty. Int J Cardiol 2004; 95 (Suppl 1): S29–33.

30. Dib N, Michler RE, Pagani FD et al. Safety and feasibility of autologous myoblast transplantation in patients with ischemic cardiomyopathy: four-year follow-up. Circulation 2005; 112: 1748–55.

31. Herreros J, Prosper F, Perez A et al. Autologous intramyocardial injection of cultured skeletal muscle-derived stem cells in patients with non-acute myocardial infarction. Eur Heart J 2003; 24: 2012–20.

32. Ince H, Petzsch M, Rehders TC, Chatterjee T, Nienaber CA. Transcatheter transplantation of autologous skeletal myoblasts in postinfarction patients with severe left ventricular dysfunction. J Endovasc Ther 2004; 11: 695–704.

33. Menasche P, Hagege AA, Vilquin JT et al. Autologous skeletal myoblast transplantation for severe postinfarction left ventricular dysfunction. J Am Coll Cardiol 2003; 41: 1078–83.

34. Siminiak T, Fiszer D, Jerzykowska O et al. Percutaneous trans-coronary-venous transplantation of autologous skeletal myoblasts in the treatment of post-infarction myocardial contractility impairment: the POZNAN trial. Eur Heart J 2005; 26: 1188–95.

35. Siminiak T, Kalawski R, Fiszer D et al. Autologous skeletal myoblast transplantation for the treatment of postinfarction myocardial injury: phase I clinical study with 12 months of follow-up. Am Heart J 2004; 148: 531–7.

36. Smits PC, van Geuns RJ, Poldermans D et al. Catheter-based intramyocardial injection of autologous skeletal myoblasts as a primary treatment of ischemic heart failure: clinical experience with six-month follow-up. J Am Coll Cardiol 2003; 42: 2063–9.

37. Bellenger NG, Davies LC, Francis JM, Coats AJ, Pennell DJ. Reduction in sample size for studies of remodeling in heart failure by the use of cardiovascular magnetic resonance. J Cardiovasc Magn Reson 2000; 2: 271–8.

38. Wackers FJ, Gibbons RJ, Verani MS et al. Serial quantitative planar technetium-99m isonitrile imaging in acute myocardial infarction: efficacy for noninvasive assessment of thrombolytic therapy. J Am Coll Cardiol 1989; 14: 861–73.

39. Gibbons RJ, Verani MS, Behrenbeck T et al. Feasibility of tomographic 99mTc-hexakis-2-methoxy-2-methylpropyl-isonitrile imaging for the assessment of myocardial area at risk and the effect of treatment in acute myocardial infarction. Circulation 1989; 80: 1277–86.

40. Crane P, Laliberte R, Heminway S, Thoolen M, Orlandi C. Effect of mitochondrial viability and metabolism on technetium-99m-sestamibi myocardial retention. Eur J Nucl Med 1993; 20: 20–5.

41. Klocke FJ, Baird MG, Lorell BH et al. ACC/AHA/ASNC guidelines for the clinical use of cardiac radionuclide imaging – executive summary: a report of the American College of Cardiology/American Heart Association Task Force on Practice Guidelines (ACC/AHA/ASNC Committee to Revise the 1995 Guidelines for the Clinical Use of Cardiac Radionuclide Imaging). Circulation 2003; 108: 1404–18.

42. Chin BB, Esposito G, Kraitchman DL. Myocardial contractile reserve and perfusion defect severity with rest and stress dobutamine (99m)Tc-sestamibi SPECT in canine stunning and subendocardial infarction. J Nucl Med 2002; 43: 540–50.

43. Wagner A, Mahrholdt H, Holly TA et al. Contrast-enhanced MRI and routine single photon emission computed tomography (SPECT) perfusion imaging for detection of subendocardial myocardial infarcts: an imaging study. Lancet 2003; 361: 374–9.

44. Schelbert HR, Schwaiger M. Positron emission tomography in human myocardial ischemia. Herz 1987; 12: 22–40.

45. Schwaiger M. Time course of metabolic findings in coronary occlusion and reperfusion and their role for assessing myocardial salvage. Eur J Nucl Med 1986; 12 (Suppl): S54–8.

46. Slart RH, Bax JJ, van Veldhuisen DJ et al. Prediction of functional recovery after revascularization in

patients with coronary artery disease and left ventricular dysfunction by gated FDG-PET. J Nucl Cardiol 2006; 13: 210–19.

47. Gambhir SS, Czernin J, Schwimmer J et al. A tabulated summary of the FDG PET literature. J Nucl Med 2001; 42 (5 Suppl): 1S–93S.

48. Wilke N, Jerosch-Herold M, Wang Y et al. Myocardial perfusion reserve: assessment with multisection, quantitative, first-pass MR imaging. Radiology 1997; 204: 373–84.

49. Lima J, Judd R, Schulman D et al. Capillary damage with human infarcts assessed by contrast-enhanced MRI indexes greater myocardial dysfunction and greater myocardial loss. Circulation 1994; 90: I410.

50. Al-Saadi N, Nagel E, Gross M et al. Noninvasive detection of myocardial ischemia from perfusion reserve based on cardiovascular magnetic resonance. Circulation 2000; 101: 1379–83.

51. Kim RJ, Shah DJ, Judd RM. How we perform delayed enhancement imaging. J Cardiovasc Magn Reson 2003; 5: 505–14.

52. Axel L, Dougherty L. Heart wall motion: improved method of spatial modulation of magnetization for MR imaging. Radiology 1989; 172: 349–50.

53. Zerhouni EA, Parish DM, Rogers WJ, Yang A, Shapiro EP. Human heart: tagging with MR imaging – a method for noninvasive assessment of myocardial motion. Radiology 1988; 169: 59–63.

54. Mahrholdt H, Wagner A, Holly TA et al. Reproducibility of chronic infarct size measurement by contrast-enhanced magnetic resonance imaging. Circulation 2002; 106: 2322–7.

55. Klem I, Heitner JF, Shah DJ et al. Improved detection of coronary artery disease by stress perfusion cardiovascular magnetic resonance with the use of delayed enhancement infarction imaging. J Am Coll Cardiol 2006; 47: 1630–8.

56. Wu K, Zerhouni E, Judd RM et al. Prognostic significance of microvascular obstruction by magnetic resonance imaging in patients with acute myocardial infarction. Circulation 1998; 97: 765–72.

57. Bengel FM, Schachinger V, Dimmeler S. Cell-based therapies and imaging in cardiology. Eur J Nucl Med Mol Imaging 2005; 32 (Suppl 2): S404–16.

58. Barnett BP, Arepally A, Karmakar PV et al. Magnetic resonance-guided real-time targeted delivery and imaging of magnetocapsules immunoprotecting pancreatic islet cells. Nat Med 2007; 18(3): 986–91.

59. Barnett BP, Kraitchman DL, Lauzon C et al. Radiopaque alginate microcapsules for x-ray visualization and immunoprotection of cellular therapeutics. Mol Pharm 2006; 3: 531–8.

60. Tannous BA, Grimm J, Perry KF et al. Metabolic biotinylation of cell surface receptors for in vivo imaging. Nat Methods 2006; 3: 391–6.

61. Chiesa R, Melissano G, Castellano R et al. Avidin and 111In-labelled biotin scan: a new radioisotopic method for localising vascular graft infection. Eur J Vasc Endovasc Surg 1995; 10: 405–14.

62. Winter PM, Morawski AM, Caruthers SD et al. Molecular imaging of angiogenesis in early-stage atherosclerosis with alpha(v)beta3-integrin-targeted nanoparticles. Circulation 2003; 108: 2270–4.

63. Winter PM, Caruthers SD, Neubauer AM et al. Magnetic resonance molecular imaging for prediction of targeted drug delivery efficacy in atherosclerosis. J Cardiovasc Magn Reson 2006; 8: 66–7.

64. Morawski AM, Winter PM, Yu X et al. Quantitative "magnetic resonance immunohistochemistry" with ligand-targeted (19)F nanoparticles. Magn Reson Med 2004; 52: 1255–62.

65. Stark DD, Weissleder R, Elizondo G et al. Superparamagnetic iron oxide: clinical application as a contrast agent for MR imaging of the liver. Radiology 1988; 168: 297–301.

66. Weissleder R. Liver MR imaging with iron oxides: toward consensus and clinical practice. Radiology 1994; 193: 593–5.

67. Frank JA, Zywicke H, Jordan EK et al. Magnetic intracellular labeling of mammalian cells by combining (FDA-approved) superparamagnetic iron oxide MR contrast agents and commonly used transfection agents. Acad Radiol 2002; 9: S484–7.

68. Kalish H, Arbab AS, Miller BR et al. Combination of transfection agents and magnetic resonance contrast agents for cellular imaging: relationship between relaxivities, electrostatic forces, and chemical composition. Magn Reson Med 2003; 50: 275–82.

69. Arbab AS, Bashaw LA, Miller BR et al. Intracytoplasmic tagging of cells with ferumoxides and transfection agent for cellular magnetic resonance imaging after cell transplantation: methods and techniques. Transplantation 2003; 76: 1123–30.

70. Bulte JW, Kraitchman DL. Monitoring cell therapy using iron oxide MR contrast agents. Curr Pharm Biotechnol 2004; 5: 567–84.

71. Kostura L, Kraitchman DL, Mackay AM, Pittenger MF, Bulte JW. Feridex labeling of mesenchymal stem cells inhibits chondrogenesis but not adipogenesis or osteogenesis. NMR Biomed 2004; 17: 513–7.

72. Bos C, Delmas Y, Desmouliere A et al. In vivo MR imaging of intravascularly injected magnetically labeled mesenchymal stem cells in rat kidney and liver. Radiology 2004; 233: 781–9.

73. Kustermann E, Roell W, Breitbach M et al. Stem cell implantation in ischemic mouse heart: a high-resolution magnetic resonance imaging investigation. NMR Biomed 2005; 18: 362–70.

74. Kraitchman DL, Heldman AW, Atalar E et al. In vivo magnetic resonance imaging of mesenchymal stem cells in myocardial infarction. Circulation 2003; 107: 2290–3.

75. Tallheden T, Nannmark U, Lorentzon M et al. In vivo MR imaging of magnetically labeled human embryonic stem cells. Life Sci 2006; 79: 999–1006.

76. Garot J, Unterseeh T, Teiger E et al. Magnetic resonance imaging of targeted catheter-based implantation of myogenic precursor cells into infarcted left ventricular myocardium. J Am Coll Cardiol 2003; 41: 1841–6.

77. Bulte JW, Kraitchman DL, Mackay AM et al. Chondrogenic differentiation of mesenchymal stem cells is inhibited after magnetic labeling with ferumoxides. Blood 2004; 104: 3410–13.

78. Arbab AS, Yocum GT, Kalish H et al. Efficient magnetic cell labeling with protamine sulfate complexed to ferumoxides for cellular MRI. Blood 2004; 104: 1217–23.

79. Walczak P, Kedziorek D, Gilad AA, Lin S, Bulte JW. Instant MR labeling of stem cells using magneto-electroporation. Magn Reson Med 2005: 769–74.

80. Ahrens ET, Flores R, Xu H, Morel PA. In vivo imaging platform for tracking immunotherapeutic cells. Nat Biotechnol 2005; 23: 983–7.

81. Giesel FL, Stroick M, Griebe M et al. Gadofluorine m uptake in stem cells as a new magnetic resonance imaging tracking method: an in vitro and in vivo study. Invest Radiol 2006; 41: 868–73.

82. Segal AW, Arnot RN, Thakur ML, Lavender JP. Indium-111-labelled leucocytes for localisation of abscesses. Lancet 1976; 2: 1056–8.

83. Lavender JP, Goldman JM, Arnot RN, Thakur ML. Kinetics of indium-III labelled lymphocytes in normal subjects and patients with Hodgkin's disease. Br Med J 1977; 2: 797–9.

84. Brenner W, Aicher A, Eckey T et al. 111In-labeled CD34+ hematopoietic progenitor cells in a rat myocardial infarction model. J Nucl Med 2004; 45: 512–18.

85. Aicher A, Brenner W, Zuhayra M et al. Assessment of the tissue distribution of transplanted human endothelial progenitor cells by radioactive labeling. Circulation 2003; 107: 2134–9.

86. Kraitchman DL, Tatsumi M, Gilson WD et al. Dynamic imaging of allogeneic mesenchymal stem cells trafficking to myocardial infarction. Circulation 2005; 112: 1451–61.

87. Zhou R, Thomas DH, Qiao H et al. In vivo detection of stem cells grafted in infarcted rat myocardium. J Nucl Med 2005; 46: 816–22.

88. Jin Y, Kong H, Stodilka RZ et al. Determining the minimum number of detectable cardiac-transplanted 111In-tropolone-labelled bone-marrow-derived mesenchymal stem cells by SPECT. Phys Med Biol 2005; 50: 4445–55.

89. Bindslev L, Haack-Sorensen M, Bisgaard K et al. Labelling of human mesenchymal stem cells with indium-111 for SPECT imaging: effect on cell proliferation and differentiation. Eur J Nucl Med Mol Imaging 2006; 33: 1171–7.

90. Leor J, Amsalem Y, Cohen S. Cells, scaffolds, and molecules for myocardial tissue engineering. Pharmacol Ther 2005; 105: 151–63.

91. Leor J, Cohen S. Myocardial tissue engineering: creating a muscle patch for a wounded heart. Ann NY Acad Sci 2004; 1015: 312–19.

92. Cosby KM, Hofmann LV, Barnett BP et al. A novel radio-opaque barium/alginate microencapsulation technique for allogeneic mesenchymal stem cell delivery and localization. J Cardiovasc Magn Reson 2007; 9: 401–2.

93. Gruber PJ, Li Z, Li H et al. In vivo imaging of MLC2v-luciferase, a cardiac-specific reporter gene expression in mice. Acad Radiol 2004; 11: 1022–8.

94. Gambhir SS, Bauer E, Black ME et al. A mutant herpes simplex virus type 1 thymidine kinase reporter gene shows improved sensitivity for imaging reporter gene expression with positron emission tomography. Proc Natl Acad Sci USA 2000; 97: 2785–90.

95. Cao F, Lin S, Xie X et al. In vivo visualization of embryonic stem cell survival, proliferation, and migration after cardiac delivery. Circulation 2006; 113: 1005–14.

96. Gilad AA, McMahon MT, Walczak P et al. Artificial reporter gene providing MRI contrast based on proton exchange. Nat Biotechnol 2007; 25: 217–19.

97. Genove G, DeMarco U, Xu H, Goins WF, Ahrens ET. A new transgene reporter for in vivo magnetic resonance imaging. Nat Med 2005; 11: 450–4.

98. Moore A, Josephson L, Bhorade RM, Basilion JP, Weissleder R. Human transferrin receptor gene as a marker gene for MR imaging. Radiology 2001; 221: 244–50.

99. Weissleder R, Moore A, Mahmood U et al. In vivo magnetic resonance imaging of transgene expression. Nat Med 2000; 6: 351–5.

100. Miyagawa M, Beyer M, Wagner B et al. Cardiac reporter gene imaging using the human sodium/iodide symporter gene. Cardiovasc Res 2005; 65: 195–202.

101. Miyagawa M, Anton M, Wagner B et al. Non-invasive imaging of cardiac transgene expression with PET: comparison of the human sodium/iodide symporter gene and HSV1-tk as the reporter gene. Eur J Nucl Med Mol Imaging 2005; 32: 1108–14.

102. Hou D, Youssef EA, Brinton TJ et al. Radiolabeled cell distribution after intramyocardial, intracoronary, and interstitial retrograde coronary venous

delivery: implications for current clinical trials. Circulation 2005; 112 (9 Suppl): I150–6.

103. Freyman T, Polin G, Osman H et al. A quantitative, randomized study evaluating three methods of mesenchymal stem cell delivery following myocardial infarction. Eur Heart J 2006; 27: 1114–22.

104. Chin BB, Nakamoto Y, Bulte JW et al. 111In oxine labelled mesenchymal stem cell SPECT after intravenous administration in myocardial infarction. Nucl Med Commun 2003; 24: 1149–54.

105. Gao J, Dennis JE, Muzic RF, Lundberg M, Caplan AI. The dynamic in vivo distribution of bone marrow-derived mesenchymal stem cells after infusion. Cell Tissues Organs 2001; 169: 12–20.

106. Hofmann M, Wollert KC, Meyer GP et al. Monitoring of bone marrow cell homing into the infarcted human myocardium. Circulation 2005; 111: 2198–202.

107. de Vries IJ, Lesterhuis WJ, Barentsz JO et al. Magnetic resonance tracking of dendritic cells in melanoma patients for monitoring of cellular therapy. Nat Biotechnol 2005; 23: 1407–13.

108. Stuckey DJ, Carr CA, Martin-Rendon E et al. Iron particles for noninvasive monitoring of bone marrow stromal cell engraftment into, and isolation of viable engrafted donor cells from, the heart. Stem Cells 2006; 24: 1968–75.

109. Dick AJ, Guttman MA, Raman VK et al. Magnetic resonance fluoroscopy allows targeted delivery of mesenchymal stem cells to infarct borders in swine. Circulation 2003; 108: 2899–904.

110. Amado LC, Salrais AP, Schuleri KH et al. Cardiac repair with intramyocardial injection of allogeneic mesenchymal stem cells after myocardial infarction. Proc Natl Acad Sci USA 2005; 102: 11474–9.

111. Hill JM, Dick AJ, Raman VK et al. Serial cardiac magnetic resonance imaging of injected mesenchymal stem cells. Circulation 2003; 11: 11.

112. Soto AV, Gilson WD, Kedziorek D et al. MRI tracking of regional persistence of feridex-labeled mesenchymal stem cells in a canine myocardial infarction model. J Cardiovasc Magn Reson 2006; 8: 89–90.

113. Limbourg FP, Ringes-Lichtenberg S, Schaefer A et al. Haematopoietic stem cells improve cardiac function after infarction without permanent cardiac engraftment. Eur J Heart Fail 2005; 7: 722–9.

114. Adonai N, Nguyen KN, Walsh J et al. Ex vivo cell labeling with 64Cu-pyruvaldehyde-bis (N4-methylthiosemicarbazone) for imaging cell trafficking in mice with positron-emission tomography. Proc Natl Acad Sci USA 2002; 99: 3030–5.

115. de Silva R, Gutierrez LF, Raval AN et al. X-ray fused with magnetic resonance imaging (XFM) to target endomyocardial Injections. Validation in a swine model of myocardial infarction. Circulation 2006; 114: 2342–50.

116. Heyn C, Bowen CV, Rutt BK, Foster PJ. Detection threshold of single SPIO-labeled cells with FIESTA. Magn Reson Med 2005; 53: 312–20.

117. Foster-Gareau P, Heyn C, Alejski A, Rutt BK. Imaging single mammalian cells with a 1.5 T clinical MRI scanner. Magn Reson Med 2003; 49: 968–71.

118. Verdijk P, Scheenen TW, Lesterhuis WJ et al. Sensitivity of magnetic resonance imaging of dendritic cells for in vivo tracking of cellular cancer vaccines. Int J Cancer 2007; 120: 978–84.

chapter 12

Genetically Engineered Stem Cells for Mechanical and Electrical Myocardial Repair

Sergey V Doronin, Irina A Potapova, Damon J Kelly, Adam J Schuldt, Amy B Rosen, Peter R Brink, Richard B Robinson, Michael R Rosen, Glenn R Gaudette and Ira S Cohen

Introduction

Clinical trials employing bone marrow-derived stem cells for treatment of myocardial infarction (MI) have shown short-term mechanical benefit.[1,2] Whether this initial improvement is translated into long-term gain remains uncertain.[3] These clinical studies were preceded by those in animal models demonstrating that stem cells delivered post-MI improve angiogenesis, myocardial wall movement, and possibly even myocyte content. However, the physiological mechanisms underlying these stem cell-induced improvements are poorly understood. It is not even certain whether the functional improvement derived from the delivered stem cells is mediated through improved active contraction or via changes in passive mechanical properties.[4] In an attempt to understand the basis of any favorable effects of stem cells, as well as to enhance their efficacy, it seems natural to genetically engineer stem cells to optimize the expression of those factors thought most likely to be beneficial. Alternatively, stem cells could be engineered for enhanced survival so that their favorable actions would be prolonged.[5]

The mechanical activity of the heart is initiated by a propagating electrical signal, the action potential, which initiates an orderly wave of activation followed by highly efficient contraction. If there is failure of either action-potential initiation (sinus arrest) or propagation through the atrioventricular (A–V) node (A–V block), an electronic pacemaker is inserted to restore electrical and contractile function. Although pacemaker therapy was a major medical advance, it is not a cure. Maintenance, battery or electrode replacement, and occasional device failures are among the difficulties. It is with these problems in mind that "biological pacemakers" were conceived. To create such a "device" it is necessary to initiate or enhance pacemaker activity in a chosen cardiac region. If stem cells are to be used as a delivery system, this requires expression of a pacemaker gene in the chosen cell type and its delivery and integration into the cardiac syncytium to change the region's electrical phenotype.

To better understand the current and potential use of genetically engineered stem cells for cardiac repair, this chapter is divided into two sections. One considers the use of genetically engineered stem cells for mechanical recovery of function while the other focuses on electrical applications. Since the field is new, there are many promising avenues of investigation that have not yet been attempted. For this reason, in each section we will consider both the current applications and potential future opportunities.

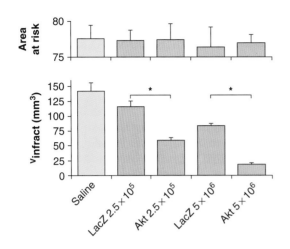

Figure 12.2 *Increasing cell survival with Akt enhances stem cell and myocyte survival. When injected into ischemic ventricular wall, adult mesenchymal stem cells transfected with Akt, a pro-survival gene, decrease infarct volume (Vinfarct) compared to the same number of cells transfected with the LacZ reporter gene. The dose-dependent response suggests that increasing the number of injected cells may further decrease infarct volume. *p < 0.01. (Reproduced with permission from reference 5.)*

marrow stem cells exposed to preconditioning via anoxia demonstrate increased *Akt* levels, and when delivered to the heart decrease myocyte apoptosis, presumably through a paracrine mechanism.[17] While preconditioning stem cells may increase their tolerance to ischemia, if the mechanism of preconditioning can be identified, the involved factors may provide another therapeutic intervention for delivery through genetically engineered stem cells with the hope of protecting endogenous myocytes from ischemia.

The combination of *Akt* and angiogenic factors such as angiopoietin 1 may result in even further improvements in cardiac function. MSCs engineered to coexpress angiopoietin 1 and *Akt* enhance cell survival, increase blood vessel density, and improve global cardiac function.[18] Although some of these cells differentiate into myocytes, there is no evidence to suggest that this occurs at a frequency nearly sufficient to be fully responsible for the documented increase in cardiac function. Thus, it is likely that

some combination of angiogenesis and enhanced myocyte survival plays an important role in the protective effect offered by these engineered stem cells.

Improved mechanical function can also be achieved by enhancing passive mechanical properties: genetic engineering can alter matrix proteins

The approaches discussed above are designed to be beneficial in ischemic tissue by enhancing myocyte survival. Improved pump function in infarcted tissue could also occur by altering the passive mechanical properties of the tissue, thereby improving global function. This approach has been tested theoretically by simulating the injection of a non-contractile passive material, which resulted in improved cardiac function.[19] An increased compliance in the infarcted region will lead to improved diastolic filling and may increase the ejection fraction. MSCs injected into the infarct border zone have just such an effect on compliance[20] (even though most of these cells do not differentiate into cardiac myocytes). Interestingly, this improvement also occurs with skeletal myoblasts,[21] suggesting a lack of specificity of the effect. This point was recently emphasized by Murry et al, who stated: "almost every cell type tested seems equipotent,"[22] suggesting that the simple addition of viable cells may be enough to improve global cardiac function. Along these lines, elastin-overexpressing endothelial cells implanted into infarcted heart tissue led to an improved ejection fraction compared to delivery of non-expressing cells.[23] The elastin-expressing cells also decreased scar size, which suggests that altering the mechanical properties of the scar may lead to decreases in infarct size. Thus, further improvements may be possible by taking advantage of the protective paracrine signals expressed in stem cells and engineering them to overexpress matrix proteins, such as elastin, to improve the passive properties of myocardial scar tissue. The optimum combination of extracellular matrix molecules would increase compliance while maintaining strength.

Improving active contraction by enhancing differentiation of stem cells into myocytes

The optimum repair substrate would contract in synchrony with the native myocardium. In order for this to occur, the cells need to form functional gap junctions, a property possessed by mesenchymal stem cells[24] (also see later section). In order to produce a contractile cell from MSCs, the mechanisms responsible for the differentiation of stem cells into cardiac myocytes need to be better understood. During cardiac differentiation from embryonic cells, a number of transcription factors are known to be activated, including *Nkx2-5*,[25] GATA4,[25], and *Mef2c*.[26] Upregulation of these genes might enhance the fraction of source cells that choose a cardiac lineage. For example, activation of the Notch receptor in MSCs may lead to differentiation of these cells along a cardiac lineage.[27]

Overexpression of cytokines and growth factors could also lead to increased cardiac differentiation. VEGF,[28] FGF,[29] and platelet derived growth factor (PDGF)[30] induce increased differentiation of embryonic stem cells into cardiac myocytes. The addition of PDGF to bone marrow cells shortens the time to the expression of α-myosin heavy chain.[31] However, since most growth factors have a short half-life, sustained delivery to the heart is difficult. Overexpression of these factors in stem cells may aid in the local delivery of these same factors in vivo that may in turn facilitate differentiation of MSCs into myocytes in situ.

Engineering stem cells to enhance myocyte proliferation

Yet another potential mechanism for genetically engineered stem cells to increase myocyte mass is the induction of native myocyte proliferation. While only a few years ago cardiac myocytes were considered to be terminally differentiated and lacking the ability to enter the cell cycle, there is now considerable evidence to suggest that adult cardiac myocytes may be able to overcome this limitation. Cell cycle markers, such as Ki67, have been found in the cardiac myocytes obtained from myocardial infarction patients,[32] and it is now generally accepted that cardiac myocytes retain an ability to synthesize DNA.[33] Endothelial progenitor cells can induce myocyte proliferation in vivo.[34] Itescu's laboratory delivered CD34+ human cells to the infarcted rat heart, and, through the use of species-specific antibodies, clearly demonstrated the presence of Ki67 in the nucleus of native rat cardiac myocytes.[34] MSCs can also induce the expression of cell cycle markers in cardiac myocytes in culture.[35] Hence, myocyte proliferation should not be overlooked as a mechanism of protection offered by stem cell-released paracrine factors. Genetically engineered stem cells that overexpress the relevant factors that induce cell cycle activity may be able to restore lost myocytes (for a list of potential factors see reference 36). One preliminary result from our group suggests that Wnt5A may play such a role.[37]

Increased homing may increase the concentration of stem cells at the site of injury

Targeting of cell delivery is almost certainly required for repair of localized areas of myocardium. It has been reported that MSCs are attracted to sites of injury in general[38–42] and specifically to sites of infarction.[43,44] Several factors such as monocyte chemoattractant protein 3 (MCP3), stromal cell derived factor 1 (SDF1), and CXCR4 and CCR5 receptors have been identified as responsible for the homing of stem cells.[45–55] In principle, it should be possible to deliver MSCs transfected with "homing receptors" that could enhance attraction to and thereby concentrate these cells at a site of injury.

Summary of approaches for mechanical recovery with genetically engineered stem cells

A variety of approaches are feasible for engineering stem cells to enhance myocardial function. The most extensively studied approaches have involved genetically engineering either pro-survival or proangiogenesis genes into stem cells to enhance myocyte survival following ischemic injury. These two approaches can limit myocardial cell loss. Another approach that can enhance mechanical function is altering the extracellular matrix to improve the passive properties of the myocardium. This has been demonstrated to have potential efficacy in a theoretical model of myocardial infarction.[19] If stem cells are to have a maximal effect, they must be concentrated at the site of injury. Engineering receptors that optimize homing may allow for enhanced or prolonged effects of delivered cells. However, ideally it would be desirable to add new contractile elements to enhance active contraction. There is some evidence that the paracrine factors released by stem cells may enhance myocyte proliferation. Active investigation of the relevant factors may be a fruitful area for future genetic engineering. Finally, stem cells have the capacity to differentiate into myocytes, although it does not occur frequently. Enhancing this native potential could be a potent solution for myocyte loss not only due to myocardial infarction but in heart failure as well.

Engineered Stem Cells for Treatment of Electrical Abnormalities

A unique requirement for the repair of electrical abnormalities with genetically engineered stem cells is functional integration with the host tissue via formation of gap junctions. These intercellular channels are the only known way in which current (or small molecules) can flow from the interior of one cell to the interior of another. The action potential (whether normal or abnormal) propagates via local circuit currents which require an intact electrical connection. Thus, the delivery cell of choice must make connexins and effectively integrate into the cardiac syncytium. The dominant connexins expressed in cardiac tissues are 40, 43, and 45, and if the genetically engineered cells are to integrate effectively then they must express connexins that can couple with the endogenous cardiac connexins.

The use of engineered stem cells to repair conduction abnormalities

Hematopoietic, mesenchymal, and embryonic stem cells are all capable of forming functional

gap junctions.[24,56–59] The existence of functional gap junctions can be demonstrated by either dual whole-cell patch clamp and direct measurement of gap junctional conductance or measurement of contraction or action-potential propagation in the delivered stem cells in synchrony with the rest of the myocardium. Durig et al used dual whole-cell patch clamping (Figure 12.3a) and Western blotting to show that CD34+ hematopoietic stem cells form functional gap junctions using connexin (Cx)43.[56] Valiunas et al, using the same techniques and immunocytochemistry, demonstrated that human MSCs expressed Cx 40 and 43 which trafficked to the cell surface.[24] The hMSCs could form functional gap junctions with each other, with heart cells, and with cell lines expressing exclusively any one of the three cardiac connexins (Figure 12.3b). Xue et al used optical mapping of action-potential propagation in a coculture of embryonic stem cells and neonatal rat ventricular myocytes to demonstrate functional integration of embryonic stem cells[59] (Figure 12.3c).

Biological pacemakers: a proof of principle for the use of genetically engineered stem cells

The initial approaches to create a biologic pacemaker elevated β receptors or downregulated K channels by delivery of naked DNA or viruses.[60,61] The results of these studies demonstrated the feasibility of affecting heart rate, but were not easily translated into cellular delivery. Overexpressing a receptor or a dominant negative construct in a delivery cell would not have an equivalent electrical effect to direct delivery of the gene to the host tissue. For a genetically engineered cell to exert a direct electrical effect, it must express a channel that results in electrical current flow across the plasma membrane which then, via current flow across gap junctions (formed between the delivery cell and a host cell), directly influences the electrical activity of the native myocardium.

A major difference between pacing regions of the heart and those that are quiescent is the presence of the current I_f in the physiologic range of membrane potentials.[62] This current is inward at

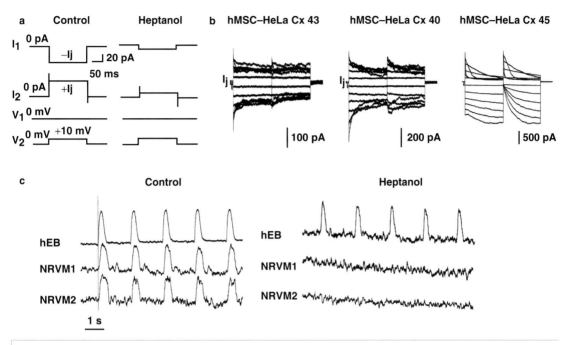

Figure 12.3 *Stem cells make functional gap junctions. (a) Hematopoietic stem cells studied with the dual whole-cell patch clamp technique are well coupled in control conditions. The magnitude of gap junctional coupling is reduced upon exposure to heptanol; an uncoupler of gap junctions.[56] (b) Human mesenchymal stem cells (hMSCs) were cocultured with HeLa cells expressing connexin 43, 40, or 45 and then studied with the whole-cell patch clamp technique. The current records recorded in response to transjunctional voltage steps indicate that the hMSCs made functional gap junctions with HeLa cells making each connexin type.[24] (c) Human embryonic stem cells (hEBs) and neonatal rat ventricular myocytes (NRVMs) were cocultured. The spontaneous electrical activity initiated by the hEBs was recorded from the neonatal myocytes at two locations in the culture dish (NVRM1 and NRVM2) in control conditions. Heptanol uncoupled the hEBs from the NRVMs and so eliminated propagation of the impulse initiated in the hEBs to NRVM1 and NRVM2.[59]*

diastolic potentials and drives the membrane to threshold. The HCN (hyperpolarization-activated nucleotide-gated cation channel) gene family encodes the I_f channel protein. It therefore made sense to deliver HCN channels to non-pacing regions of the heart in order to create pacemaker activity.

Potapova et al created the first cell-based biological pacemaker using genetically engineered human MSCs transfected with the HCN2 gene (Figure 12.4) by delivering about 1 million of these genetically engineered cells to the left ventricular free wall of the canine heart.[63] Figure 12.5 shows schematically how such a pacemaker would work. The delivery cell would form a two-cell functional syncytium with native myocardium via gap junction formation. Because of this functional coupling, the membrane potential in the hMSC would closely follow

the membrane potential of the myocyte. During diastole, when the myocyte's membrane potential is most negative, the HCN channels would open, generating an inward current which would flow through the gap junction channels, depolarizing the myocyte towards threshold. The two-cell functional syncytium is spontaneously active, a property not shared by either the host myocyte (which lacks the HCN channels) or the transfected hMSC (which lacks all the myocyte channels). Figure 12.6 illustrates the rhythm generated by the genetically engineered hMSCs. This activity occurred upon stimulation of both vagi 7 days after stem cell implantation, which temporarily allowed escape pacemaker activity.

Human MSCs are not the only cells to be used as biological pacemakers. They have also been generated by embryonic stem cells (ESCs)

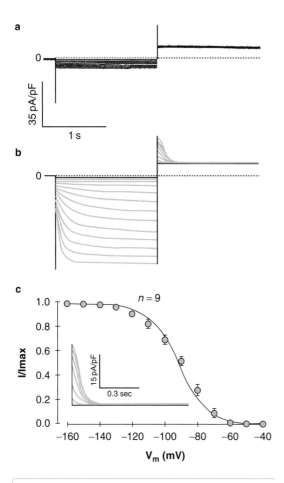

Given the efficacy of electronic pacemakers, it is likely that the first-generation clinical application of biological pacemakers will include an electronic backup. Such a tandem conformation should have the improved physiologic responsiveness of the biologic pacemaker and prolong the battery life of its electronic counterpart. The first steps in that direction were taken recently in two publications in *Circulation*.[64,65] Our group compared native and mutant forms of HCN2 in tandem with an electronic pacemaker,[64] while Tse et al employed a deletion mutant of HCN1.[65] Both groups showed that their biological pacemakers demonstrated responsiveness to catecholamines. In these experiments the genes were directly delivered to myocytes via adenovirus. These experiments also presented the first uses of mutant HCN genes which can be engineered to optimize pacemaker function. In fact, it may even be possible to re-engineer potassium channels to open on hyperpolarization as a substitute gene for members of the HCN gene family. The first such attempt was made by Kashiwakura et al who modified the potassium channel Kv1.4 to activate on hyperpolarization by site directed mutagenesis.[66] One disadvantage of this synthetic gene approach is that it lacks the cyclic adenosine monophosphate (cAMP) responsiveness which is an integral part of HCN genes.

Figure 12.4   *Human mesenchymal stem cells can be transfected with the murine HCN2 (mHCN2) pacemaker gene. Current records from a patch clamp protocol in which the hMSCs were hyperpolarized from a holding potential (V_m) of –40 mV in 10-mV increments to a maximum negative potential of –160 mV. (a) Nontransfected hMSC; (b) transfected hMSC; (c) activation curve for the mHCN2-induced current in hMSCs shows that the current activates in the diastolic range of potentials.*[63]

Genetically engineered stem cells as a therapy for arrhythmias?

Although stem cell therapy has been used successfully exclusively for the creation of biological pacemakers, viral gene transfer has also been focused on a number of re-entrant arrhythmias including atrial fibrillation[67] and postinfarct ventricular tachycardia.[68] It is worth examining these approaches to determine whether similar cellular therapies may be developed.

differentiated along a cardiac lineage and delivered to either the pig[58] or guinea-pig heart.[59] Xue et al also infected these ESCs with lentivirus carrying the green fluorescent protein (GFP) gene and showed that the infection did not alter their ability to differentiate into pacemaker cells, providing the proof of principle for genetic engineering of ESCs with viruses.[59]

Some targets do not translate to cell therapy but functional outcomes might: an example in atrial fibrillation

Donohue et al delivered an inhibitory G protein (G_{ai2}) to the A–V node in circumstances of acutely induced atrial fibrillation.[67] The expression of this gene, which decreases adenylyl cyclase activity and downregulates cAMP levels, resulted in a reduced safety

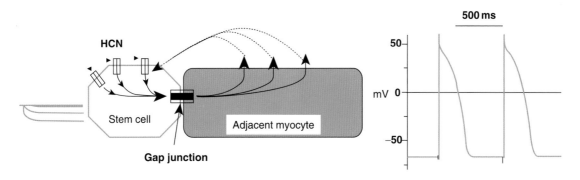

Figure 12.5   *Schematic illustrating the two-cell functional syncytium that generates pacemaker activity upon delivery and integration of transfected hMSCs. The hMSCs contribute the HCN2-induced inward current at diastolic potentials. The ventricular cell contributes all other components of the electrical activity. The action-potential to the right of the ventricular cell illustrates the normal ventricular action-potential in the absence of the HCN2-induced current. (Adapted from reference 62.)*

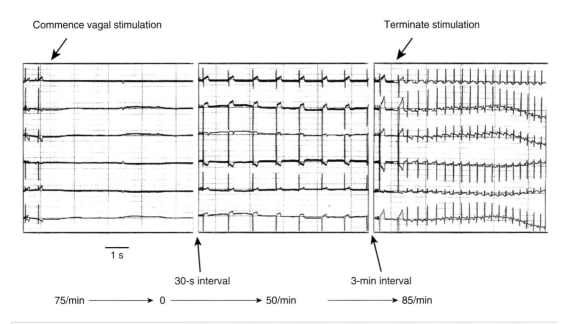

Figure 12.6   *Transfected hMSCs generate a spontaneous rhythm in the canine heart. Approximately one million hMSCs transfected with the* mHCN2 *gene were injected into the canine left ventricular free wall. Seven days later, the dog was anesthetized, the electrocardiogram (ECG) recorded, and both vagi were stimulated, resulting in cessation of activity in the sinoatrial (SA) node (left panel). After a period of time, a spontaneous rhythm initiated (middle panel). Upon cessation of vagal stimulation, the normal sinus rhythm returned (right panel). Additional experiments demonstrated that the spontaneous activity originates at the site of the hMSC injection.*[63]

factor for conduction through the A–V node and a reduced ventricular rate by 20%. Later studies by the same group in a model of persistent atrial fibrillation in the setting of severe congestive heart failure demonstrated that a constituitively active *G205L* mutant of the $G_{\alpha i2}$ protein could exert a similar ventricular rate reduction, and that this was a sufficient change in rate to reverse the

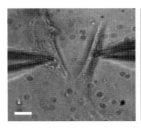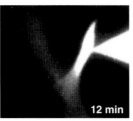

12 min

Figure 12.7 *Human MSCs (hMSCs) can pass RNA via gap junctions. (a) Phase contrast record of three hMSCs that are coupled by gap junctions. (b) Fluorescent image of the same cells indicates the passage of a 12-base-long morpholino tagged with a fluorescent probe from a donor hMSC to the recipient hMSCs.*[72]

tachycardia-induced myopathy caused by the disease. This is an example of a gene therapy that is not easily translated into cell therapy. Overexpressing the G protein construct in a cellular delivery system would not result in dramatic reductions in cAMP in the myocytes. Instead, the success with the approach should encourage those interested in cell therapy to focus on the functional outcome that yielded success: reducing the safety factor for conduction in the A–V node. One way in which cells might achieve a similar effect is to deliver them with no excitable membrane currents but the ability to couple to the resident A–V nodal cells, thus reducing the net inward current density (and safety factor) in the conduction pathway. Indeed, in an analogous approach, Bunch et al injected fibroblasts with or without transforming growth factor β1 (TGFβ1) into the peri-A–V nodal region of canines and demonstrated an increased A–H interval in normal sinus rhythm and an increased R–R interval 4 weeks after recovery from induction of atrial fibrillation.[69] The mechanism of the slowing remains uncertain, but might involve attendant additional membrane and reduced safety factor for conduction.

Dominant negative constructs might translate to cellular delivery of siRNA: an example in postinfarction ventricular tachycardia

Recently, Sasano et al terminated postinfarction ventricular tachycardia in the pig by the focal delivery of a dominant negative construct of the KCNH2 channel.[70] This construct reduced the

magnitude of the rapid component of the delayed rectifier (I_{kr}) in the region at risk, lengthening the action-potential and preventing re-entry. Delivery of a dominant negative construct in a genetically engineered cell is not likely to result in downregulation of the ion channel in the host tissue, as neither the message nor the protein would permeate gap junction channels. Although at first glance this would seem another target poorly suited to genetically engineered cell therapy because of the size of the RNA and the protein, there is a viable alternative. Small interfering RNAs (siRNAs) are pieces of RNA of 18–22 bases in length which are complementary to mRNA. When expressed they hybridize with mRNA, targeting the mRNA to RISCs (RNA-induced silencing complexes) where the mRNA is degraded and the gene effectively silenced.[71] Valiunas et al demonstrated that oligonucleotides up to 24 bases in length permeate gap junction channels composed of Cx 43 at observable rates on a tens of minutes time scale.[72] Figure 12.7 shows that hMSCs which express this connexin can be used as a delivery system. Further, when cells overexpressing an siRNA for a DNA repair enzyme (polymerase β) were cocultured with fluorescently labeled wild type cells and then later sorted, gene knockdown for polymerase β could be demonstrated in the wild type cells. Since siRNA is available for all known genes, its cellular delivery represents a viable alternative to viral delivery of dominant negative constructs.

Summary of prospects for electrical repair with genetically engineered stem cells

For successful cell-based therapy for cardiac arrhythmias, it is necessary for the genetically engineered stem cell to electrically integrate into the host myocardium. All three types of stem cells (hematopoietic, mesenchymal, and embryonic) have demonstrated the capacity for gap junction formation and electrical integration. Proof of principle for this type of therapy has been demonstrated. Biological pacemakers with sustained activity have been reported using both hMSCs and ESCs. Gene therapy has demonstrated success in the treatment of animal models of atrial fibrillation and postinfarction ventricular tachycardias. The approaches in these gene therapy experiments employed focal delivery of adenoviruses with limited persistence. Focal treatments are amenable to adaptation to cellular therapies. However, some targets accessible to gene therapy have no cellular correlate (i.e. $G_{\alpha i2}$ in atrial fibrillation). Instead, adaptation to cellular therapy in these cases should focus on the functional outcome. Other therapies for cardiac arrhythmias rely on delivery of a dominant negative construct (mutant *HERG* (human ether-a-go-go-related gene) in postinfarction ventricular tachycardia). While dominant negative mRNA or the protein it encodes is incapable of permeating gap junctions, recent studies have demonstrated that siRNA can. Cells delivering a construct for making an appropriate siRNA could, in principle, be the equivalent of dominant negative gene therapy.

However, significant barriers remain for an electrical therapy to be successful. In the long term, the electrical characteristics of the delivery system must not change. Thus, it will be important to have stable transfections in stem cells that do not divide, do not differentiate, and do not die. Much remains to be done before short-term successes can be translated into long-term therapies.

Acknowledgments

This work was supported by HL28958 and HL67101 from the National Heart, Lung, and Blood Institute (NHLBI), and a grant from Boston Scientific Corporation. GRG and SVD are recipients of National Scientist Development Grants from the American Heart Association (AHA).

References

1. Wollert KC, Meyer GP, Lotz J et al. Intracoronary autologous bone-marrow cell transfer after myocardial infarction: the BOOST randomised controlled clinical trial. Lancet 2004; 364: 141–8.
2. Schachinger V, Erbs S, Elsasser A et al. Intracoronary bone marrow-derived progenitor cells in acute myocardial infarction. N Engl J Med 2006; 355: 1210–21.
3. Meyer GP, Wollert KC, Lotz J et al. Intracoronary bone marrow cell transfer after myocardial infarction: eighteen months' follow-up data from the randomized, controlled BOOST (BOne marrOw transfer to enhance ST-elevation infarct regeneration) trial. Circulation 2006; 113: 1287–94.
4. Gaudette GR, Cohen IS. Cardiac regeneration: materials can improve the passive properties of myocardium, but cell therapy must do more. Circulation 2006; 114: 2575–7.
5. Mangi AA, Noiseux N, Kong D et al. Mesenchymal stem cells modified with *Akt* prevent remodeling and restore performance of infarcted hearts. Nat Med 2003; 9: 1195–201.
6. Haynesworth SE, Baber MA, Caplan AI. Cytokine expression by human marrow-derived mesenchymal progenitor cells in vitro: effects of dexamethasone and IL-1 alpha. J Cell Physiol 1996; 166: 585–92.
7. Liu CH, Hwang SM. Cytokine interactions in mesenchymal stem cells from cord blood. Cytokine 2005; 32: 270–9.
8. Kinnaird T, Stabile E, Burnett MS et al. Marrow-derived stromal cells express genes encoding a broad spectrum of arteriogenic cytokines and promote in vitro and in vivo arteriogenesis through paracrine mechanisms. Circ Res 2004; 94: 678–85.
9. Kinnaird T, Stabile E, Burnett MS et al. Local delivery of marrow-derived stromal cells augments collateral perfusion through paracrine mechanisms. Circulation 2004; 109: 1543–9.
10. Gruber R, Kandler B, Holzmann P et al. Bone marrow stromal cells can provide a local environment that favors migration and formation of tubular structures of endothelial cells. Tissue Eng 2005; 11: 896–903.
11. Matsumoto R, Omura T, Yoshiyama M et al. Vascular endothelial growth factor-expressing mesenchymal stem cell transplantation for the treatment of acute myocardial infarction. Arterioscler Thromb Vasc Biol 2005; 25: 1168–73.
12. Wang X, Hu Q, Mansoor A, Lee J et al. Bioenergetic and functional consequences of stem cell-based VEGF delivery in pressure-overloaded swine hearts. Am J Physiol Heart Circ Physiol 2006; 290: H1393–405.
13. Wang Y, Haider HK, Ahmad N et al. Combining pharmacological mobilization with intramyocardial delivery of bone marrow cells over-expressing VEGF is more effective for cardiac repair. J Mol Cell Cardiol 2006; 40: 736–45.
14. Yang J, Zhou W, Zheng W et al. Effects of myocardial transplantation of marrow mesenchymal stem cells transfected with vascular endothelial growth factor for the improvement of heart function and angiogenesis after myocardial infarction. Cardiology 2007; 107: 17–29.
15. Nagaya N, Kangawa K, Itoh T et al. Transplantation of mesenchymal stem cells improves cardiac function in a rat model of dilated cardiomyopathy. Circulation 2005; 112: 1128–35.
16. Gnecchi M, He H, Noiseux N et al. Evidence supporting paracrine hypothesis for *Akt*-modified

mesenchymal stem cell-mediated cardiac protection and functional improvement. FASEB J 2006; 20: 661–9.

17. Uemura R, Xu M, Ahmad N, Ashraf M. Bone marrow stem cells prevent left ventricular remodeling of ischemic heart through paracrine signaling. Circ Res 2006; 98: 1414–21.

18. Jiang S, Haider H, Idris NM, Salim A, Ashraf M. Supportive interaction between cell survival signaling and angiocompetent factors enhances donor cell survival and promotes angiomyogenesis for cardiac repair. Circ Res 2006; 99: 776–84.

19. Wall ST, Walker JC, Healy KE, Ratcliffe MB, Guccione JM. Theoretical impact of the injection of material into the myocardium: a finite element model simulation. Circulation 2006; 114: 2627–35.

20. Berry MF, Engler AJ, Woo YJ et al. Mesenchymal stem cell injection after myocardial infarction improves myocardial compliance. Am J Physiol Heart Circ Physiol 2006; 290: H2196–203.

21. Mills WR, Mal N, Kiedrowski MJ et al. Stem cell therapy enhances electrical viability in myocardial infarction. J Mol Cell Cardiol 2007; 42: 304–14.

22. Murry CE, Reinecke H, Pabon LM. Regeneration gaps: observations on stem cells and cardiac repair. J Am Coll Cardiol 2006; 47: 1777–85.

23. Mizuno T, Yau TM, Weisel RD, Kiani CG, Li RK. Elastin stabilizes an infarct and preserves ventricular function. Circulation 2005; 112: I81–8.

24. Valiunas V, Doronin S, Valiuniene L et al. Human mesenchymal stem cells make cardiac connexins and form functional gap junctions. J Physiol 2004; 555: 617–26.

25. Monzen K, Shiojima I, Hiroi Y et al. Bone morphogenetic proteins induce cardiomyocyte differentiation through the mitogen-activated protein kinase kinase kinase TAK1 and cardiac transcription factors Csx/Nkx-2.5 and GATA-4. Mol Cell Biol 1999; 19: 7096–105.

26. Lin Q, Schwarz J, Bucana C, Olson EN. Control of mouse cardiac morphogenesis and myogenesis by transcription factor MEF2C. Science 1997; 276: 1404–7.

27. Li H, Yu B, Zhang Y et al. Jagged1 protein enhances the differentiation of mesenchymal stem cells into cardiomyocytes. Biochem Biophys Res Commun 2006; 341: 320–5.

28. Chen Y, Amende I, Hampton TG et al. Vascular endothelial growth factor promotes cardiomyocyte differentiation of embryonic stem cells. Am J Physiol Heart Circ Physiol 2006; 291: H1653–8.

29. Dell'Era P, Ronca R, Coco L et al. Fibroblast growth factor receptor-1 is essential for in vitro cardiomyocyte development. Circ Res 2003; 93: 414–20.

30. Sachinidis A, Gissel C, Nierhoff D et al. Identification of plateled-derived growth factor-BB as cardiogenesis-inducing factor in mouse embryonic stem cells

under serum-free conditions. Cell Physiol Biochem 2003; 13: 423–9.

31. Xaymardan M, Tang L, Zagreda L et al. Platelet-derived growth factor-AB promotes the generation of adult bone marrow-derived cardiac myocytes. Circ Res 2004; 94: E39–45.

32. Beltrami AP, Urbanek K, Kajstura J et al. Evidence that human cardiac myocytes divide after myocardial infarction. N Engl J Med 2001; 344: 1750–7.

33. Pasumarthi KB, Field LJ. Cardiomyocyte cell cycle regulation. Circ Res 2002; 90: 1044–54.

34. Schuster MD, Kocher AA, Seki T et al. Myocardial neovascularization by bone marrow angioblasts results in cardiomyocyte regeneration. Am J Physiol Heart Circ Physiol 2004; 287: H525–32.

35. Doronin S, Kochupura P, Azeloglu E et al. Canine heart regeneration. Presented at Keystone Symposium: Molecular Biology of Cardiac Diseases and Regeneration, 2005, Streamboat Springs, Colorado, USA.

36. Dowell JD, Field LJ, Pasumarthi KB. Cell cycle regulation to repair the infarcted myocardium. Heart Fail Rev 2003; 8: 293–303.

37. Doronin S, Kelly D, Schuldt A et al. Stem cells induce myocardial proliferation in vivo and in vitro by release of paracrine factors. Presented at Keystone Symposium: Molecular Pathways in Cardiac Development and Disease, 2007, Breckenridge, Colorado, USA.

38. Agung M, Ochi M, Yanada S et al. Mobilization of bone marrow-derived mesenchymal stem cells into the injured tissues after intraarticular injection and their contribution to tissue regeneration. Knee Surg Sports Traumatol Arthrosc 2006; 14: 1307–14.

39. Chapel A, Bertho JM, Bensidhoum M et al. Mesenchymal stem cells home to injured tissues when co-infused with hematopoietic cells to treat a radiation-induced multi-organ failure syndrome. J Gene Med 2003; 5: 1028–38.

40. Ji JF, He BP, Dheen ST, Tay SS. Interactions of chemokines and chemokine receptors mediate the migration of mesenchymal stem cells to the impaired site in the brain after hypoglossal nerve injury. Stem Cells 2004; 22: 415–27.

41. Ramirez M, Lucia A, Gomez-Gallego F et al. Mobilisation of mesenchymal cells into blood in response to skeletal muscle injury. Br J Sports Med 2006; 40: 719–22.

42. Satake K, Lou J, Lenke LG. Migration of mesenchymal stem cells through cerebrospinal fluid into injured spinal cord tissue. Spine 2004; 29: 1971–9.

43. Jiang WH, Ma AQ, Zhang YM et al. Migration of intravenously grafted mesenchymal stem cells to injured heart in rats. Sheng Li Xue Bao 2005; 57: 566–72.

44. Kraitchman DL, Tatsumi M, Gilson WD et al. Dynamic imaging of allogeneic mesenchymal

stem cells trafficking to myocardial infarction. Circulation 2005; 112: 1451–61.

45. Kastrup J, Ripa RS, Wang Y, Jorgensen E. Myocardial regeneration induced by granulocyte-colony-stimulating factor mobilization of stem cells in patients with acute or chronic ischaemic heart disease: a non-invasive alternative for clinical stem cell therapy? Eur Heart J 2006; 27: 2748–54.

46. Schenk S, Mal N, Finan A et al. Monocyte chemotactic protein-3 is a myocardial mesenchymal stem cell homing factor. Stem Cells 2007; 25: 245–51.

47. Rossi L, Manfredini R, Bertolini F et al. The extracellular nucleotide UTP is a potent inducer of hematopoietic stem cell migration. Blood 2007; 109: 533–42.

48. Aghi M, Cohen KS, Klein RJ, Scadden DT, Chiocca EA. Tumor stromal-derived factor-1 recruits vascular progenitors to mitotic neovasculature, where microenvironment influences their differentiated phenotypes. Cancer Res 2006; 66: 9054–64.

49. Lombaert IM, Wierenga PK, Kok T et al. Mobilization of bone marrow stem cells by granulocyte colony-stimulating factor ameliorates radiation-induced damage to salivary glands. Clin Cancer Res 2006; 12: 1804–12.

50. Robertson P, Means TK, Luster AD, Scadden DT. CXCR4 and CCR5 mediate homing of primitive bone marrow-derived hematopoietic cells to the postnatal thymus. Exp Hematol 2006; 34: 308–19.

51. Jung Y, Wang J, Schneider A et al. Regulation of SDF-1 (CXCL12) production by osteoblasts; a possible mechanism for stem cell homing. Bone 2006; 38: 497–508.

52. Mahmud N, Patel H, Hoffman R. Growth factors mobilize CXCR4 low/negative primitive hematopoietic stem/progenitor cells from the bone marrow of nonhuman primates. Biol Blood Marrow Transplant 2004; 10: 681–90.

53. Ceradini DJ, Kulkarni AR, Callaghan MJ et al. Progenitor cell trafficking is regulated by hypoxic gradients through HIF-1 induction of SDF-1. Nat Med 2004; 10: 858–64.

54. Konakahara S, Ohashi K, Mizuno K, Itoh K, Tsuji T. CD29 integrin- and LIMK1/cofilin-mediated actin reorganization regulates the migration of haematopoietic progenitor cells underneath bone marrow stromal cells. Genes Cells 2004; 9: 345–58.

55. Hattori K, Heissig B, Rafii S. The regulation of hematopoietic stem cell and progenitor mobilization by chemokine SDF-1. Leuk Lymphoma 2003; 44: 575–82.

56. Durig J, Rosenthal C, Halfmeyer K et al. Intercellular communication between bone marrow stromal cells and CD34+ haematopoietic progenitor cells is mediated by connexin 43-type gap junctions. Br J Haematol 2000; 111: 416–25.

57. Gepstein L, Feld Y, Yankelson L. Somatic gene and cell therapy strategies for the treatment of cardiac arrhythmias. Am J Physiol Heart Circ Physiol 2004; 286: H815–22.

58. Kehat I, Khimovich L, Caspi O et al. Electromechanical integration of cardiomyocytes derived from human embryonic stem cells. Nat Biotechnol 2004; 22: 1282–9.

59. Xue T, Cho HC, Akar FG et al. Functional integration of electrically active cardiac derivatives from genetically engineered human embryonic stem cells with quiescent recipient ventricular cardiomyocytes: insights into the development of cell-based pacemakers. Circulation 2005; 111: 11–20.

60. Edelberg JM, Aird WC, Rosenberg RD. Enhancement of murine cardiac chronotropy by the molecular transfer of the human beta2 adrenergic receptor cDNA. J Clin Invest 1998; 101: 337–43.

61. Miake J, Marban E, Nuss HB. Biological pacemaker created by gene transfer. Nature 2002; 419: 132–3.

62. Rosen MR, Brink PR, Cohen IS, Robinson RB. Genes, stem cells and biological pacemakers. Cardiovasc Res 2004; 64: 12–23.

63. Potapova I, Plotnikov A, Lu Z et al. Human mesenchymal stem cells as a gene delivery system to create cardiac pacemakers. Circ Res 2004; 94: 952–9.

64. Bucchi A, Plotnikov AN, Shlapakova I et al. Wild-type and mutant HCN channels in a tandem biological-electronic cardiac pacemaker. Circulation 2006; 114: 992–9.

65. Tse HF, Xue T, Lau CP et al. Bioartificial sinus node constructed via in vivo gene transfer of an engineered pacemaker HCN channel reduces the dependence on electronic pacemaker in a sick-sinus syndrome model. Circulation 2006; 114: 1000–11.

66. Kashiwakura Y, Cho HC, Barth AS, Azene E, Marban E. Gene transfer of a synthetic pacemaker channel into the heart: a novel strategy for biological pacing. Circulation 2006; 114: 1682–6.

67. Donahue JK, Heldman AW, Fraser H et al. Focal modification of electrical conduction in the heart by viral gene transfer. Nat Med 2000; 6: 1395–8.

68. Donahue JK, Kikuchi K, Sasano T. Gene therapy for cardiac arrhythmias. Trends Cardiovasc Med 2005; 15: 219–24.

69. Bunch TJ, Mahapatra S, Bruce GK et al. Impact of transforming growth factor-beta1 on atrioventricular node conduction modification by injected autologous fibroblasts in the canine heart. Circulation 2006; 113: 2485–94.

70. Sasano T, McDonald AD, Kikuchi K, Donahue JK. Molecular ablation of ventricular tachycardia after myocardial infarction. Nat Med 2006; 12: 1256–8.

71. Filipowicz W. RNAi: the nuts and bolts of the RISC machine. Cell 2005; 122: 17–20.

72. Valiunas V, Polosina YY, Miller H et al. Connexin-specific cell-to-cell transfer of short interfering RNA by gap junctions. J Physiol 2005; 568: 459–68.

chapter 13

Cell Transplantation in Patients with Acute Myocardial Infarction: Current Status and Future Applications

Kai C Wollert

Introduction

Modern reperfusion strategies and advances in pharmacological management of acute myocardial infarction (AMI) have resulted in an increasing proportion of patients surviving the acute event. Many of these patients eventually develop adverse left ventricular remodeling and heart failure. None of our current therapies addresses the underlying cause of the remodeling process, i.e. the damage to the cardiomyocytes and the vasculature in the infarcted area. The alleged transdifferentiation capacity of adult stem cells and the recent discovery of endogenous cardiac repair mechanisms have suggested that cardiac repair (i.e. replacement of necrotic or scarred tissue with viable myocardium) might be achieved in the clinical setting.[1]

Stem cells are capable of self-renewal, transformation into dedicated progenitor cells, and differentiation into specialized progeny. Traditionally, adult stem cells were believed to differentiate only within tissue lineage boundaries (e.g. hematopoietic stem cells giving rise to mature hematopoietic cells). The fairly recent concept of adult stem cell plasticity implies that stem cells can transdifferentiate into cell types outside their original lineage.[2] Along this line, it has been reported that hematopoietic stem cells when transplanted into infarcted mouse myocardium transdifferentiate into cardiomyocytes and vascular cells.[3] Another hypothesis that has created some excitement recently predicts that limited myocardial regeneration can occur after tissue injury through the recruitment of resident and cardiac stem cells.[4] Ironically, while these new ideas have already triggered clinical trials, fusion of transplanted stem cells with resident cardiomyocytes has been offered as an alternative explanation for previous claims of transdifferentiation.[5–8] Moreover, it has been proposed that stem cells secrete cytokines and growth factors which may promote angiogenesis, suppress cell death of resident cardiomyocytes, modulate interstitial matrix composition, and maybe even recruit cardiac stem cells.[9,10] Regardless of the mechanisms, it appears that stem cell therapy has the potential to improve perfusion and contractile performance of the injured heart (Figure 13.1).

Potential Donor Cells

Conceptually, a variety of stem and progenitor cell populations could be used for cardiac repair after AMI, and many of these potential donor cells are discussed in detail in this book. Each cell type has its own profile of advantages, limitations, and practicability issues. Studies comparing the regenerative capacity of distinct cell populations are scarce. Most investigators have therefore chosen a

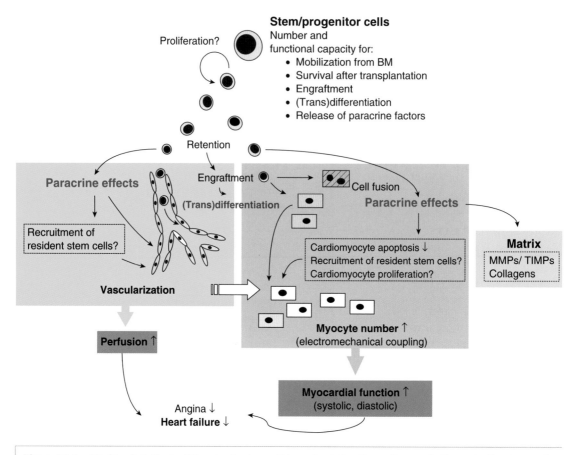

Figure 13.1 *Working hypothesis of therapeutic stem cell transplantation for cardiac repair. Conceptually, stem and progenitor cell transplantation may have a favorable impact on tissue perfusion and contractile performance by promoting vascularization and myocyte formation. Depending on the stem cell type and local milieu, the relative contribution of cell incorporation (transdifferentiation and/or fusion) versus paracrine effects may vary. Stem and progenitor cell numbers and functional capacity are influenced by a patient's age, gender, cardiovascular risk factors, and underlying disease state. BM, bone marrow; MMP, matrix metalloproteinase; TIMP, tissue inhibitor of metalloproteinase. (Adapted from reference 1.)*

pragmatic approach by using unfractionated nucleated bone marrow cells, which contain different stem and progenitor cell populations, including hematopoietic stem cells, endothelial progenitor cells, and mesenchymal stem cells.

Endothelial progenitor cells

Endothelial progenitor cells (EPCs) have been defined by their cell surface expression of the hematopoietic marker proteins CD133 and CD34 and the endothelial marker vascular endothelial growth factor receptor 2, and their capacity to incorporate into sites of neovascularization and to differentiate into endothelial cells in situ. The cell

surface antigen CD133 is expressed on early hematopoietic stem cells and EPCs, both of which collaborate to promote vascularization of ischemic tissues. There is increasing evidence that culture-expanded EPCs contain a CD14+/CD34−/CD133−-mononuclear cell population with "EPC capacity", which mediates its angiogenic effects by releasing paracrine factors.[11]

Mesenchymal stem cells

Mesenchymal stem cells represent a rare population of CD34− and CD133− cells present in bone marrow stroma and other mesenchymal tissues.[12] Mesenchymal stem cells can differentiate into osteocytes, chondrocytes, adipocytes, and cardiomyocyte-like cells under specific culture conditions. When injected into infarct tissue, mesenchymal stem cells may enhance regional wall motion and prevent adverse remodeling. It has been suggested that these effects may be related to paracrine effects rather than differentiation of mesenchymal stem cells into cardiomyocytes.[13,14] Since mesenchymal stem cells can be expanded in vitro, and reportedly have a low immunogenicity, they might be used in an allogeneic setting in the future.[12]

Skeletal myoblasts

Skeletal myoblasts (satellite cells) are progenitor cells which normally lie in a quiescent state under the basal membrane of mature muscular fibers. Myoblasts can be isolated from skeletal muscle biopsies and expanded in vitro. Myoblasts differentiate into myotubes and retain skeletal muscle properties when transplanted into an infarct scar. Although grafted myotubes may contract in response to electrical stimulation, they do not express intercalated disc proteins, indicating that the majority are not electromechanically coupled to their host cardiomyocytes. Nevertheless, myoblast transplantation has been shown to augment systolic and diastolic performance in animal models, possibly through the release of paracrine factors.[15]

Resident cardiac stem cells

Recently, several groups have detected stem and progenitor cells within the heart that are capable of differentiating into cardiomyocytes and/or vascular lineages. It has been suggested that these cells can be clonally expanded and used for cardiac repair in an autologous setting.[4] Clearly, independent confirmation of these provocative findings is required. If confirmed, cardiac resident stem and progenitor cells hold great promise for clinical applications, although it is conceivable that the bone marrow contains a pluripotent stem cell population with similar properties.[16,17]

Embryonic stem cells

Embryonic stem cells (ESCs) are totipotent stem cells derived from the inner cell mass of blastocysts. Under specific culture conditions, ESCs differentiate into multicellular embryoid bodies containing differentiated cells from all three germ layers including cardiomyocytes. Human ESC-derived cardiomyocytes display structural and functional properties of early-stage cardiomyocytes that couple with host cardiomyocytes when transplanted into normal or infarcted myocardium.[18,19] In theory, infinite numbers of cardiomyocytes could be obtained from human ESC clones. However, unresolved ethical and legal issues, concerns about the tumorigenicity of residual ESCs in ESC-derived cardiomyocyte preparations, and the need to use allogeneic cells for transplantation currently hamper their use in clinical studies. Eventually, nuclear transfer techniques may provide a means of generating an unlimited supply of histocompatible ESCs for the treatment of cardiac disease.

Multipotent adult germline stem cells

A recent study has highlighted the pluripotency and plasticity of murine spermatogonial stem cells, which are responsible for maintaining spermatogenesis throughout life in the male. In culture, adult spermatogonial stem cells acquire ESC properties. These multipotent adult germline stem cells spontaneously differentiate into derivatives of the three embryonic germ layers in vitro, including cardiomyocytes and vascular cells.[20] Eventually, establishment of human multipotent adult germline stem cells from testicular biopsies may allow individual cell-based therapy without the ethical and immunological problems associated with human ESCs.[20]

Modes of Cell Delivery in the Setting of Acute Myocardial Infarction

The goal of any cell delivery strategy is to transplant sufficient numbers of cells into the myocardial region of interest and to achieve maximum retention of cells within that area. Retention may be defined as the fraction of transplanted cells retained in the myocardium for a short period of time (hours). The local

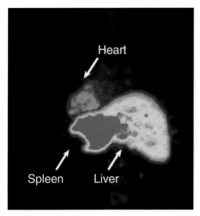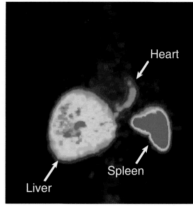

Figure 13.2 *Myocardial homing and biodistribution of unfractionated bone marrow cells after intracoronary transfer. Nine days after primary angioplasty and stent implantation for AMI, this patient received an intracoronary infusion of autologous nucleated bone marrow cells into the stented left circumflex coronary artery. A small fraction of the cells was radiolabeled with [^{18}F]fluorodeoxyglucose ([^{18}F]FDG) just prior to intracoronary transfer. Positron emission tomography (PET) imaging was performed 65 min after cell transfer. Left posterior oblique (a) and left anterior oblique (b) views of the chest and upper abdomen are shown. Approximately 3% of the cells homed to the lateral wall of the heart; most remaining activity is detected in liver and spleen. (Adapted from reference 23.)*

milieu is an important determinant of cell retention, as it will influence short-term cell survival and, if a transvascular approach is used, cell adhesion, transmigration through the vascular wall, and tissue invasion. Transvascular strategies are especially suited for the treatment of recently infarcted and reperfused myocardium when chemoattractants are highly expressed.[21] Direct injection techniques have been used in patients presenting late in the disease process when an occluded coronary artery precludes transvascular cell delivery (e.g. patients with chronic myocardial ischemia) or when cell homing signals are expressed at low levels in the heart (scar tissue). However, cell delivery by direct injection may not be safe in patients with AMI and friable necrotic tissue.

Selective intracoronary application delivers a maximum concentration of cells homogeneously to the site of injury. Unselected bone marrow cells, circulating blood-derived progenitor cells, and mesenchymal stem cells have been delivered via the intracoronary route in patients with AMI. In these studies, cells were delivered through the central lumen of an over-the-wire balloon catheter during transient balloon inflations to maximize the contact time of the cells with the microcirculation of the infarct-related artery.[22] In experimental models, intravenous delivery of endothelial progenitor cells and mesenchymal stem cells has been shown to improve cardiac function after AMI. However, cell homing to non-cardiac organs limits the applicability of this approach. Indeed, in a recent clinical study, homing of unselected bone marrow cells to the infarct region was observed only after intracoronary stop-flow delivery but not after intravenous infusion (Figure 13.2).[23] Considering that the acutely infarcted myocardium recruits circulating stem and progenitor cells to the site of injury, mobilization of stem and progenitor cells by cytokines may offer a non-invasive strategy for cardiac regeneration. Indeed, it has been reported that the stem cell mobilizing cytokines stem cell factor (SCF) and granulocyte colony stimulating factor (G-CSF) improve cardiac function after AMI in mice.[24,25] Notably, G-CSF can accelerate infarct healing directly by enhancing macrophage infiltration and matrix metalloproteinase activation, and suppressing cardiomyocyte apoptosis, suggesting that stem cell-independent mechanisms may contribute to the favorable effects of G-CSF post-AMI.[26,27]

Current Status of Cell Therapy in Patients with Acute Myocardial Infarction

Inspired by experimental data suggesting that functional recovery after AMI can be augmented by stem cell transfer, clinical trials were initiated to assess the therapeutic potential of cell therapy in patients post-AMI. All clinical studies have included patients who had undergone primary angioplasty and stent implantation to reopen the infarct-related artery and who received optimal medical treatment during the acute phase and follow-up, and cells were infused intracoronarily by using the stop-flow balloon-catheter approach. Current trials may be categorized into studies using unselected bone marrow cells or selected stem cell populations.

Unselected bone marrow cells

Following initial safety and feasibility studies, four larger randomized trials of bone marrow cell therapy after AMI have now been completed (Table 13.1).[28–31] The combined experience from these trials indicates that intracoronary delivery of unselected bone marrow cells is feasible and safe in the short and mid-term (up to 18 months). Bone marrow harvest and intracoronary cell delivery are not associated with bleeding complications or ischemic damage to the myocardium. No increased rates of in-stent restenosis have been observed. Clinical surveillance, Holter monitoring, and data from an electrophysiological study indicate that bone marrow cell transfer is not associated with an increased propensity to ventricular arrhythmias; moreover, intramyocardial calcifications or tumor formation were not observed after intracoronary bone marrow cell delivery.[28–32]

In the BOne marrOw transfer to enhance ST-elevation infarct regeneration (BOOST) trial, intracoronary transfer of nucleated bone marrow cells resulted in an improvement of global left ventricular ejection fraction of 6 percentage points after 6 months as compared to the control group. This improvement of ejection fraction was due mostly to improved regional wall motion in the infarct border zone.[28] For comparison, improvements of 3–4 percentage points are achieved by primary angioplasty and stent implantation in AMI, suggesting that the further improvement of ejection fraction by cell therapy may be clinically meaningful.

The beneficial effects of intracoronary bone marrow cell transfer were confirmed in the recent Reinfusion of Enriched Progenitor cells And Infarct Remodeling in Acute Myocardial Infarction (REPAIR-AMI) trial. In this study, mononucleated bone marrow cell transfer promoted an increase in left ventricular ejection fraction of 2.5 percentage points after 4 months as compared to a control group that also underwent bone marrow aspiration but received an intracoronary infusion of a placebo.[29]

In contrast to BOOST and REPAIR-AMI, two other randomized studies did not report significant improvements of left ventricular ejection fraction after intracoronary cell transfer.[30,31] While the exact reasons for the differing results remain elusive, it is worthwhile to take a closer look at the design of these studies (Table 13.1). In one of the negative studies, cells were delivered already 24 hours after coronary reperfusion.[30] In BOOST and REPAIR-AMI, cells were transplanted several days later. Subgroup analyses in REPAIR-AMI indicate that the timing of cell delivery may be important, and that the beneficial effects on ejection fraction are lost when the cells are delivered too early.[29] The Autologous Stem cell Transplantation in Acute Myocardial Infarction (ASTAMI) trial also did not find a significant effect of bone marrow cell transfer on left ventricular ejection fraction recovery.[31] While the cells were delivered late after reperfusion in ASTAMI (after 4–6 days), a particular cell preparation method that leads to an enrichment of lymphocytic bone marrow cells was employed. It is not clear whether this method actually recovers the bone marrow cell populations that are required to achieve functional improvements after AMI. Together, these data remind us that

Table 13.1 Randomized bone marrow cell trials in patients with acute myocardial infarction

Study	Design	n	Cell type	Dose	Time of delivery post-AMI	Outcomes Improved	No change
BOOST[28]	Randomized controlled	30 treated 30 controls	Nucleated BMCs	128 ml	6 ± 1 days	Global LVEF	LVEDV
REPAIR-AMI[29]	Placebo-controlled	95 treated 92 controls	Mononucleated BMCs	50 ml	3–6 days	Global LVEF	LVEDV
Janssens[30]	Placebo-controlled	32 treated 34 controls	Mononucleated BMCs	130 ml	1 day	—	Global LVEF LVEDV
ASTAMI[31]	Randomized controlled	47 treated 50 controls	Lymphocytic BMCs	50 ml	6 ± 1 days	—	Global LVEF LVEDV

BMC, bone marrow cell; AMI, acute myocardial infarction; LVEF, left ventricular ejection fraction; LVEDV, left ventricular end-diastolic volume. In BOOST, cells were prepared by gelatine-polysuccinate density gradient sedimentation which retrieves all nucleated cell types from the bone marrow; REPAIR-AMI and Janssens employed a Ficoll® gradient, which recovers the mononuclear cell fraction. In ASTAMI, lymphocytic bone marrow cells were enriched. Dose refers to the average amount of bone marrow that was harvested.

procedural issues, such as the cell preparation method and timing of cell transfer, need to be further refined.

It should be noted that none of the trials so far has revealed a significant effect of bone marrow cell transfer on left ventricular end-diastolic volumes, an index of left ventricular remodeling. However, larger studies may be required to settle this issue. Moreover, few data are available regarding the long-term effects of bone marrow cell transfer after AMI. Follow-up data from the BOOST trial indicate that the improvements of left ventricular ejection fraction are maintained 18 months after cell transfer;[32] however, ejection fraction also increased somewhat in the control group during long-term follow-up,[32] which would be expected in AMI patients on chronic angiotensin converting enzyme inhibitor and β-blocker therapy. Tissue Doppler echocardiography analyses in BOOST indicate that bone marrow cell transfer may prevent the development of diastolic dysfunction during long-term follow-up. Significant effects of cell transfer on E/A ratio (peak early diastolic/late diastolic velocities) and tissue Doppler E_a/A_a (annular velocities) ratio, but not on isovolumic relaxation time, suggest that cell therapy positively affects left ventricular stiffness but not active relaxation.[33]

Selected bone marrow cell populations

The Transplantation Of Progenitor Cells And Regeneration Enhancement in Acute Myocardial Infarction (TOPCARE-AMI) trial compared mononucleated bone marrow cells with circulating blood-derived progenitor cells (mostly EPCs) in post-AMI patients a few days after reperfusion. Both cell types appeared to have similar safety and efficacy profiles.[34] However, since TOPCARE-AMI was not randomized, firm conclusions regarding the efficacy of endothelial progenitor cells post-AMI cannot be drawn at the present time. In the recent randomized Transplantation Of Progenitor Cells And Regeneration Enhancement in Chronic Heart Failure (TOPCARE-CHF) trial, patients received an intracoronary infusion of unselected mononucleated bone marrow cells or circulating blood-derived progenitor cells months or years after an AMI. Notably, a significant

improvement in left ventricular ejection fraction was observed only in patients receiving mononucleated bone marrow cells in this setting.[35] The effects of culture-expanded mesenchymal stem cells after AMI have been investigated in one randomized clinical trial.[36] While no serious side-effects were reported, it is not known whether intracoronary mesenchymal stem cell delivery promoted ischemic damage to the myocardium,[36] a complication that has occurred after intracoronary mesenchymal stem cell infusions in dogs.[37] Six months after cell transfer, regional wall motion and global left ventricular ejection fraction were improved and left ventricular end-diastolic volumes were decreased.[36] These striking effects need to be confirmed by additional studies. In another trial, CD133+ enriched bone marrow cells were infused into the infarct-related artery in post-AMI patients. Higher luminal losses within the stented segment and the distal, non-stented segments of the infarct-related artery were observed, raising the concern that CD133+ cells may promote in-stent restenosis and atherosclerosis progression.[38] As these data were obtained from retrospective analysis and lacked randomized controls, future studies need to define the risk and mechanisms of such adverse effects on the epicardial coronary circulation (which were not observed in any of the trials using unfractionated nucleated bone marrow cells).[38]

Stem and progenitor cell mobilization

The Front-Integrated Revascularization and Stem Cell Liberation in Evolving Acute Myocardial Infarction by Use of Granulocyte-Colony-Stimulating Factor (FIRSTLINE-AMI) trial randomized 50 patients with AMI to a control group or a 6-day open-label course of G-CSF that was initiated within 1–2 hours after primary angioplasty and stenting.[39] G-CSF therapy after stent implantation was not associated with an enhanced rate of in-stent restenosis or other serious adverse events, and promoted significant improvements in left ventricular ejection fraction and metabolic activity in the infarct territory.[39] Critics have pointed out that the beneficial effects of G-CSF in FIRSTLINE-AMI were magnified by an unexpected decrease in ejection fraction in the control group.[40] The favorable safety profile of G-CSF post-AMI was confirmed in two other recent trials which, however, did not observe a beneficial effect on left ventricular ejection fraction.[41,42] It remains to be seen whether differences in study design, e.g. later start of G-CSF injections in the negative trials, account for the discrepant results.

The Foreseeable Future of Cell Therapy in Patients with Acute Myocardial Infarction

We advocate to no longer perform studies involving small numbers of patients, but rather to conduct larger, double-blind, randomized controlled clinical trials to firmly establish the effects of cell therapy on surrogate markers, such as left ventricular ejection fraction and remodeling, myocardial perfusion, or exercise capacity.[43] Most important, upcoming trials should address procedural issues such as the optimal cell type, cell dosage, and timing of cell transfer. While these trials may also look at combined morbidity and mortality endpoints, they may be too small to be conclusive in this regard. Some of the ongoing trials of intracoronary bone marrow cell transfer after AMI are summarized in Table 13.2. Ultimately, outcome trials and cost–benefit analyses will be required.

Notably, the absolute number of transplanted bone marrow cells did not correlate with subsequent improvements in ejection fraction in previous post-AMI studies. This may be because the cell numbers infused were within a narrow range, or because differences in the functional capacity of the cells, such as the ability to home to and engraft in the infarcted area, to undergo transdifferentiation, and/or to produce paracrine factors, may override differences in cell numbers. Intriguingly, cell labeling studies indicate that fewer than 5% of unselected nucleated bone marrow cells are retained in the infarcted area after intracoronary delivery in patients (Figure 13.2).[23] Although this rate of cell retention was sufficient to improve left ventricular systolic and

diastolic function in the BOOST trial, it is conceivable that pharmacological strategies might be used to enhance the homing capacity or other functional parameters of the cells. Experimental studies are already pointing in this direction.[44] Post-hoc analyses of the BOOST trial database suggest that the effects of bone marrow cell transfer are consistent across several subgroups defined according to sex, age, infarct territory, and time from symptom onset to reperfusion.[28] However, patient subgroups that derive the greatest benefit from cell transfer need to be identified prospectively in future trials (e.g. patients presenting late after symptom onset in whom little myocardial salvage can be expected from reperfusion therapy). In this regard, data from REPAIR-AMI indicate that the effects of bone marrow cell transfer may be more pronounced in patients with more severely depressed baseline left ventricular ejection fraction.[29] Cytokines with stem-cell mobilizing and/or direct cardioprotective properties should be further evaluated as stand alone therapy or in combination with cell transfer after AMI. Eventually, cytokines may emerge as a non-invasive alternative or as an adjunct to cell therapy.

Meanwhile, fundamental questions need to be addressed experimentally. What is the fate of the injected cells after transplantation? Genetic and transgenic markers should be employed to determine lineage commitment of engrafted cells. Cell labeling and imaging techniques need to be developed to track stem cell fate in patients and correlate cell retention and engraftment with functional outcomes. Can the regenerative capacity of transplanted stem cells be enhanced by drugs, cytokines, or gene therapy approaches? Pharmacological and genetic strategies may help to enhance stem cell retention, engraftment, differentiation, and paracrine capability.[45,46]

For the time being, cardiac repair remains the holy grail of cell therapy. While unselected bone marrow cells may have a favorable impact on systolic function, they probably do not make new myocardium. This should stimulate further basic research into the prospects of cell types with transdifferentiation capacity, such as ESCs,

Table13.2   Ongoing randomized cell therapy trials in patients with acute myocardial infarction

Study	Country	Design	n	Groups	Primary endpoints	Principal investigators
REGENT	Poland	Randomized, multicenter	200	Mononucleated BMCs vs CD34+/CXCR4+ cells	Global LVEF, LV volumes (by MRI)	Michal Tendera
HEBE	The Netherlands	Randomized, multicenter	200	Mononucleated BMCs vs peripheral mononucleated cells vs standard therapy	Regional function in dysfunctional segments (by MRI)	Alexander Hirsch Jan J Piek
BOOST-2	Germany, Norway, Bulgaria	Randomized, multicenter, placebo-controlled, factorial design	200	Placebo vs nucleated BMCs (low-dose vs high-dose, pretreated vs not pretreated)	Global LVEF (by MRI)	Kai C Wollert Gerd P Meyer Helmut Drexler

n, expected total enrollment; MRI, magnetic resonance imaging.

multipotent adult germline stem cells, and, possibly, multipotent bone marrow-derived stem cells and resident cardiac stem cells.

References

1. Wollert KC, Drexler H. Clinical applications of stem cells for the heart. Circ Res 2005; 96: 151–63.
2. Wagers AJ, Weissman IL. Plasticity of adult stem cells. Cell 2004; 116: 639–48.
3. Orlic D, Kajstura J, Chimenti S et al. Bone marrow cells regenerate infarcted myocardium. Nature 2001; 410: 701–5.
4. Torella D, Ellison GM, Mendez-Ferrer S, Ibanez B, Nadal-Ginard B. Resident human cardiac stem cells: role in cardiac cellular homeostasis and potential for myocardial regeneration. Nat Clin Pract Cardiovasc Med 2006; 3 (Suppl 1): S8–13.
5. Alvarez-Dolado M, Pardal R, Garcia-Verdugo JM et al. Fusion of bone-marrow-derived cells with Purkinje neurons, cardiomyocytes and hepatocytes. Nature 2003; 425: 968–73.
6. Nygren JM, Jovinge S, Breitbach M et al. Bone marrow-derived hematopoietic cells generate cardiomyocytes at a low frequency through cell fusion, but not transdifferentiation. Nat Med 2004; 10: 494–501.
7. Murry CE, Soonpaa MH, Reinecke H et al. Haematopoietic stem cells do not transdifferentiate into cardiac myocytes in myocardial infarcts. Nature 2004; 428: 664–8.
8. Balsam LB, Wagers AJ, Christensen JL et al. Haematopoietic stem cells adopt mature haematopoietic fates in ischaemic myocardium. Nature 2004; 428: 668–73.
9. Kamihata H, Matsubara H, Nishiue T et al. Implantation of bone marrow mononuclear cells into ischemic myocardium enhances collateral perfusion and regional function via side supply of angioblasts, angiogenic ligands, and cytokines. Circulation 2001; 104: 1046–52.
10. Kinnaird T, Stabile E, Burnett MS et al. Marrow-derived stromal cells express genes encoding a broad spectrum of arteriogenic cytokines and promote in vitro and in vivo arteriogenesis through paracrine mechanisms. Circ Res 2004; 94: 678–85.
11. Urbich C, Dimmeler S. Endothelial progenitor cells: characterization and role in vascular biology. Circ Res 2004; 95: 343–53.

12. Pittenger MF, Martin BJ. Mesenchymal stem cells and their potential as cardiac therapeutics. Circ Res 2004; 95: 9–20.

13. Dai W, Hale SL, Martin BJ et al. Allogeneic mesenchymal stem cell transplantation in postinfarcted rat myocardium: short- and long-term effects. Circulation 2005; 112: 214–23.

14. Wollert KC, Drexler H. Mesenchymal stem cells for myocardial infarction: promises and pitfalls. Circulation 2005; 112: 151–3.

15. Dowell JD, Rubart M, Pasumarthi KB, Soonpaa MH, Field LJ. Myocyte and myogenic stem cell transplantation in the heart. Cardiovasc Res 2003; 58: 336–50.

16. Yoon YS, Wecker A, Heyd L et al. Clonally expanded novel multipotent stem cells from human bone marrow regenerate myocardium after myocardial infarction. J Clin Invest 2005; 115: 326–38.

17. Mouquet F, Pfister O, Jain M et al. Restoration of cardiac progenitor cells after myocardial infarction by self-proliferation and selective homing of bone marrow-derived stem cells. Circ Res 2005; 97: 1090–2.

18. Kehat I, Khimovich L, Caspi O et al. Electromechanical integration of cardiomyocytes derived from human embryonic stem cells. Nat Biotechnol 2004; 22: 1282–9.

19. Menard C, Hagege AA, Agbulut O et al. Transplantation of cardiac-committed mouse embryonic stem cells to infarcted sheep myocardium: a preclinical study. Lancet 2005; 366: 1005–12.

20. Guan K, Nayernia K, Maier LS et al. Pluripotency of spermatogonial stem cells from adult mouse testis. Nature 2006; 440: 1199–203.

21. Frangogiannis NG. The mechanistic basis of infarct healing. Antioxid Redox Signal 2006; 8: 1907–39.

22. Strauer BE, Brehm M, Zeus T et al. Repair of infarcted myocardium by autologous intracoronary mononuclear bone marrow cell transplantation in humans. Circulation 2002; 106: 1913–18.

23. Hofmann M, Wollert KC, Meyer GP et al. Monitoring of bone marrow cell homing into the infarcted human myocardium. Circulation 2005; 111: 2198–202.

24. Orlic D, Kajstura J, Chimenti S et al. Mobilized bone marrow cells repair the infarcted heart, improving function and survival. Proc Natl Acad Sci USA 2001; 98: 10344–9.

25. Ohtsuka M, Takano H, Zou Y et al. Cytokine therapy prevents left ventricular remodeling and dysfunction after myocardial infarction through neovascularization. FASEB J 2004; 18: 851–3.

26. Minatoguchi S, Takemura G, Chen XH et al. Acceleration of the healing process and myocardial regeneration may be important as a mechanism of improvement of cardiac function and remodeling by postinfarction granulocyte colony-stimulating factor treatment. Circulation 2004; 109: 2572–80.

27. Harada M, Qin Y, Takano H et al. G-CSF prevents cardiac remodeling after myocardial infarction by activating the Jak-Stat pathway in cardiomyocytes. Nat Med 2005; 11: 305–11.

28. Wollert KC, Meyer GP, Lotz J et al. Intracoronary autologous bone-marrow cell transfer after myocardial infarction: the BOOST randomised controlled clinical trial. Lancet 2004; 364: 141–8.

29. Schachinger V, Erbs S, Elsasser A et al. Intracoronary bone marrow-derived progenitor cells in acute myocardial infarction. N Engl J Med 2006; 355: 1210–21.

30. Janssens S, Dubois C, Bogaert J et al. Autologous bone marrow-derived stem-cell transfer in patients with ST-segment elevation myocardial infarction: double-blind, randomised controlled trial. Lancet 2006; 367: 113–21.

31. Lunde K, Solheim S, Aakhus S et al. Intracoronary injection of mononuclear bone marrow cells in acute myocardial infarction. N Engl J Med 2006; 355: 1199–209.

32. Meyer GP, Wollert KC, Lotz J et al. Intracoronary bone marrow cell transfer after myocardial infarction: eighteen months' follow-up data from the randomized, controlled BOOST (BOne marrOw transfer to enhance ST-elevation infarct regeneration) trial. Circulation 2006; 113: 1287–94.

33. Schaefer A, Meyer GP, Fuchs M et al. Impact of intracoronary bone marrow cell transfer on diastolic function in patients after acute myocardial infarction: results from the BOOST trial. Eur Heart J 2006; 27: 929–35.

34. Schachinger V, Assmus B, Britten MB et al. Transplantation of progenitor cells and regeneration enhancement in acute myocardial infarction: final one-year results of the TOPCARE-AMI Trial. J Am Coll Cardiol 2004; 44: 1690–9.

35. Assmus B, Honold J, Schachinger V et al. Transcoronary transplantation of progenitor cells after myocardial infarction. N Engl J Med 2006; 355: 1222–32.

36. Chen SL, Fang WW, Ye F et al. Effect on left ventricular function of intracoronary transplantation of autologous bone marrow mesenchymal stem cell in patients with acute myocardial infarction. Am J Cardiol 2004; 94: 92–5.

37. Vulliet PR, Greeley M, Halloran SM, MacDonald KA, Kittleson MD. Intra-coronary arterial injection of mesenchymal stromal cells and microinfarction in dogs. Lancet 2004; 363: 783–4.

38. Mansour S, Vanderheyden M, De Bruyne B et al. Intracoronary delivery of hematopoietic bone marrow stem cells and luminal loss of the infarct-related artery in patients with recent myocardial infarction. J Am Coll Cardiol 2006; 47: 1727–30.

39. Ince H, Petzsch M, Kleine HD et al. Preservation from left ventricular remodeling by front-integrated revascularization and stem cell liberation in evolving acute myocardial infarction by use of granulocyte-colony-stimulating factor (FIRSTLINE-AMI). Circulation 2005; 112: 3097–106.

40. de Muinck ED, Simons M. Calling on reserves: granulocyte colony stimulating growth factor in cardiac repair. Circulation 2005; 112: 3033–5.

41. Zohlnhofer D, Ott I, Mehilli J et al. Stem cell mobilization by granulocyte colony-stimulating factor in patients with acute myocardial infarction: a randomized controlled trial. JAMA 2006; 295: 1003–10.

42. Ripa RS, Jorgensen E, Wang Y et al. Stem cell mobilization induced by subcutaneous granulocyte-colony stimulating factor to improve cardiac regeneration after acute ST-elevation myocardial infarction: result of the double-blind, randomized, placebo-controlled stem cells in myocardial infarction (STEMMI) trial. Circulation 2006; 113: 1983–92.

43. Bartunek J, Dimmeler S, Drexler H et al. The consensus of the task force of the European Society of Cardiology concerning the clinical investigation of the use of autologous adult stem cells for repair of the heart. Eur Heart J 2006; 27: 1338–40.

44. Sasaki K, Heeschen C, Aicher A et al. Ex vivo pretreatment of bone marrow mononuclear cells with endothelial NO synthase enhancer AVE9488 enhances their functional activity for cell therapy. Proc Natl Acad Sci USA 2006; 103: 14537–41.

45. Kawamoto A, Murayama T, Kusano K et al. Synergistic effect of bone marrow mobilization and vascular endothelial growth factor-2 gene therapy in myocardial ischemia. Circulation 2004; 110: 1398–405.

46. Gnecchi M, He H, Liang OD et al. Paracrine action accounts for marked protection of ischemic heart by Akt-modified mesenchymal stem cells. Nat Med 2005; 11: 367–8.

chapter 14

Cell Transplantation in Chronic Heart Failure: Proof of Concept and Early Clinical Experience

Philippe Menasché

Introduction

After receiving a diagnosis of congestive heart failure, one in five patients will be dead within 12 months.[1] This condition affects at least 10 million people in Western Europe and approximately half this number in the United States,[2] and in 2004, the cost of treating cardiovascular disease and stroke in this country was estimated to reach $368 billion. These statistics alone clearly outline that despite advances in drug and device therapies, new approaches to heart failure are eagerly needed. In this setting, the recognition that endogenous repair mechanisms are inadequate to repair extensively damaged hearts led, more than a decade ago, to testing the concept of repopulating areas of non-viable myocardium with cells. The results of the seminal experiments showing that cells injected into failing hearts could create new tissue and improve function then generated an escalating interest in cell transplantation as a potential new means of treating heart failure. Indeed, the current field of cardiac cell therapy also encompasses acute myocardial infarction and refractory angina in "no-option" patients, but replacement of chronically akinetic scars by new functional myocardium probably remains the most challenging indication because of the limited blood supply to the transplanted cells and the absence of local cues required for driving them towards a cardiomyogenic differentiation pathway.[3] The

present review focuses on this heart failure setting exclusively. It will summarize the main preclinical data that have established the proof of concept, the results of the initial clinical trials, and the major hurdles that still need to be overcome.

Proof of Concept

Chronologically, the proof that transplanted cells could contribute to the repair of postinfarction myocardial tissue was brought by the use of fetal cardiomyocytes. Groundbreaking experiments showed that these cells could engraft in postinfarction fibrotic scars, express gap junction proteins enabling their coupling with host cardiomyocytes, and improve left ventricular (LV) function.[4,5] However, the anticipated difficulties in exploiting these cells for therapeutic purposes then led to expanding the proof of concept by investigating skeletal myoblasts, which feature more clinically appealing characteristics such as an autologous origin, a high degree of scalability in culture, a myogenic lineage restriction reducing the risk of tumor formation, and a strong resistance to ischemia. A large number of experimental studies in small and large animal models of myocardial infarction, and subsequently of non-ischemic cardiomyopathy (reviewed in reference 6), unequivocally demonstrated the differentiation of myoblasts transplanted in postinfarction chronic scars into myotubes and an associated improvement in LV function. More recently, the beneficial effects of myoblast transplantation have been further supported by sonomicrometry data in a dog model of heart failure,[7] while the limitation of remodeling was documented by magnetic resonance imaging (MRI) in rabbit hearts[8] and pressure–volume loops in sheep.[9] Additional proof of concept has been brought by bone marrow cell transplantation studies which have shown that mononuclear cells, mesenchymal stem cells, and hematopoietic progenitors are all able to improve the functional outcome of chronically infarcted hearts at varying degrees, although most of these experiments have rather entailed the use of these cells in the acute setting of a myocardial infarction (reviewed in references 10 and 11).

Of note, a common feature of all these experiments was the consistent recognition that cell engraftment was quantitatively limited because of an initial leakage of the cells[12] and the superimposed high rate of death of those retained in the target tissue. The initial injection-associated washout[13] has two detrimental effects: it reduces the efficacy expected from the transplantation and leads to an extracardiac cell dissemination with still unknown consequences. Interestingly, the magnitude of this procedure-associated cell loss does not seem to be influenced by the route of delivery, since, at least in the case of skeletal myoblasts, engraftment has been shown to be equivalent after surgical and catheter-based injections.[14] Furthermore, different tracking methods (immunolabeling, genetic tags, and more recently MRI of cells loaded with superparamagnetic iron particles) have shown that a huge proportion of the successfully engrafted cells (up to 90%) then die over the first weeks.[15] This high rate of graft attrition results from the interplay of multiple factors including inflammation, apoptosis, hypoxia, and loss of survival signals from extracellular matrix attachments and cell–cell interactions. Overall, myoblasts appear to be more resistant than other cells, although their number also declines over time.[16] As discussed at the end of this review, strategies that increase

both cell transfer and survival are thus mandatory to optimize the benefits of cell transplantation and enable an engraftment rate high enough to translate to a clinically meaningful improvement in functional outcome.

The proof-of-concept that cell therapy may be an effective means of alleviating heart failure, however, is somewhat weakened by our persisting uncertainty about the puzzling mechanistic discrepancy between the poor long-term engraftment rate and the functional benefits of the procedure. Although an improvement in pump function due to a graft-induced cardiac "regeneration" has been postulated as a primary mechanism, this hypothesis is now increasingly challenged by two types of observation. First, the number of surviving cells is too small to directly account for an augmented contractility. To cause heart failure, an infarct needs to kill approximately 25% of the left ventricle, which represents a myocyte deficit in the order of one billion,[17] and it is clear that such an objective cannot be currently achieved. Second, there is little, if any, evidence that adult stem cells, whether myogenic or bone marrow-derived, can convert into cardiomyocytes, and most of the heretofore reported transdifferentiation events are now recognized as fluorescence-related artifacts, or fusion of donor cells with the native ones leading the former to adopt the phenotype of the latter.[18,19] Furthermore, the histological finding that some scattered cells may occasionally express cardiac-specific surface markers does not automatically imply that they have turned into cardiomyocytes, as such a conclusion requires the still missing demonstration that these cells have recapitulated the molecular, electrophysiological, and functional patterns of the cardiomyogenic lineage. Indeed, newly created cardiomyocytes electromechanically coupled with those of the host myocardium should be demonstrated to prove that cardiac regeneration has been achieved, and, so far, the opposite has rather been shown, i.e. neither skeletal myoblasts[20] nor bone marrow cells[21] express in vivo the gap junction proteins supporting an effective coupling with the native cardiomyocytes. This statement, however, does not apply to fetal cardiac cells or cardiac-committed embryonic stem cells, which, so far, are the only cells that have been convincingly shown to differentiate along the cardiomyogenic pathway following their in-scar engraftment.[22-24] This discrepancy between the magnitude of cell engraftment and that of functional recovery has thus raised the alternative hypothesis that cells do not act via some intrinsic contractile properties but rather through the release of a wide array of cytokines and growth factors that favorably influence the surrounding myocardium. This paracrine paradigm is currently supported by two lines of evidence. First, bone marrow cells have been shown in vitro to secrete large amounts of these soluble factors,[25,26] and their biological relevance is exemplified by the observation that the benefit of *Akt*-transduced mesenchymal stem cells can be reproduced by the cell-free supernatant recovered from their cultures;[27] the involvement of locally released signaling molecules is also suggested by the ability of bone marrow cells to reduce both necrosis and apoptosis of the human myocardium in an in vitro model of simulated ischemia[28] through protein kinase signaling. Likewise, microarray studies conducted in collaboration with Professor Felipe Prosper, University of Navarra, Spain suggest that skeletal myoblasts could similarly behave as vehicles for local signaling molecules. Second, there are now several in vivo observations that bone marrow cells and myoblasts can increase angiogenesis directly by releasing angiogenic proteins[29] or indirectly by enhancing homing of circulating endothelial progenitors in injured tissue through the stromal cell derived factor 1 (SDF1)–CXCR4 pathway,[30,31] or regulating the myocardial balance of angiogenic cytokines.[32] Additional cell-induced effects include reduction of apoptosis,[33] possibly through increased *Akt* expression,[26] and changes in the expression of metalloproteinases,[34,35] resulting in the reduction of extracellular matrix fibrosis.[14,31,35,36] Put together, these data are consistent with paracrine effects that trigger repair mechanisms, and could explain why these mechanisms may still be manifest beyond the physical presence of the cells that have initiated them. Although mobilization of tissue-resident cardiac stem cells has also been invoked as a potential target for cell-released factors,[37] this hypothesis still remains largely speculative in view of our ignorance about

the persistence of these stem cells in adult human beings, at least at a significant level. Indeed, the preliminary results of an ongoing study in our department indicate that the very rare c-*kit*-positive cells that can be found in either right ventricular biopsies taken in heart transplant recipients or right appendage tissue specimens collected during coronary artery bypass surgery express hematopoietic markers, and, more specifically, those of mast cells without evidence for expression of markers of the cardiac lineage such as *Nkx2-5*. A last mechanistic hypothesis assumes a buttressing effect of cells on the infarcted segment, which would improve scar elasticity and translate into a limitation of ventricular dilatation. A recent study using a finite element model simulation has elegantly shown that when a non-contractile material is added to an infarcted LV wall, the resulting increase in wall volume, although small, translates into a reduction in border zone myofiber stress which can contribute to reduced remodeling and increased ejection fraction (EF) through volume changes and not functional regeneration.[38] The beneficial effects of cells on ventricular dimensions reported in chronically infarcted models also suggest the abovementioned paracrinally induced changes in extracellular matrix composition, a hypothesis consistent with the correlation between elevation of metalloproteinase 9 (which indirectly contributes to enhanced fibrosis and is downregulated following myoblast transplantation[34]) and LV end-diastolic volumes in postinfarction patients.[39] The recent observation that cell commitment to a given lineage can itself be specified by the degree of matrix elasticity[40] emphasizes the complexity and biological importance of the graft–matrix relationship. It also raises a word of caution about the use of mesenchymal stem cells,[41] which are unlikely to convert into cardiomyocytes but could, at best, adopt a myogenic phenotype (with no obvious advantage over true myoblasts) or respond to a rigid matrix by differentiating along an unwanted osteogenic pathway.[42]

Taken together, these data provide compelling evidence that transplantation of skeletal myoblasts, or bone marrow-derived cells (and actually other cell types), induces local, yet incompletely identified, microenvironmental changes which translate into a better preservation of left ventricular function more likely related to the cell-released products than to the contractile properties of the cells themselves (except for fetal and embryonic stem cells). These considerations have thus paved the way for the first clinical trials which will now be discussed.

Early Clinical Experience

So far, two types of adult cells have undergone clinical testing in patients with heart failure: skeletal myoblasts and bone marrow cells.

Skeletal myoblast studies

They started in June 2000, when we performed the first human transplantation of autologous myoblasts in a patient with severe ischemic heart failure.[43] This case initiated a series of 10 patients with a low left ventricular ejection fraction (LVEF) ($\leq 35\%$), a history of myocardial infarction with a residual non-viable scar, and an indication for coronary artery bypass grafting (CABG) in areas remote from the transplanted regions. Overall, 871 million cells, of which 87% were myoblasts, were injected. At an average follow-up of 52 months (range 18–58), the patients are symptomatically improved and the incidence of hospitalizations for heart failure has been relatively low (0.13/patient-years). Echocardiographically measured LVEF and volumes have remained stable over time. Early ventricular arrhythmias prompted the implantation of an internal cardioverter-defibrillator (ICD) in five patients, of whom three have demonstrated new arrhythmic events at later time points (6, 7, and 18 months after implantation).[44] One patient died 17.5 months after his surgery from a presumed stroke, and the pathologic examination of his heart could identify clusters of myotubes embedded in scar tissue.[45]

Overall, these findings are consistent with those of the three other adjunct-to-CABG phase I trials which have been reported. The study of Gavira and co-workers[46] included 12 patients who received an average of 221 million myoblasts, and demonstrated, at the 1-year postoperative follow-up, a significant increase in global and regional contractility along with an improvement in the viability and perfusion of the myoblast-transplanted segments, as assessed by positron emission tomography (PET). Of note, none of the patients experienced cardiac arrhythmias, which was speculatively attributed by the authors to the use of autologous, instead of fetal calf, serum for culturing the cells. In the study of Siminiak et al,[47] 10 patients were injected with varying doses of cells (from 4 ± 10^5 to 5 ± 10^7), which resulted in a significant increase in EF that was maintained throughout the 12-month follow-up period. Four episodes of sustained ventricular tachycardia were documented (two during the early postoperative period and two others after 2 weeks). The third study was reported by Dib and co-workers[48] and included two cohorts. A first group of 24 patients underwent a dose-escalating trial of skeletal myoblast transplantation in conjunction with CABG (four three-patient groups were treated with 1, 3, 10, and 30×10^7 cells while the remaining 12 patients received a fixed dose of 3×10^8). As in the previous studies, the procedure resulted in an increase of the echocardiographically measured EF which was sustained until the 2-year study point. In some patients, PET and MRI also documented improved viability in the transplanted areas. Non-sustained ventricular tachycardia was reported in three cases. The second cohort of this study included six patients in whom skeletal myoblasts were injected during implantation of a left ventricular assist device (LVAD) as a bridge to transplantation. In four cases, the heart was then available (after device explantation or death) for pathological study, which demonstrated patterns of myofiber engraftment very similar to those described in our autopsy study. Importantly, these three studies basically differed from ours in that the cell-implanted area was consistently revascularized.

In parallel to these surgical trials, three catheter-based studies have been reported. In one of them, myoblasts were delivered by a catheter introduced into the coronary sinus route, featuring an extendable needle allowing injection of cells directly into the infarct area under endovascular ultrasound guidance. Experimentally, this system results in an effective myoblast engraftment,[49] and the 10-patient study has confirmed both the technical feasibility and safety of this approach.[50] The other two percutaneous trials entailed myoblast injections by endoventricular catheter after electromechanical mapping. One of the studies (10 patients) reported a 1-year improvement in the contractility of cell-injected segments and an increase in EF during low-dose dobutamine infusion.[51] The second study also demonstrated an improved function in the six treated patients compared with six case-matched controls.[52]

Put together, these studies allow some conclusions to be drawn on the feasibility and safety of the procedure. The feasibility is now well demonstrated by the fact that a small muscular biopsy (approximately 10 g) can be grown under Good Manufacturing Practice (GMP) conditions in a 2–3-week period to yield several hundred million cells with a high percentage of viability and purity (as assessed by CD56 staining on flow cytometry). Regarding safety, the multiple cell injections in the postinfarction scar and along its borders have not been a concern. The only safety issue has been the increased risk of ventricular arrhythmias because of the occurrence of sustained ventricular tachycardias reported in some patients during the early post-transplantation period.[44,47] The prevailing hypothesis to explain these events is that myoblast engraftment features clusters which remain electrically insulated from the surrounding host cardiomyocytes, a pattern expected to cause slowing of the conduction velocity and subsequent re-entry circuits.[53] Support for this hypothesis comes from the observation made in coculture experiments that genetically induced overexpression of connexin 43 on myoblasts improves electrical impulse propagation and decreases arrhythmogenesis.[53] However, other mechanisms have been invoked, including delayed cardiac repolarization and myoblast automaticity, which could induce stretch-mediated fibrillation-like contractions of

the neighboring cardiomyocytes.[54] The in vivo experimental data have been more divergent, as one study reported that myoblast-transplanted rat hearts demonstrated an increased incidence of sustained ventricular tachycardia,[55] while in another set of experiments conducted in canine left ventricular wedge preparations, abnormal impulse propagation and arrhythmia inducibility were primarily related to the infarct and not worsened by additional myoblast injections.[56] These discrepant data could be explained by the various factors that may influence the prevalence and severity of ventricular arrhythmias such as the graft size,[53] the exact location of myoblast injections (those performed in the core of the scar seem less arrhythmogenic than those lining the border zone[57]), and the extent of the procedure-induced inflammatory reaction. The situation of the human infarcted heart is complexified by the intrinsically arrhythmogenic nature of the underlying heart failure disease, which has made uncontrolled phase I studies unable to conclusively establish a causal relationship between myoblast engraftment and arrhythmias. The difficulty in establishing such a relationship is magnified by the fact that a spatial standardization of injections is difficult to achieve from one patient to the other because of the patchy pattern of scars, which feature islands of near-normal myocardium interspersed with foci of fibrosis so that cells may be randomly delivered in non-viable and viable tissue, and, as such, result in a variable arrhythmogenic potential. In an attempt to clarify this issue, all patients included in the randomized MAGIC trial (see below) have been instrumented with an ICD, not only for safety reasons (most of the included patients met the MADIT (Multicenter Automatic Defibrillator Implantation Trial II criteria) but also for using ICD readouts as an objective means of comparing the prevalence of arrhythmias between myoblast-transplanted patients and placebo-injected ones. At the 6-month study point, the time-to-first arrhythmia was not found to be statistically different between the placebo and treated groups, which is reassuring even though the small sample size calls for a cautious interpretation of these data.

In view of the number of arrhythmic episodes observed in the placebo-injected patients, these results also provide an additional confirmation of the benefits of ICD implantation in this high-risk patient population, irrespective of any cell therapy.

Although the abovementioned phase I trials have been useful for providing feasibility and safety data, they have been neither designed nor powered to allow a meaningful assessment of the putative functional benefits of the procedure. To address this issue, we then implemented a multicenter randomized, double-blind, placebo-controlled dose-ranging trial (MAGIC, for Myoblast Autologous Grafting in Ischemic Cardiomyopathy). Patients basically meeting the same inclusion criteria as in the previous studies (severe LV dysfunction, postinfarction non-viable scar, and indication for CABG) underwent a muscular biopsy followed, 3 weeks later, by injection of either cells (at two different doses: 400 and 800 million) or a placebo solution in the core and at the margins of the infarct area. Cells were prepared in two centralized manufacturing facilities working under tightly harmonized procedures. As previously mentioned, all patients were implanted with an ICD prior to hospital discharge. The primary endpoints of the study were safety (occurrence of major adverse cardiac events and ventricular arrhythmias over the first 6 postoperative months) and efficacy (changes in regional and global LV function, as assessed by echocardiograms read in a primary laboratory by blinded investigators). The results obtained in the 97 patients were presented at the 2006 Scientific Sessions of the American Heart Association. In brief, safety data did not differ between groups. Myoblast transplantation failed to increase regional or global LV function beyond what was seen in the placebo group, but the highest dose of cells resulted in a significant reversal of LV remodeling, which was a prespecified secondary endpoint. This finding is consistent with the previously discussed paracrine hypothesis whereby myoblasts elicit favorable changes in the composition of the extracellar matrix by reducing fibrosis[14] and, if sustained over time, might be clinically relevant

in view of the prognosis impact of LV dimensions.

In parallel to the MAGIC trial, a percutaneous open-label single-center study[58] has included 23 patients with EF below 40% and old (>10 years) infarcts, who were randomized to myoblast injections by endoventricular catheter according to a dose-escalating protocol (12 patients divided into four three-patient blocks ranging from 30 to 600 million cells) or optimal medical management alone (11 patients). The 6-month interim results, as assessed by echocardiography and single photon emission computed tomography (SPECT), confirm reassuring safety outcomes (only one arrhythmic episode in the 300-million cell subgroup) and also suggest a trend towards smaller LV dimensions in the myoblast-treated patients, but the limited amount of available data still preclude any definite conclusion.

Bone marrow studies

Comparatively fewer studies have looked at the effects of bone marrow cell transplantation in patients with heart failure (reviewed in reference 2). In the surgical setting, cells have always been injected epicardially in scar areas, except for one study in which they were also infused directly into the coronary artery through the bypass graft.[59] Apart from the numerous small-sized uncontrolled trials reported so far, two studies deserve greater consideration. Thus, Mocini et al[60] have studied 36 patients with a recent (<6 months) myocardial infarction and reasonably well preserved EF (in the range of 50%) referred for CABG. Eighteen of them received additional injections of autologous bone marrow mononuclear cells (mean number 292×10^6) in the border zone of the infarct area, while the remaining 18 subjects served as controls. There were no safety concerns, with the caveat of an initially higher troponin I peak after cell therapy. Three months after the procedure, echocardiographic studies showed that the transplanted patients incurred a significant improvement of the wall motion score index and EF compared with respective baseline values, but the difference of endpoint values compared with those of the control group was not significant. The interpretation of these data is further complicated by the non-randomized design of the trial (control and treated patients were consecutively included in blocks of six) and the unexpected finding that there was no change in EF over time in the control patients, which is unusual following successful bypass surgery, and could have artifactually skewed the results in favor of the treated group. Based on the results of the BOOST trial (where the initial benefit of bone marrow cell intracoronary infusions waned over time because of a "catch-up" in the control group[61]), it is clear that a longer follow-up than 3 months is required to validate this trial outcome. The study by Hendrikx et al[62] featured a more rigorous design. Twenty patients with EF in the region of 40% were randomized to receive in-scar injections of autologous bone marrow mononuclear cells (mean number 60×10^6) or saline in addition to CABG. Four months later, magnetic resonance imaging (MRI) demonstrated a significant improvement in wall thickening in cell-transplanted patients, whereas this index remained unchanged in the control group. However, this pattern failed to translate into a better recovery of EF, which was similar in the two groups, and the decrease in defect score, as assessed by thallium scintigraphy, was not different either between the control and cell-treated patients. Of note, when the treated patients were stratified as responders versus non-responders, only the number and percentage of CD34+ progenitors was found to be predictive of a positive outcome. Overall, these results are consistent with previous experimental data showing that transplantation of unfractionated bone marrow in infarcted fibrotic areas does not provide a functional benefit,[63] probably because the cells fail to find the appropriate cues for survival, proliferation, and differentiation. The efficacy of bone marrow cell therapy is likely to be further decreased by the reduced neovascularization capacity of these cells when they are harvested from patients with chronic ischemic cardiomyopathy and depressed LV function.[64]

In an attempt to improve the outcome of the procedure, some investigators have tested the effects of transplanting a select population of bone marrow-derived progenitors primarily credited for their angiogenic potential. In one study, 20 patients with EF $\leq 35\%$ were randomized to off-pump single left internal mammary–left anterior descending coronary artery bypass alone or completed by peri-infarct injections of a median number of 22×10^6 CD34+ cells.[65] After 6 months, EF was significantly higher in the treated patients, but the lack of perfusion studies makes it impossible to know whether this outcome was related to increased angiogenesis, while the increase in absolute EF in CD34+-treated patients is so tremendous (17%!) and outside the order of magnitude usually reported after stem cell therapy that it requires to be reproduced and validated by other groups. Another study has extended the use of CD34+ cells by preinjection stem cell mobilization by granulocyte colony stimulating factor (G-CSF) and subsequent apheresis.[66] Five patients were then injected with an average of 12×10^6 cells (a figure surprisingly lower than that used in the previous study, which did not entail any mobilization) delivered from the center of the scar to its periphery. Despite the claim that the procedure resulted in a sustained improvement in LV function (until 7 months postoperatively), these results are virtually impossible to interpret because of the concomitant revascularization of the cell-transplanted area and the lack of a true control group. Indeed, in the setting of these studies that have tested defined populations of bone marrow cells, one of the most promising appears to be that of Steinhoff and co-workers[67] who injected CD133+ progenitors during CABG. Based on the sound rationale that these cells feature an angiogenic potential, their trial, although not strictly randomized, yet provides encouraging hints in favor of the capacity of the CD133+ population to improve LV function at 6 months postoperatively, particularly in patients with the lowest preoperative LVEF.

In parallel, a limited number of studies have assessed the effects of bone marrow cells delivered percutaneously. One open-label non-randomized trial[68] entailed mononuclear cell delivery by endoventricular catheter in 11 patients, and reported improved exercise capacity and reduced perfusion defects at a 12-month follow-up; interestingly, the 6-month improvement in reversible perfusion defects was found to be correlated with some subpopulations (monocytes, B cells, hematopoietic progenitor cells, and early hematopoietic progenitor cells), thereby supporting the concept of selecting discrete lineages rather than using unfractionated bone marrow. The other study recently published by Assmus et al[69] featured a more elaborate cross-over type of design, and included 75 patients allocated to receive no cell infusion or intracoronary infusions of either circulating progenitor cells or mononuclear cells (isolated from venous blood and bone marrow, respectively). The major result is that at the 3-month study point, bone marrow cells yielded a significant increase in both global and regional LV function, regardless of whether patients crossed over from the control or the circulating progenitor cell group. Although still limited, these data open interesting perspectives for the catheter-based treatment of chronic heart failure by bone marrow cells. Furthermore, in light of the previous experimental findings that skeletal myoblasts and bone marrow cells improve postinfarction function to a similar extent,[70] they strengthen a paracrine mechanism of action since none of these cell types is expected to directly participate in the heart's contractile function. The IACT study (which claims a totally unproven and actually unlikely "regeneration" of infarcted muscle following intracoronary delivery of bone marrow mononuclear cells) falls beyond the scope of this review in that the included patients had chronic infarcts but relatively well preserved LV function (11 of them had EF ≥ 50%).[71]

Summary and Conclusions

Put together, the above considerations convey the encouraging message that there is a consistent trend for cell therapy to become a potentially useful new adjunct to existing therapies for heart failure. However, to extend beyond the boundaries of controlled clinical trials to enter the real world of large-scale medical practice, three major types of hurdle still remain to be overcome.

Adult cell-specific issues

The most serious limitation of skeletal myoblasts is probably their lineage restriction which precludes, among others, the in vivo expression of connexin 43, and leads engrafted myoblast clusters to remain electrically insulated from the surrounding myocardium.[20,72] Even though the differentiated myotubes may respond to the cardiomyocyte-triggered stretch by contractions, these events do not allow the formation of a true functional syncytium whereby the donor cells beat in synchrony with those of the recipient. Engineering myoblasts to make them overexpress connexin 43 is conceptually appealing and technically possible.[53,73] The clinical applicability of this approach remains, however, more problematic, since in addition to the safety problems common to gene therapy, it raises the question of the spatial distribution of gap junction proteins expressed by transduced myoblasts; currently, it remains uncertain whether this distribution would be homogeneous enough to allow an effective electromechanical integration and the attendant improvement in function without causing arrhythmias. The same limitations apply to bone marrow cells, which are equally unable to couple with host cardiomyocytes.[21] More generally, the basic question is then whether a true myocardial regeneration based on the provision of new donor-derived cardiomyocytes is mandatory, or whether the paracrine effects of the grafted cells are sufficient to improve function irrespective of the graft phenotype. Indeed, in a recent study which has compared different cell types in a mouse model of myocardial infarction, only skeletal myoblasts and embryonic stem cells proved to be functionally effective compared with fibroblasts, and transplanted and cytokine-mobilized bone marrow cells.[74] One could then argue that if both presumably non-contracting lineage-restricted myoblasts and potentially contracting pluripotent embryonic stem cells are equally effective in improving the functional outcome, the contractile properties are less important than the paracrine effects. However, these experiments entailed cell injections in acutely ischemic myocardium. In heart failure, where a key patho-physiological factor is the loss of a critical mass of cardiomyocytes and its replacement by non-functional fibrosis, we still believe that, although more challenging, the ultimate goal should be regeneration. The results initially obtained with fetal cardiomyocyte transplantation then suggest that only cells programmed toward a cardiac lineage are able to effect a true myocardial remuscularization, and, in this setting, cardiac-specified human embryonic stem cells currently hold the greatest promise.[23,24]

Autologous cell-specific issues

As previously mentioned, one of the strong arguments favoring the use of skeletal myoblasts and, later on, of bone marrow-derived cells has been their autologous origin. However, with accumulated experience, the limitations of patient-specific products have become increasingly evident. They include: (1) the naturally occurring individual variability between patients which makes it difficult to end up with a reproducible and well characterized cell therapy product; this may account for the discrepant results yielded by clinical trials supposed to use the same type of cells which, for a given similar number, can actually exhibit quite different functional capacities influenced by age and risk factors; and (2) the cost of personalized quality controls which need to be repeated for each patient-specific batch. In the case of skeletal myoblasts, additional constraints include the delay in treatment required for upscaling the muscular biopsy and the logistical complexity related to back-and-forth shipments of the cellular products when the processing is centralized in a core laboratory (the latter limitation may also apply to bone marrow-derived cells except in the case of extemporaneous on-site use). Thus, from the perspective of large-scale treatment, the implementation of cardiac cell therapy would be greatly simplified by the constitution of cell banks, allowing the almost immediate availability of an "off-the-shelf" tightly controlled and accurately characterized product. It is clear that such an allogeneic product raises, in turn, the major concern of immunogenicity, which could possibly be addressed by an immunosuppressive treatment (with its attendant risks), knockout of some major histocompatibility genes, induction of chimerism, or even perhaps coadministration of allogeneic mesenchymal stem cells if their tolerogenicity was unambiguously demonstrated.[75] Additional studies are thus warranted to thoughtfully compare the risk–benefit and cost–effectiveness ratios of autologous and allogeneic cell therapy products.

Cell-specific issues

We have previously emphasized that the therapeutic efficacy of cell therapy was likely hampered by the poor efficiency of current delivery techniques and the subsequently high rate of cell death. These observations provide a convenient framework for developing strategies that could successfully address these issues.

Thus, the increase in initial cell transfer requires new delivery devices targeted at improving the accuracy of targeting while reducing cell leakage. The optimization of graft survival can then be accomplished through at least two types of approaches which have already proved to be effective: (1) an increase in blood supply to the grafted area which can be obtained by various methods (surgical or percutaneous revascularization, coinjected,[76] or transfected[29] angiogenic growth factors, cotransplantation of angiogenic bone marrow-derived cells[77]); and (2) the incorporation of cells in a bioinjectable scaffold (particularly hydrogels and nanofibers) designed to restore a three-dimensional microenvironment. Alternative cell-survival enhancing strategies also need to be considered, and particularly include transfection of the cells to be grafted with genes encoding pro-survival factors,[78] or their preconditioning by physical[15,16] or pharmacological (potassium channel agonists) methods.[79] Clearly, the development of these techniques cannot be dissociated from that of tracking cells for providing quantitative data on engraftment. Currently, much enthusiasm is generated by cell labeling with iron superparamagnetic iron particles to allow non-invasive monitoring of graft fate by MRI,[80] but some concerns are yet expressed about the reliability of this method and its potentially harmful effects on cell functionality.[81] Additional practical issues to address include the optimal route of administration and cell dosing.

The number of still unknown factors surrounding cardiac cell therapy fuels the case for slowing or even stopping clinical trials until we have a more thorough understanding of the mechanistic underpinning of stem cells. Although we fully concur with the idea that a "reasonable" degree of mechanistic understanding and the validation of preclinical data in a large animal model are mandatory,[82] we also believe that it is fair to acknowledge that there is no animal model that can fully replicate the complexity and multiplicity of biological and mechanical factors involved in the pathophysiology of heart failure. The report of arrhythmias after the first cases of myoblast transplantation is a strong demonstration of how clinical trials are essential in identifying potential safety concerns, orienting additional basic research, developing strategies aimed at optimizing the risk–benefit ratio, and, ultimately, moving the field forward. The prerequisite, however, is that these trials be designed, powered, conducted, and analyzed in such a way that they generate clinically relevant data really allowing the determination of whether and to what extent cardiac cell therapy may affect the outcome of patients with heart failure.

References

1. Boyle AJ, Schulman SP, Hare JM, Oettgen P. Is stem cell therapy ready for patients? Stem cell therapy for cardiac repair. Ready for the next step. Circulation 2006; 114: 339–52.
2. Ang KL, Shenje LT, Srinivasan L, Galinanes M. Repair of the damaged heart by bone marrow cells: from experimental evidence to clinical hope. Ann Thorac Surg 2006; 82: 1549–58.
3. Wollert KC, Drexler H. Cell-based therapy for heart failure. Curr Opin Cardiol 2006; 21: 234–9.
4. Leor J, Patterson M, Quinones MJ et al. Transplantation of fetal myocardial tissue into the infarcted myocardium of rat. A potential method for repair of infarcted myocardium? Circulation 1996; 94 (9 Suppl): II332–6.
5. Scorsin M, Hagege AA, Marotte F et al. Does transplantation of cardiomyocytes improve function of infarcted myocardium? Circulation 1997; 96 (9 Suppl): II188–93.
6. Dowell JD, Rubart M, Pasumarthi KB, Soonpaa MH, Field LJ. Myocyte and myogenic stem cell transplantation in the heart. Cardiovasc Res 2003; 58: 336–50.
7. He KL, Yi GH, Sherman W et al. Autologous skeletal myoblast transplantation improved hemodynamics and left ventricular function in chronic heart failure dogs. J Heart Lung Transplant 2005; 24: 1940–9.
8. Van den Bos EJ, Thompson RB, Wagner A et al. Functional assessment of myoblast transplantation for cardiac repair with magnetic resonance imaging. Eur J Heart Fail 2005; 7: 435–43.
9. McConnell PI, del Rio CL, Jacoby DB et al. Correlation of autologous skeletal myoblast survival with changes in left ventricular remodeling in dilated ischemic heart failure. J Thorac Cardiovasc Surg 2005; 130: 1001–9.
10. Dimarakis I, Habib NA, Gordon MY. Adult bone marrow-derived stem cells and the injured heart: just the beginning? Eur J Cardiothorac Surg 2005; 28: 665–76.
11. Rubart M, Field LJ. Cardiac regeneration: repopulating the heart. Annu Rev Physiol 2006; 68: 29–49.
12. Teng CJ, Luo J, Chiu RC, Shum-Tim D. Massive mechanical loss of microspheres with direct intramyocardial injection in the beating heart: implications for cellular cardiomyoplasty. J Thorac Cardiovasc Surg 2006; 132: 628–32.
13. Dow J, Simkhovich BZ, Kedes L, Kloner RA. Washout of transplanted cells from the heart: a potential new hurdle for cell transplantation therapy. Cardiovasc Res 2005; 67: 301–7.
14. Gavira JJ, Perez-Ilzarbe M, Abizanda G et al. A comparison between percutaneous and surgical transplantation of autologous skeletal myoblasts in a swine model of chronic myocardial infarction. Cardiovasc Res 2006; 71: 744–53.
15. Zhang M, Methot D, Poppa V et al. Cardiomyocyte grafting for cardiac repair: graft cell death and anti-death strategies. J Mol Cell Cardiol 2001; 33: 907–21.
16. Maurel A, Azarnoush K, Sabbah L et al. Can cold or heat shock improve skeletal myoblast engraftment in infarcted myocardium? Transplantation 2005; 80: 660–5.
17. Murry CE, Reinecke H, Pabon LM. Regeneration gaps: observations on stem cells and cardiac repair. J Am Coll Cardiol 2006; 47: 1777–85.
18. Murry CE, Soonpaa MH, Reinecke H et al. Haematopoietic stem cells do not transdifferentiate into cardiac myocytes in myocardial infarcts. Nature 2004; 428: 664–8.

19. Balsam LB, Wagers AJ, Christensen JL et al. Haematopoietic stem cells adopt mature haematopoietic fates in ischaemic myocardium. Nature 2004; 428: 668–73.

20. Leobon B, Garcin I, Menasche P et al. Myoblasts transplanted into rat infarcted myocardium are functionally isolated from their host. Proc Natl Acad Sci USA 2003; 100: 7808–11.

21. Lagostena L, Avitabile D, De Falco E et al. Electrophysiological properties of mouse bone marrow c-kit+ cells co-cultured onto neonatal cardiac myocytes. Cardiovasc Res 2005; 6: 482–92.

22. Rubart M, Pasumarthi KB, Nakajima H et al. Physiological coupling of donor and host cardiomyocytes after cellular transplantation. Circ Res 2003; 92: 1217–24.

23. Hodgson DM, Behfar A, Zingman LV et al. Stable benefit of embryonic stem cell therapy in myocardial infarction. Am J Physiol Heart Circ Physiol 2004; 287: H471–9.

24. Menard C, Hagege AA, Agbulut O et al. Transplantation of cardiac-committed mouse embryonic stem cells to infarcted sheep myocardium: a preclinical study. Lancet 2005; 366: 1005–12.

25. Kinnaird T, Stabile E, Burnett MS et al. Marrow-derived stromal cells express genes encoding a broad spectrum of arteriogenic cytokines and promote in vitro and in vivo arteriogenesis through paracrine mechanisms. Circ Res 2004; 94: 678–85.

26. Uemura R, Xu M, Ahmad N, Ashraf M. Bone marrow stem cells prevent left ventricular remodeling of ischemic heart through paracrine signaling. Circ Res 2006; 98: 1414–21.

27. Gnecchi M, He H, Liang OD et al. Paracrine action accounts for marked protection of ischemic heart by Akt-modified mesenchymal stem cells. Nat Med 2005; 11: 367–8.

28. Kubal C, Sheth K, Nadal-Ginard B, Galinanes M. Bone marrow cells have a potent anti-ischemic effect against myocardial cell death in humans. J Thorac Cardiovasc Surg 2006; 132: 1112–18.

29. Yau TM, Kim C, Ng D et al. Increasing transplanted cell survival with cell-based angiogenic gene therapy. Ann Thorac Surg 2005; 80: 1779–86.

30. Askari AT, Unzek S, Popovic ZB et al. Effect of stromal-cell-derived factor 1 on stem-cell homing and tissue regeneration in ischaemic cardiomyopathy. Lancet 2003; 362: 697–703.

31. Misao Y, Takemura G, Arai M et al. Bone marrow-derived myocyte-like cells and regulation of repair-related cytokines after bone marrow cell transplantation. Cardiovasc Res 2006; 69: 476–90.

32. Fazel S, Cimini M, Chen L et al. Cardioprotective c-kit+ cells are from the bone marrow and regulate the myocardial balance of angiogenic cytokines. J Clin Invest 2006; 116: 1865–77.

33. Tang YL, Zhao Q, Qin X et al. Paracrine action enhances the effects of autologous mesenchymal stem cell transplantation on vascular regeneration in rat model of myocardial infarction. Ann Thorac Surg 2005; 80: 229–36; discussion 236–7.

34. Murtuza B, Suzuki K, Bou-Gharios G et al. Transplantation of skeletal myoblasts secreting an IL-1 inhibitor modulates adverse remodeling in infarcted murine myocardium. Proc Natl Acad Sci USA 2004; 101: 4216–21.

35. Xu X, Xu Z, Xu Y, Cui G. Effects of mesenchymal stem cell transplantation on extracellular matrix after myocardial infarction in rats. Coron Artery Dis 2005; 16: 245–55.

36. Kudo M, Wang Y, Wani MA et al. Implantation of bone marrow stem cells reduces the infarction and fibrosis in ischemic mouse heart. J Mol Cell Cardiol 2003; 35: 1113–19.

37. Anversa P, Leri A, Kajstura J. Cardiac regeneration. J Am Coll Cardiol 2006; 47: 1769–76.

38. Wall ST, Walker JC, Healy KE, Ratcliffe MB, Guccione JM. Theoretical impact of the injection of material into the myocardium: a finite element model simulation. Circulation 2006; 114: 2627–35.

39. Webb CS, Bonnema DD, Ahmed SH et al. Specific temporal profile of matrix metalloproteinase release occurs in patients after myocardial infarction: relation to left ventricular remodeling. Circulation 2006; 114: 1020–7.

40. Engler AJ, Sen S, Sweeney HL, Discher DE. Matrix elasticity directs stem cell lineage specification. Cell 2006; 126: 677–89.

41. Berry MF, Engler AJ, Woo YJ et al. Mesenchymal stem cell injection after myocardial infarction improves myocardial compliance. Am J Physiol Heart Circ Physiol 2006; 290: H2196–203.

42. Yoon YS, Park JS, Tkebuchava T, Luedeman C, Losordo DW. Unexpected severe calcification after transplantation of bone marrow cells in acute myocardial infarction. Circulation 2004; 109: 3154–7.

43. Menasche P, Hagege AA, Scorsin M et al. Myoblast transplantation for heart failure. Lancet 2001; 357: 279–80.

44. Hagege AA, Marolleau JP, Vilquin JT et al. Skeletal myoblast transplantation in ischemic heart failure: long-term follow-up of the first phase I cohort of patients. Circulation 2006; 114 (1 Suppl): I108–13.

45. Hagege AA, Carrion C, Menasche P et al. Viability and differentiation of autologous skeletal myoblast grafts in ischaemic cardiomyopathy. Lancet 2003; 361: 491–502.

46. Gavira JJ, Herreros J, Perez A et al. Autologous skeletal myoblast transplantation in patients with nonacute myocardial infarction: 1-year follow-up. J Thorac Cardiovasc Surg 2006; 131: 799–804.

Index

Note: Page references *in italic* to tables or figures

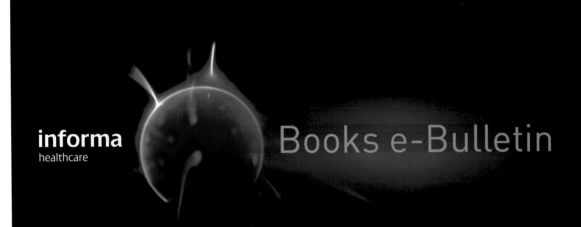
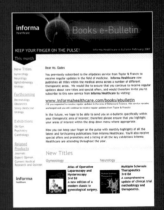

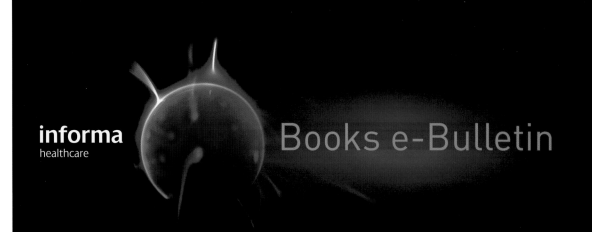
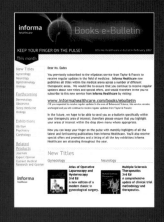